Congenital Heart Disease

Serena Francesca Flocco · Angelo Lillo
Federica Dellafiore · Eva Goossens
Editors

Congenital Heart Disease

The Nursing Care Handbook

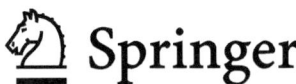 Springer

Editors
Serena Francesca Flocco
Pediatric and Adult Congenital Heart
Disease Center
IRCCS Policlinico San Donato University
Hospital
San Donato Milanese (MI)
Italy

Federica Dellafiore
Health Professions Research and
Development Unit
IRCCS Policlinico San Donato
San Donato Milanese (MI)
Italy

Angelo Lillo
Policlinico S.Orsola-Malpighi
Bologna
Italy

Eva Goossens
Department of Public Health and Primary Care
Academic Center for Nursing and
Midwifery, KU Leuven
Leuven
Belgium

Research Foundation Flanders (FWO)
Brussels
Belgium

ISBN 978-3-319-78421-2   ISBN 978-3-319-78423-6   (eBook)
https://doi.org/10.1007/978-3-319-78423-6

Library of Congress Control Number: 2018960933

This Springer imprint is published by the registered company Springer Nature Switzerland AG
The registered company address is: Gewerbestrasse 11, 6330 Cham, Switzerland

Foreword

It is our great delight and distinct honor to write the foreword to this book dedicated to the nursing care of the patient with congenital heart disease. To the best of our knowledge, this is the first book that is dedicated to nursing for the emergent population of patients with congenital heart disease. Indeed, advances in medicine have resulted in increased life expectancy, which yields a growing number of patients in need for lifelong care. In addition to the numerous medical issues that are associated with the management of people with congenital heart disease, these patients and families also face a lot of nonmedical problems. Nurses typically play an important role on the verge of both areas and are complementary to other healthcare professionals involved in the care for these patients.

The authors are to be congratulated for their prescience in editing this important contribution to the body of knowledge. This book assembles a large panel of authors with expertise in the different aspects of nursing care for patients with congenital heart disease. Doing so, well-known topics are covered, but also issues that are sometimes underestimated are addressed. The importance of this book is that it tries to make sure that such aspects are not ignored in the care of our patients.

Some chapters in this book pertain to technical aspects in nursing care for afflicted patients. They address the different paths of a daily clinical work-up. Other chapters focus on nonmedical aspects. Not surprisingly, a chapter on transfer and transition is included. Indeed, nurses play a key role in the transition of young patients and their families and in the preparation for the transfer to adult care. The book concludes with a chapter on nursing research and quality improvement initiatives, showing how deeply involved nurses are in the improvement of care to patients with congenital heart disease.

Never before has such a concentrated effort been made to provide the reader with a state-of-the-art review of nursing care in congenital heart disease. It is our pleasure and privilege to warmly recommend this textbook to all nurses who want to improve their skills in managing the problems of these patients.

Massimo Chessa
Pediatric and Adult Congenital Heart Centre
I.R.C.S.S.-Policlinico San Donato-University Hospital
Milan, Italy

Philip Moons
Department of Public Health and Primary Care
KU Leuven—University of Leuven
Leuven, Belgium

Institute of Health and Care Science
University of Gothenburg
Gothenburg, Sweden

Contents

Congenital Heart Disease Classification, Epidemiology, Diagnosis, Treatment, and Outcome

Angelo Micheletti

Abstract

Congenital heart disease (CHD) is a problem in the structure of the heart that is present at birth. CHD is still the most common inborn defect with an approximate prevalence at birth of 5–11 per 1000 live births and incidence of 1%. The aim of this chapter is to give both a general overview on CHD and to address just a few specific issues for each type of structural disease. Congenital cardiac malformations may be classified in different ways; to highlight the underlying anatomy and pathophysiology, the diseases could be grouped as follows: (a) CHD with shunt between systemic and pulmonary circulation, (b) left heart CHD, (c) right heart CHD, (d) CHD with anomalous origin of great arteries, and (e) miscellanea.

1.1 Introduction

Congenital heart disease (CHD) is still the most common inborn defect with an approximate prevalence at birth of 5–11 per 1000 live births and incidence of 1% [1]. By definition, CHD means a disease that has been present since birth but not necessary "clinically" evident since birth: this is the case, for example, of moderate size atrial septal defect of unobstructive subaortic stenosis.

Taking into account the pathophysiology and diagnosis of CHD, it is helpful to highlight three key points: (1) the presence of shunt between arterial and venous blood, (2) the presence of cyanosis, and (3) the changes in circulation after birth [2]. A shunt consists of an abnormal communication between two cardiac chambers or vessels allowing blood to go from one side to the other. Shunting may be described

A. Micheletti
Department of Paediatric Cardiology and Cardiac Surgery, Adult with Congenital Heart Disease, IRCCS—San Donato University Hospital, Milan, Italy
e-mail: a.micheletti@libero.it

© Springer International Publishing AG, part of Springer Nature 2019
S. F. Flocco et al. (eds.), *Congenital Heart Disease*,
https://doi.org/10.1007/978-3-319-78423-6_1

as left-to-right, right-to-left, or bidirectional. The direction is strictly dependent on pressure gradient across the shunt; most commonly blood goes from high-pressure left-sided heart to low-pressure right-sided heart. Therefore shunt direction affects the status of pulmonary blood flow which can vary from normal, increased, or decreased. Any large left-to-right (L-R) shunt results in increased blood flow into the lungs associated with shortness of breath and prominent vascular markings on chest x-ray, volume overload of left ventricle (LV) associated with chamber dilatation, and subsequently heart failure; if untreated, it will eventually result in pulmonary artery (PA) pressure overload which, by time, will cause irreversible structural arterial wall changes ending up with pulmonary hypertension (PH), with increased pulmonary vascular resistance (PVR), and, later on, in pulmonary vascular obstructive disease (PVOD). High and fixed PVR is the feature of pulmonary vascular obstructive disease. When PVR approaches or even exceeds systemic vascular resistance, direction of the shunting becomes bidirectional or mainly right-to-left (R-L), condition known as Eisenmenger syndrome. Generally, in presence of right-to-left shunt, venous poor-oxygenated blood mixes with arterial high-oxygenated blood, causing cyanosis. Cyanosis is a bluish discoloration of the skin and mucous membranes resulting from presence of 5.0 g/dL or greater of deoxyhemoglobin in the blood.

Presence of shunts is crucial during fetal life when the placenta provides the exchange of gases and nutrients and lungs receive only about 15% of combined ventricular output. Fetal circulation is characterized by four sites of shunting: the placenta, ductus venosus through which umbilical vein drains into inferior vena cava, foramen ovale within the interatrial septum, and the arterial duct through which blood in the PA flows into descending aorta. Just after birth, placental circulation disappears and pulmonary circulation is established. Interruption of the umbilical cord results in an increase in systemic vascular resistance and closure of the ductus venosus. Concomitant lung expansion results in reduction of pulmonary artery pressure and PVR, an increase in pulmonary blood flow, functional closure of the foramen ovale, and closure of patent arterial duct due to increased arterial oxygen saturation.

With lung expansion and the resulting increase of alveolar oxygen tension, an initial significant rapid fall in PVR occurs mainly due to the vasodilating oxygen effect on pulmonary vasculature. Later on, between 4 and 8 weeks after birth, there is another slower fall in the PVR and PA pressure secondary to wall changes in pulmonary arterioles. Many neonatal conditions associated with different forms of CHD, causing inadequate oxygenation, may interfere with the normal pulmonary arteriole maturation, resulting in persistent pulmonary hypertension or delay in usual PVR fall.

Ductus arteriosus usually closes spontaneously within the first 48 h after birth, by constriction of the medial smooth muscle; after this functional closure, an anatomical closure occurs, by 2–3 weeks of age, by permanent changes in the endothelium and subintimal layers. Many factors may interfere with ductal closure such as oxygen, maturity of the newborn, prostaglandin E_2 levels, and acidosis [3].

To achieve a precise diagnosis of CHD, even in very complex cases, along with an accurate physical examination, many both noninvasive and invasive tools are currently available. Transthoracic echocardiography (TTE) is the first-line diagnostic technique in terms of anatomical and functional information in all CHD, whereas cardiac catheterization still constitutes the final definitive diagnostic test for many of them. Over the last decade, due to the significant improvement of interventional cardiology in dealing with several forms of CHD, a new "multimodality" imaging approach has been promoted aiming at the integration rather than at the selection of the necessary details. 3D echocardiography, cardiac computed tomography (CT), and magnetic resonance (MR) have become of great interest due to their ability to generate both 3D anatomical and hemodynamic functional information.

Effective treatment of all the spectrum of CHD is currently feasible due to the amazing improvement in medical care, catheter-based interventions, and surgical procedures which have dramatically extended survival and life expectancy. Survival through childhood is now common even in the most complex and lethal malformations, such as hypoplastic left heart syndrome. As a consequence of these advances, there have been major demographic shifts, so that adult patients with CHD now outnumber children even with complex forms of CHD [4].

The aim of this chapter is to give both a general overview on CHD and to address just a few specific issues for each type of structural disease. Congenital cardiac malformations may be classified in different ways; to highlight the underlying anatomy and pathophysiology, the diseases could be grouped as follows: (a) CHD with shunt between systemic and pulmonary circulation, (b) left heart CHD, (c) right heart CHD, (d) CHD with anomalous origin of great arteries, and (e) miscellanea.

1.1.1 CHD with Shunt Between Systemic and Pulmonary Circulation

1.1.1.1 Atrial Septal Defect
Atrial septal defect (ASD) is a communication between the atrial chambers permitting left-to-right shunting (Fig. 1.1).

It is the second most common type of CHD, accounting for about 7–10% of all CHD patients, more prevalent in women (2:1), and most likely to be diagnosed in late childhood or adults. There are different types of ASD (Fig. 1.2) [5]:

– Ostium secundum ASD: The most frequent variant of ASD, 70–80% of all ASDs, results from deficiency of the flap valve of the oval fossa, ranging from incomplete development, with failed overlapping to the septum secundum, to the presence of multiple fenestrations to complete absence. Anomalous pulmonary venous return is present in about 10% of cases.
– Ostium primum ASD: Occurs in about 15% of all ASDs and is a part of atrioventricular septal defect; it is placed near the crux.
– Sinus venosus defect: 5–10%, located superiorly and posteriorly, near the entry of superior vena cava (SVC) or inferiorly and posteriorly near the entry of inferior vena cava (IVC), commonly associated with anomalous drainage of right pulmonary veins.
– Coronary sinus ASD: 1%, located in the roof of the coronary sinus which could be partially or completely missing and often associated with left SVC that drains to the left atrium.

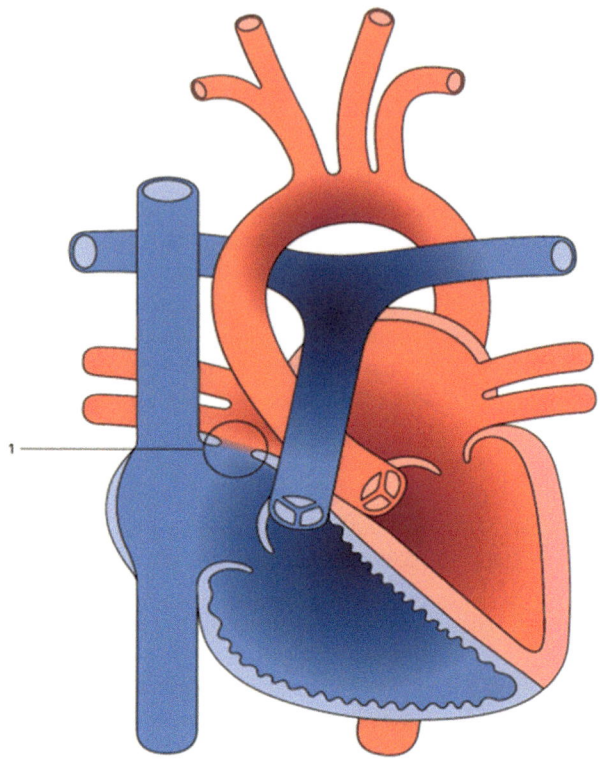

Fig. 1.1 Atrial septal defect (1)

Fig. 1.2 Different types of ASD

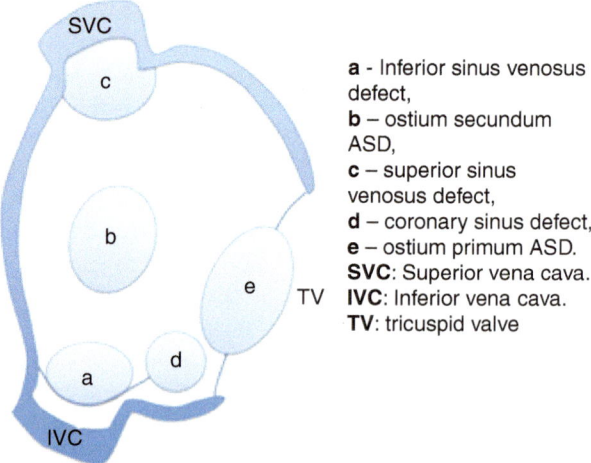

a - Inferior sinus venosus defect,
b – ostium secundum ASD,
c – superior sinus venosus defect,
d – coronary sinus defect,
e – ostium primum ASD.
SVC: Superior vena cava.
IVC: Inferior vena cava.
TV: tricuspid valve

The L-R shunt causes volume overload of the right chambers and pulmonary circulation; the entity of shunt is related to defect size, right ventricle (RV) and LV compliance and pressure. Usually volume overload is well tolerated allowing some to go undetected until adulthood; when the shunt is significant, however, with age, symptoms can occur such as exertional dyspnea, pulmonary infections, and atrial arrhythmias [6].

Foramen ovale is an interatrial communication, during fetal life, between septum secundum (limbus of fossa ovalis) and septum primum (the valve of fossa ovalis) which allows venous return from IVC to shunt across to the left atrium. Normally it closes at birth functionally, whereas a complete anatomic closure occurs in 70–75% of adults [7]. Patent foramen ovale (PFO) refers to persistence of this normal communication postnatally; it assumes clinical importance in certain CHD and in patients with cerebral vascular accident due to paradoxical emboli [8].

Diagnosis. From childhood, the classic clinical findings include widely split and fixed second heart sound associated with a low-pitched systolic ejection murmur. TTE is the diagnostic test of choice. In case of PH, diagnostic cardiac catheterization is mandatory to calculate pulmonary vascular resistance and to assess pulmonary circulation vasoreactivity.

Treatment. The presence of hemodynamically significant L-R shunt (a ratio of pulmonary blood flow to systemic blood flow of >1.5:1.0) and/or right chamber volume overload without significant PH represents the indication for ASD closure. Closure can be accomplished by surgery or, in case of secundum ASD and adequate anatomic rims, by device implantation during interventional catheterization [9].

Outcome. Atrial arrhythmias are the most frequent late complication, and the risk increases with advancing age at repair. PH is another late complication affecting survival but is rare in patients operated before 25 years of age, and the risk increases with advancing age at repair as well [10]. If closure is performed in adolescence or childhood, life expectancy returns to normal [11].

1.1.1.2 Ventricular Septal Defect

Ventricular septal defect (VSD) is defined as a communication between the two ventricles (Fig. 1.3). It is the most common CHD, almost 20% of all defects, and may occur in isolation or as a part of a complex cardiac malformation [10]. According to the anatomical position, different types of VSD can be described (Fig. 1.3):

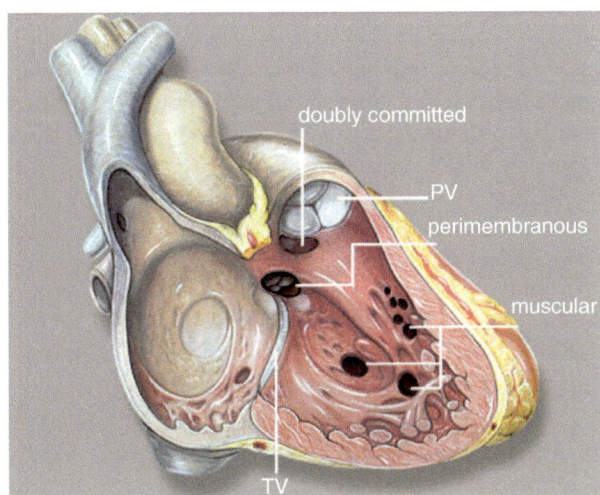

Fig. 1.3 Different types of VSD according to anatomical position within the septum viewed from RV side. *TV* tricuspid valve. *PV* pulmonary valve

- Perimembranous VSD: The most frequent variant, placed within the membranous septum with variable anatomical extension toward the other components of interventricular septum (IVS), inlet, outlet, and apical. It is in close relationship with the septal leaflet of the tricuspid valve (TV) and the his bundle of electrical conduction system. Aneurysm of membranous septum is frequently associated and may result, over time, in partial or complete closure.
- Muscular VSD: About 15–18% of all VSDs, could be placed within any muscular component of IVS, and is surrounded by complete muscular rims. Quite often small defects close spontaneously; rarely the defects can be multiple, the so-called "Swiss-cheese" septum.
- Doubly committed, juxta-arterial VSD: More frequent in Asian countries, it is localized just beneath the arterial valves which are, as a consequence, in fibrous continuity.
- Inlet defect: Located in the inlet component of the septum, immediately inferior to the atrioventricular valve apparatus; typically occurring in down syndrome.

Shunt direction and magnitude are determined by the size of the defect, ventricular systolic and diastolic function, the presence of right ventricular outflow tract obstruction (RVOT), and PVR.

The clinical spectrum of this defect is wide: large L-to-R shunt causes high pulmonary blood flow, LV volume overload presenting with heart failure, and, particularly in infancy and childhood, failure to thrive and repeated respiratory infections. Large VSD with large L-R shunt is associated with PH and, if untreated, ends up in pulmonary vascular disease as in Eisenmenger syndrome. In case of doubly committed VSD, less common perimembranous, there is a risk for prolapse of the right coronary or noncoronary cusp of the aortic valve, resulting in progressing aortic regurgitation [12]. Subaortic discrete obstruction and/or right mid-ventricular discrete stenosis (double-chambered RV) may develop, the latter being the result of a high-velocity VSD jet lesion on RV endothelium. Finally arrhythmias can occur although less frequently than other forms of CHD.

Diagnosis. The classic pansystolic murmur, which is best audible along the left mid to lower sternal border, may not be heard until a few weeks of age when the shunt becomes maximal. Generally, the smaller is the defect, the higher is the murmur intensity. A second sound physiologically split with respiration is indicative of normal pulmonary pressure. In POVD associated with VSD, varying degrees of cyanosis may be noted. On chest x-ray, the degree of cardiomegaly and the increase in pulmonary vascular markings directly relate to the magnitude of the L-R shunt. TTE is mandatory to assess all the characteristics in terms of position, size, number, association with other congenital defects or aortic valve dysfunction, direction of the shunting, relationship with tricuspid valve and its cordal apparatus, the presence of aneurysmal tissue, and the distance between VSD and aortic valve [13]. In some selected cases, a diagnostic cardiac catheterization is needed to calculate PVR and to assess pulmonary circulation vasoreactivity.

Treatment. Spontaneous closure of small, restrictive VSD may occur. Closing moderate to large VSD by open heart surgery is usually performed during infancy to prevent complications later [14]. Although surgery remains the treatment of choice, with low operative mortality, transcatheter closure has become a valid and alternative procedure to be considered only in selected cases either in children or in adults [15].

Outcome. The long-term prognosis for a patient with a successful surgically repaired VSD is excellent with life expectancy as good as in the general population [16]. Acute and/or late-onset complete atrioventricular block (cAVB) due to conduction system injury remains a crucial issue after surgical or transcatheter closure of perimembranous VSD; the incidence of cAVB, after device closure, requiring permanent pacemaker implantation is 2.6%, and the risk is higher in children aged <6 years [17–19]. The prognosis for patients with Eisenmenger syndrome is the worst among the VSD population.

1.1.1.3 Atrioventricular Septal Defect

Atrioventricular septal defect (AVSD) refers to a spectrum of cardiac malformations characterized by abnormal development of atrioventricular junction which normally derives from endocardial cushion tissue. It is clearly associated with chromosomal abnormalities, mainly trisomy 21, Down syndrome.

The key anatomic feature is the presence of common AV junction guarded by a 5-leaflet common AV valve, associated with deficient septation. Arrangement of common AV valve leaflets differs significantly from the normal tricuspid and mitral valves. Anatomy can vary from:

- Partial AVSD, with an ostium primum ASD and two separate valve orifices and without inlet VSD
- Complete AVSD, with an ostium primum ASD, single valve orifice, and inlet VSD

The predominant hemodynamic consequence of this abnormal anatomy is the presence of intracardiac shunting between either the atriums or the ventricles or from ventricles to atriums. This will result in volume and/or pressure overload of cardiac chambers which may be exacerbated by the regurgitation of one or more components of the common AV valve. The incidence of associated lesions is high, approaching 50% of the cases. Symptoms are usually the result of intracardiac left-to-right shunting and/or regurgitation of AV valve; patients with only an atrial level shunt are rarely symptomatic, whereas signs of congestive heart failure (CHF) as tachypnea, dyspnea, diaphoresis, failure to thrive, and frequent chest infections are typical of significant ventricular level shunt and/or significant AV valve regurgitation.

Diagnosis. Due to the presence of a common AV junction, the AV conduction system is typically displaced posteriorly and inferiorly. On ECG, it results in superior and rightward QRS axis deviation frequently associated with prolonged PR interval and QRS duration.

On chest x-ray, cardiomegaly and increased pulmonary vascular markings reflect significant left-to right intracardiac shunting and/or left AV valve regurgitation; the presence of prominent central pulmonary arteries combined with peripheral "pruning" and right heart enlargement reflects Eisenmenger syndrome.

Comprehensive and sequential 2D and 3D TTE [20] should be focused on all the anatomical details and to rule out unbalanced ventricles, outflow tract obstructions, and associated lesions.

Diagnostic cardiac catheterization is usually reserved for all the cases in whom there is concern about PVR.

Treatment. Medical management with diuretics and ACE inhibitors is usually required for complete AVSD while waiting for surgical repair although the use of afterload reduction with ACE inhibitors is still controversial. In most infants, failure to thrive is an indication for repair which is usually performed within the first 3–6 months. Patients with unrepaired AVSD and Eisenmenger syndrome respond to pulmonary vasodilator therapy after diagnostic catheterization [21].

Outcome. Currently, excellent short-term survival after AVSD repair is the norm.

In the postoperative AVSD patients, the most common causes of late morbidity and mortality and consequently need of reoperation are dysfunction of the left AV valve (mainly regurgitation), subaortic stenosis, residual septal defects, and heart block [22]. Early mortality has been reported at 4% after reoperation during childhood; the highest risk is in those patients requiring left AV valve replacement [23]. Atrial arrhythmias appear to have an earlier age of onset after AVSD repair than in other atrial shunts, likely due to concomitant left AV valve dysfunction [24].

1.1.1.4 Patent Ductus Arteriosus

Patent ductus arteriosus (PDA) is a vascular structure which connects the descending aorta to the roof of pulmonary arterial trunk near the origin of left pulmonary artery. Usually it closes spontaneously within the first 48 h after birth, by constriction of the medial smooth muscle due to the acute increase in oxygen tension and reduction in prostaglandin E_2 and I_2 levels. Subsequently, during the following 2–3 weeks, muscle fibers are replaced by connective tissue resulting in formation of ligamentum arteriosum. If this does not occur, there is a patent ductus arteriosus (PDA). It accounts for 5–10% of all CHD in children, more frequent in females than in males [25]. Considering the anatomy, it can vary significantly in its shape, size, and attachment to the aorta; usually its narrowest part is the pulmonary arterial end. The most common type is a funnel-shaped duct with a localized narrowing at the pulmonary artery junction. PDA results in L-R shunt with potential left heart volume overload and pulmonary artery pressure overload. Clinical features depend on size, length, and age at presentation; especially the size should be correlated to the age and weight of the patient. Small PDA is usually not associated with either symptoms or signs of volume/pressure overload. Moderate and large PDA may present predominantly with left heart failure due to volume overload or right heart failure due to PA and RV pressure overload. Large PDA, if not closed in time, generally develops in Eisenmenger syndrome.

Diagnosis. In case of large PDA, peripheral arterial pulses are bounding with a rapid upstroke; pulse pressure is wide because of rapid runoff of the blood from the systemic circulation to the pulmonary circulation. In a patient with small to moderate PDA, only a systolic murmur may be heard, whereas, in a large shunt, a continuous machinery-type murmur is audible at the upper left sternal edge; the systolic component sound is a crescendo, and the diastolic component sound is a decrescendo. A normal ECG or left ventricular hypertrophy (LVH) is seen with small to moderate PDA. Biventricular hypertrophy is seen with large PDA and pulmonary hypertension. Classically, chest x-ray reveals enlarged cardiac silhouette when the relative pulmonary-to-systemic flow ratio is >2:1; cardiomegaly occurs with the enlargement of left atrium (LA) and left ventricle and ascending aorta. Pulmonary vascular markings are increased. TTE evaluation gives accurate information about ductal anatomy and physiology and is practically feasible in almost all infants, in children, and in many adults.

Treatment. PDA should be closed in patients with signs of LV volume overload even if asymptomatic and in patients with PAH but PAP < 2/3 of systemic pressure or PVR < 2/3 of systemic vascular resistance (SVR). Closure should be avoided in "silent" duct, very small with no murmur, and in PDA-Eisenmenger. Percutaneous closure can be performed in those cases who meet certain criteria concerning body weight and ductal size; it is feasible and safe in children weighing more than 5 kg with PDA diameter of 2.5–3 mm. In smaller-weight babies, this option is still under debate [26, 27], whereas larger PDAs are currently best managed with surgery (via thoracotomy).

Percutaneous closure is the first choice treatment in adults, even if cardiac surgery is indicated due to other concomitant cardiac lesions, because calcification of the duct increases surgical complications. The PDA anatomical characteristics guide the choice of proper occlusion device because different types are worldwide currently available. Small ducts can be closed using coils such as Cook detachable coil, whereas large PDAs (Fig. 1.4) can be addressed, according to the anatomy, using different devices such as an Amplatzer Duct Occluder (ADO) I device or its modification ADO II (Fig. 1.5) [28] or a mVSD Amplatzer Occluder or an ASD Amplatzer Occluder [29] or the new Occlutech(®) PDA Occluder [30].

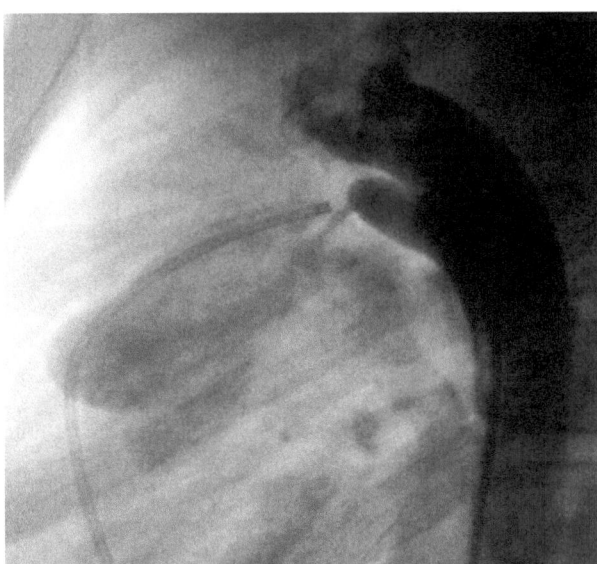

Fig. 1.4 Fluoroscopy, lateral view, aortic angiogram: PDA

Fig. 1.5 Percutaneous closure with Amplatzer Duct Occluder II device

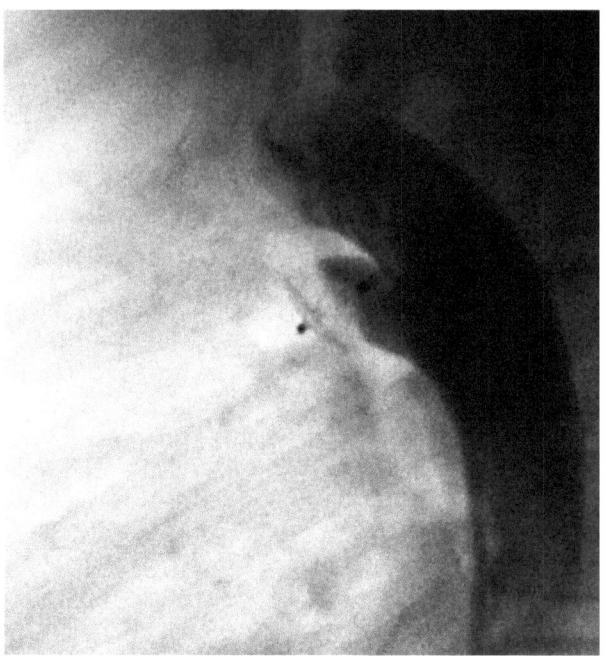

Outcome. Early and mid-term complications after transcatheter closure may include device embolization or dislocation. Embolization can occur more often after coil release; according to the size, coil can embolize in the pulmonary arteries or in the aorta and subsequently in all the arterial vessels as the intracranial arteries. In case of dislocation or malposition, device can cause left pulmonary artery stenosis or aortic stenosis associated, quite often, to residual shunting. Hemolysis is another rare and serious complication usually after coil PDA occlusion, related to a residual flow at the end of the procedure. If it happens, it is difficult to eliminate as long as the residual shunt is closed. At present, overall device occlusion rate is about 95%. Early complications after surgical closure may include recurrent laryngeal nerve palsy, chylothorax, pneumothorax, and immediate LV dysfunction. Untreated PDA may lead to POVD and Eisenmenger condition. Aneurysm of the ductus is a rare complication that develops gradually.

1.1.1.5 Aortopulmonary Window

Aortopulmonary window (APW) is a large defect between the ascending aorta and the main PA which results from failure of the spiral septum to completely divide the embryonic truncus arteriosus (Fig. 1.6). It represents 0.2–0.6% of all CHDs. In approximately half of the patients, there are associated cardiac abnormalities, most commonly VSD, interrupted aortic arch, aortic coarctation, and tetralogy of Fallot [31]. In isolated APW, clinical features are similar to those of large PDA.

Diagnosis. In isolated APW, peripheral pulses are bounding, but the heart murmur is of the systolic ejection type rather than continuous murmur at the base. On

Fig. 1.6 Aortopulmonary window (1)

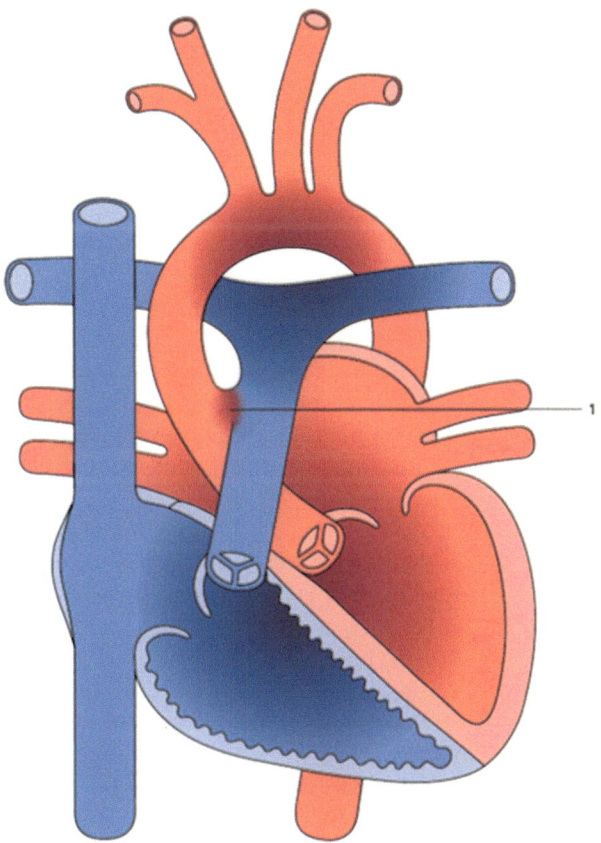

ECG, biventricular hypertrophy is seen. Classically, chest x-ray reveals enlarged cardiac silhouette due to the enlargement of left chambers; pulmonary vascular markings are markedly increased. TTE evaluation gives accurate information about the anatomy of APW which always should be ruled out in case of unexplained pulmonary hypertension. Diagnostic cardiac catheterization is usually reserved for all the cases in whom there is concern about PVR.

Treatment. This defect has no tendency to reduce or close spontaneously; therefore prompt surgical closure is indicated when the diagnosis is made as long as PVR is normal. In some selected cases of isolated APW with favorable anatomy, percutaneous device closure can be achieved [32].

Outcome. Without intervention, 40–50% of all patients will die due to congestive heart failure during the first year of life, and a large number of survivors will suffer from sequelae of congestive heart failure or pulmonary vascular disease later on. Outcomes of early repair of APW are excellent, including infants with complex associated cardiac lesions which should contemporarily be repaired. Cardiac reoperation can be required in complex APW, mainly with concomitant arch repair, and is usually related to aortic obstruction [33].

1.1.2 Left-Heart Congenital Heart Disease

1.1.2.1 With Inflow Obstruction

Cor Triatriatum Sinister

Cor triatriatum sinister (CTS) is a rare congenital abnormality characterized by the left atrium being divided into two chambers by a fibrous membrane, a proximal chamber that receives the pulmonary venous drainage and a distal chamber that contains the mitral valve and the left atrial appendage. CTS can occur in isolation (classic) or in association with other congenital cardiac anomalies (atypical) such as an ASD [34]. The atypical form occurs in 50–85% of all patients with CTS, although it is rare in adolescents and adults. Older patients more often have an isolated type of CTS. Symptoms are related to the size of fenestrations within the fibrous membrane and therefore to the degree of obstruction; presenting symptoms can mimic those seen in mitral stenosis and are related to both pulmonary venous and pulmonary arterial hypertension [35].

Diagnosis. Physical findings include dyspnea, a loud S2 and basal lung crackles. ECG usually shows right axis deviation and right ventricular hypertrophy (RVH). On chest x-ray, there is evidence of pulmonary venous congestion or pulmonary edema, prominent PA, and varying degree of right heart enlargement. TTE is mandatory to assess the intra-atrial membrane characteristics and the presence of associated CHD. In the differential diagnosis, a supramitral membrane is distinguished from the CTS membrane by its location below the left atrial appendage. This is an important differentiation, because, as a result of its proximity to the mitral valve and left circumflex coronary artery, the resection of a supramitral membrane is more difficult than in case of CTS membrane.

Treatment. Surgery is the definitive treatment and should be considered at any age if there are any associated symptoms or complications.

Outcome. Surgery in patients with CTS is performed with good outcomes. Mortality and reoperation rate are nearly 0% in patients with classic CTS and are determined by the repair of associated anomalies in atypical CTS [36]. The risk of recurrent intra-atrial obstruction postoperatively is low [37]. Pulmonary hypertension regresses rapidly in survivors if the correction is made early.

Congenital Mitral Valve Stenosis

Different anatomic types are described [38]:

- Congenital mitral valve (MV) stenosis: Extremely rare, it usually involves abnormalities of one or more components of the valve apparatus (Fig. 1.7).
- Supravalvar mitral ring: A thin fibrous membrane partially or completely encircles the mitral orifice and adheres to the leaflets. It is most commonly associated with "shone complex" which comprises parachute MV, subaortic stenosis, and coarctation of the aorta.
- Parachute MV: In the most typical and frequent form, all the chordal attachments are to a single papillary muscle (Fig. 1.8).

Fig. 1.7 Congenital mitral
valve dysplasia and
stenosis (1)

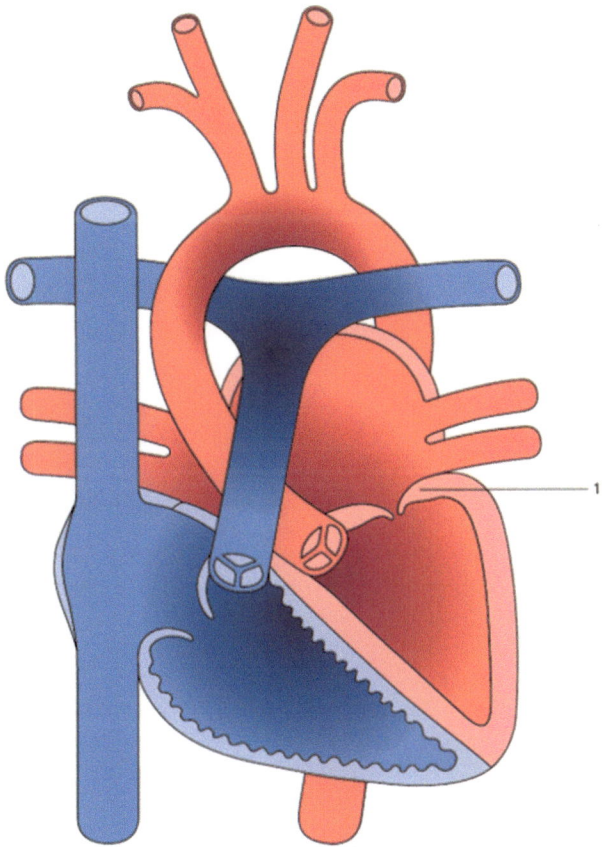

- Double-orifice MV: Two complete mitral orifices are supported by their own tension apparatus. The orifices are usually unbalanced with the smaller one directed to the anterolateral commissure. Rarely it may be associated with AVSD or VSD and coarctation.
- Arcade MV: The leaflets insert directly into the papillary muscles or the ventricular wall without chordal attachments, resulting in stenosis and regurgitation.

Symptoms and clinical signs clearly reflect the degree of pulmonary venous congestion, pulmonary hypertension, and right heart failure. The onset strictly depends on the severity of the stenosis: severe stenosis becomes evident in the neonatal period (failure to thrive, diaphoresis, cough, and recurrent respiratory infections), whereas mild or moderate disease usually presents later on in infancy, childhood, or adolescence.

Diagnosis. The typical murmur is an apical low-pitched rumbling mid-diastolic murmur. In presence of PH, a right ventricular heave is usually palpable. ECG during infancy may be normal; as the disease progresses, LA enlargement, RVH, and RA enlargement gradually appear. With ongoing atrium dilatation, atrial

Fig. 1.8 Parachute mitral valve (1)

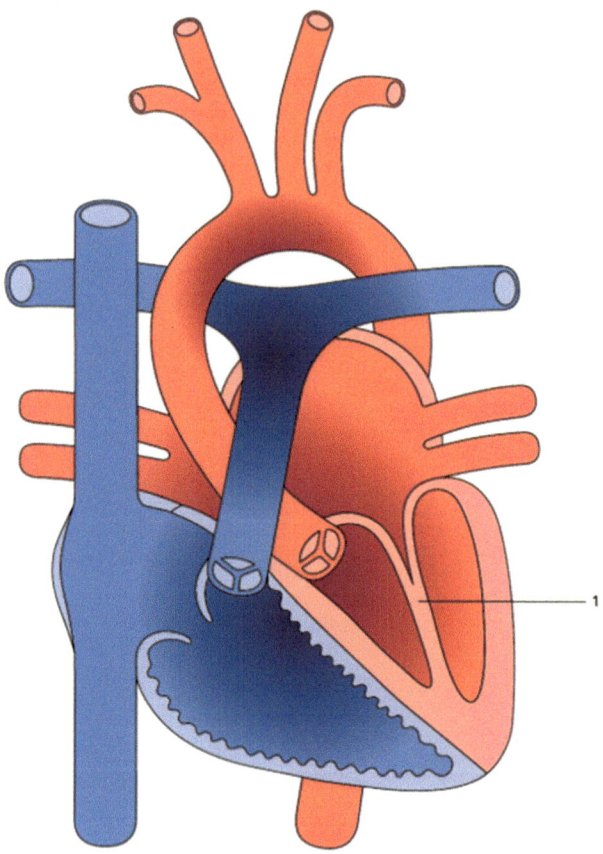

arrhythmias may occur. Chest x-ray shows dilatation of LA, PA, and RV; in severe disease, Kerley's B lines may be evident. TTE is diagnostic of the condition in terms of anatomic and functional MV details. Cardiac catheterization is indicated when there is discrepancy between echo measurements, hemodynamics, and clinical status or to ascertain the presence of POVD and its reversibility.

Treatment. Patients may require diuretics to alleviate pulmonary venous congestions. In case of severe obstruction, surgical valve repair or replacement with a prosthetic valve may be indicated but carries morbidity and mortality [39]. Only a few selected patients with hypoplastic annulus may benefit from balloon angioplasty which delays the need for surgical valve repair or replacement [40]. Valve choices for infants are limited: a mechanical valve is preferred with the caveat that long-term anticoagulation is necessary. For supravalvar mitral ring, early surgical repair should be considered in the presence of severe heart failure. Isolated double-orifice MV may never require intervention. MV arcade is usually repairable making the need of replacement quite rare.

Outcome. The prognosis after valve repair or replacement depends on many factors: patient age and size, the degree of annual hypoplasia, ventricular size and performance, severity of PH, and presence of other lesions [41]. MV replacement in neonates and infants is associated with an early mortality rate of approximately 10–20% at 6 months [42]; furthermore, prosthetic valves need to be replaced within 5–10 years due to the infant's growth and prosthetic stenosis or pannus formation. Similar data are reported in children: 50% of patients require prosthesis replacement by 10 years post-valve implantation [43].

In adults following percutaneous valvuloplasty, the survival rate is 80–90% in those with favorable MV morphology. Bioprosthetic valves last approximately 5–10 years, whereas mechanical valves last a lifetime. Five-year survival rate in adults after valve replacement exceed 70% unless they have coinciding complex CHD.

1.1.2.2 Congenital Mitral Valve Regurgitation

It is most often associated with other congenital cardiac abnormalities. Mitral valve prolapse (MVP) is rare in infants and extremely rare in neonates; exceptions are cases associated with Marfan syndrome or other connective tissue disorders as Ehlers-Danlos syndrome or osteogenesis imperfecta [44]. In MVP leaflets extend beyond the annular plane during ventricular systole; any portion of MV leaflets can be affected resulting in varying degrees of regurgitation.

Along with aortic dilation, MVP is the cardiovascular abnormality typical of Marfan syndrome which is a heritable autosomal dominant connective tissue disorder causing histologic and morphologic changes in fibrillin structure. Both the anterior and posterior leaflets become elongated and redundant; chordal rupture, progressive annular dilation, and calcification may occur.

Timing of MVP presentation is variable and depends on the degree of regurgitation. Due to left atrial dilation, left main stem bronchial compression, elevated pulmonary capillary hydrostatic pressure, atrial arrhythmias, and respiratory symptoms occur. Children with severe MV regurgitation may present with orthopnea, dyspnea, chest pain, palpitations, reduced exercise tolerance, or syncope.

Diagnosis. A regurgitant holosystolic murmur is audible at the apex with radiation to the left axilla and left back. A loud S3 and an apical rumble may be present as well. In case of moderate to severe regurgitation, ECG and CXR may show hypertrophy and dilation of left chambers. The main tool used for diagnosing congenital MV regurgitation is echocardiography for both qualitative and quantitative assessment.

Treatment. Patients presenting with congestive heart failure require diuretics and ACE inhibitors to reduce afterload and to improve cardiac output [45]. Isolated MVP and cleft mitral valve rarely require intervention in infants or children unless Marfan syndrome coexists; in this case, MV replacement may be indicated depending on the severity of regurgitation. Percutaneous MV repair has been emerging as an option for the treatment of MV regurgitation in adults; current modalities include MV repair by placing metal clip on the leaflets and MV annuloplasty by placing into the coronary sinus to the great cardiac vein in order to circle three-fourths of the entire annulus [46].

MV is typically repaired prior to the need for replacement; multiple techniques are nowadays available for repair. Replacement is most commonly performed using mechanical valves, necessitating lifelong anticoagulation.

Outcome. Cleft MV and MVP, without intervention, have excellent short-term outcomes because they feature no progression of insufficiency except in the presence of connective tissue abnormalities. Short- and immediate-term outcomes after repairing a cleft MV are excellent, and most patients require no additional interventions. Patients with Marfan syndrome and MV involvement should be closely monitored keeping in mind the associated complications, in particular of the aortic valve, aorta, ventricular function, and arrhythmias; aortic aneurysm dissection or rupture is rare in childhood and more typically occurs in the third and fourth decades of life [47].

1.1.2.3 With Outflow Obstruction

Aortic Stenosis
Aortic stenosis (AS) represents 3–6% of all patients with CHD, and it occurs more often in males (male-female ratio of 4:1). Stenosis may be at the valvular (70%), subvalvular (23%), or supravalvular (7%) level.

Valvular AS is usually caused by bicuspid aortic valve with a fused commissure and an eccentric orifice [48] (Fig. 1.9). Less common is the unicuspid valve with

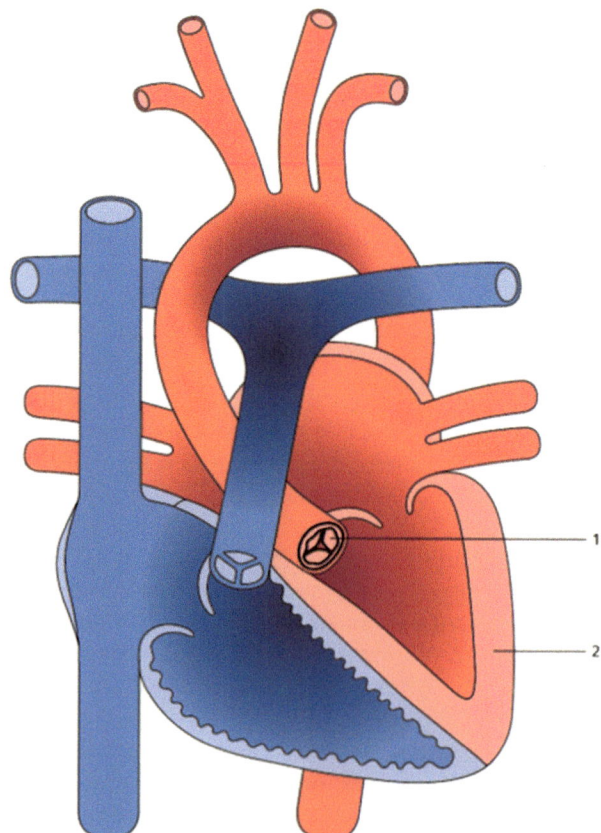

Fig. 1.9 Congenital aortic valve stenosis: (1) Valvular AS. (2) Left ventricular hypertrophy

Fig. 1.10 Supravalvular aortic stenosis: (1) Supravalvular AS. (2) LV hypertrophy

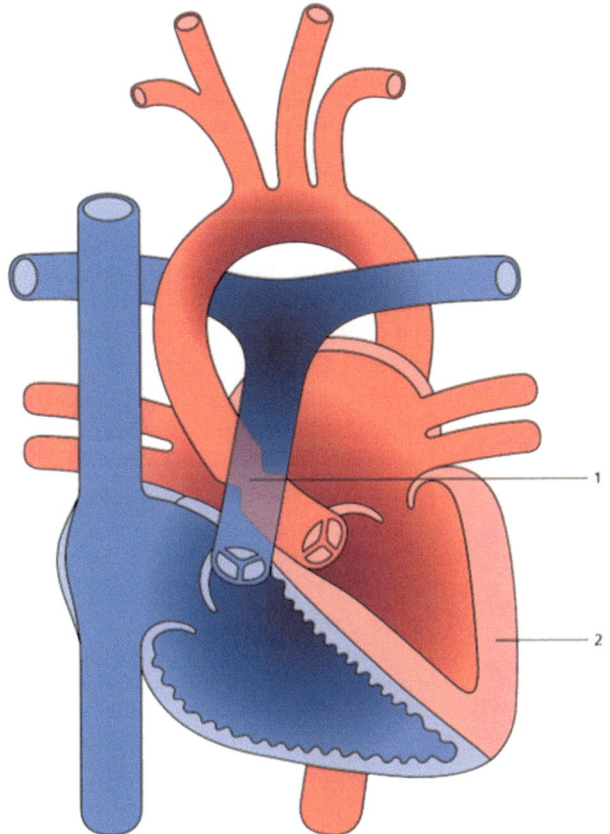

one lateral attachment, while a tricuspid valve with a central stenotic orifice is the least common form.

Subvalvular stenosis may result from discrete membranous diaphragm, usually associated with other CHDs like VSD, PDA, or coarctation, or, less commonly, from tunnel-like fibromuscular narrowing of left ventricular outflow tract. The latter is usually associated with other LV anomalies including Shone complex.

In supravalvular AS the constriction occurs at the upper margin of the sinus of Valsalva, and aorta narrows in an hourglass deformity (Fig. 1.10). This is often associated with Williams-Beuren syndrome, an elastin protein gene disorder, which includes characteristic facies, mental retardation, and multiple PA stenoses.

Patients with AS are usually asymptomatic throughout childhood, even when stenosis is severe. Only 5% of children develop congestive heart failure in the neonatal period due to critical AS. Some children, as they approach adolescence, may become symptomatic for exercise intolerance; episodes of chest pain, due to myocardial ischemia; and syncope on exertion. Both chest pain and syncope are serious symptoms which may precede sudden death.

Aortic valvular stenosis is a progressive disease; two processes probably account for this: the development of myocardial fibrosis and the decrease in size of the stenotic valvar orifice by fibrosis and, later on, calcification of the valve. Bicuspid aortic valves often go undetected in early life; however, up to 70% of the cases develop some degree of stenosis or regurgitation by age 30.

Diagnosis. Infants with critical AS usually present in poor general condition, poor pulses, S3 and/or S4, and hyperdynamic precordium with a right ventricular tap. They may have either no murmur or a soft systolic ejection-type murmur due to the severe cardiac function impairment; differential oxygen saturations between the right arm (higher) and lower limbs (lower) are often detected.

In children and adolescents with severe valvular AS, a harsh grade 3–4/6, ejection systolic murmur is best heard at the second right or left intercostal space with good transmission to the neck and apex. In case of stenotic and regurgitant bicuspid valve, a high-pitched, early diastolic decrescendo murmur may be audible as well. Correlation of the severity of AS and the ECG abnormalities is relatively poor; LVH with or without strain pattern may be present in severe cases. Echocardiography is the preferred method for diagnosis and decision-making; it allows one to visualize directly the valve, to quantify the degree of stenosis, to assess cardiac function, and to detect associated CHD. In infant with severe AS, endocardial fibroelastosis can be visualized by the presence of a bright white layer in the endocardial tissue. Cardiac catheterization is rarely performed solely for diagnostic purposes; low cardiac output state can underestimate the degree of AS; therefore the aortic valve area can be calculated using the Gorlin and Hakki equations which include cardiac output and pressure gradient.

Treatment. For critical, neonatal valvular AS, inotropic agents and diuretics should be started to treat CHF; prostaglandin E_1 infusion should be given to reopen the arterial duct. Relief of the AS, either by percutaneous balloon valvuloplasty (PBV) or surgical valvotomy, should be achieved as soon as possible. Percutaneous valvuloplasty has become the preferred treatment at many centers, also in children and young adults [49]. Children who have undergone aortic valvotomy may require valve replacement later on if the valve becomes calcified or rigid or, sooner, if important regurgitation occurs; no currently available replacement valve is perfect: mechanical prostheses are long-lived but thrombogenic so anticoagulation is required; homograft valves, although free from thrombogenic complications, are often shorter-lived because of destruction by calcification at an unpredictable rate. Another option for aortic valve replacement, even in neonates and especially in small children with dysplastic and obstructed aortic valves, is the Ross operation [50] in which the patient's native pulmonary valve is excised and placed in aortic position and a homograft valve is placed in pulmonary position. The major advantages are related to the neoaortic valve which, being the patient's own tissue, degenerates very slowly, continues to grow with the patient, and does not require anticoagulation. Major disadvantages are high operative rates of acute and chronic morbidity and mortality when performed in neonates and infant, RV-PA conduit degeneration and dysfunction, and the potential dilation of the neoaorta with subsequent development of aortic regurgitation.

In subvalvar AS, surgical obstruction removal is indicated to relieve the LV pressure overload and to reduce the mechanical trauma to the aortic valve. The operative risk approaches that of operation for valvular AS; the major hazard is the possibility of damage to the mitral valve anterior leaflet since the membrane is quite often attached to that.

In supravalvular AS, surgery may be indicated for a lesser pressure gradient compared with valvular AS due to the potential concomitant disease of coronary arteries. Surgical obstruction relief is accomplished by different techniques: patch enlargement of the narrowing or slide aortoplasty techniques, according to the anatomy and the degree of ascending aorta hypoplasia.

Outcome. Mortality rate for infants and small children with valvular AS ranges from 15 to 20%. Sick neonates with poor preoperative general conditions have a mortality rate as high as 40%. The hospital mortality in older children is 1–2%.

Overall, PBV achieves a 60% reduction in the aortic valve gradient with a procedure-related mortality of 1.9% and complication rate strongly correlated with the age of the child. Repeat PBV and valve replacement occurred in 15% of patients after initial PBV [51], whereas 25% of patients require valve replacement 15–20 years after the original surgery.

Subaortic membrane has a high recurrence rate after surgical removal mainly in patients operated sooner and with high peak pressure gradients, suggesting a more severe form of disease [52].

Over the long term after supravalvular stenosis surgical relief, reobstruction and aortic valve progressive regurgitation can occur [53].

Coarctation of the Aorta

Coarctation of the aorta (CoA) is considered part of a generalized arteriopathy and not only a circumscript narrowing of the aorta. It occurs as a discrete stenosis most commonly seen in periductal region or as a long, hypoplastic segment (Fig. 1.11). It accounts for 5–8% of all CHD and may occur in isolation or in association with other anomalies: bicuspid aortic valve (up to 80%); subvalvular, valvular, or supravalvular AS; MV stenosis (as seen in Shone complex); hypoplastic left heart syndrome; and aberrant subclavian artery. CoA can be associated with Turner, Williams-Beuren [54], and congenital rubella syndromes or neurofibromatosis.

CoA causes significant increase in LV afterload resulting in increased wall stress, compensatory hypertrophy, and LV dysfunction; from the aorta a variable degree of arterial collateral circulation can develop. Elastic fiber rupture and fibrosis are typical of cystic medial necrosis which is found in the ascending and descending aorta determining an increased arterial stiffness [55]. Clinical signs and symptoms depend on the severity of CoA; when severe, closure of the arterial duct after birth will result in critical aortic obstruction, LV dilatation and dysfunction, low cardiac output state, and, if untreated, death. In less severe forms, CoA may be picked up during childhood when a murmur may be heard and femoral pulses found to be weak; in adulthood the most common sign is systemic hypertension [56]. Symptoms may include nosebleeds, dizziness, headache, shortness of breath, abdominal angina, leg cramps, claudication, exertional leg fatigue, and cold feet. Some life-threatening

Fig. 1.11 Aortic isthmic coarctation (1)

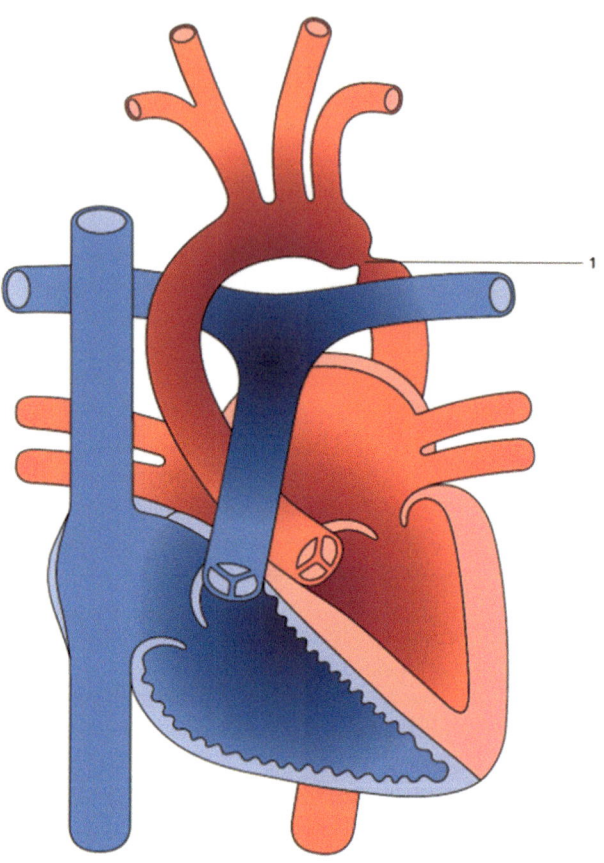

conditions may occur during "natural history" of CoA: left heart failure, intracranial hemorrhage (from berry aneurysm of circle of Willis), aortic rupture/dissection, premature coronary and cerebral artery disease, and infective endocarditis.

Diagnosis. Neonates with severe CoA are pale and experience varying degree of respiratory distress and low cardiac output state; differential cyanosis may be present due to a right-to-left ductal shunt causing cyanosis only in the lower half of the body. Peripheral pulses may be weak and thready; the S2 is single and loud; a gallop is usually present, whereas a heart murmur is not audible in 50% of sick babies as long as the cardiac function improves. On ECG, RVH or right bundle branch block (RBBB) is often seen rather than LVH. On x-ray, marked cardiomegaly and pulmonary venous congestion are usually present.

In adolescent and adult patients, a significant CoA is diagnosed when there is a systolic blood pressure gradient between the upper and lower limb of at least 20 mmHg or less than 20 mmHg in the presence of systemic hypertension; common physical findings are weak or absent lower limb pulses. A continuous murmur in the left back near the scapula signals the presence of large collateral arteries; a systolic murmur sometimes can be heard in the left infraclavicular area or in the left upper back. ECG generally shows LVH in patients with chronic hypertension. In some cases, chest-x-ray shows some typical findings which strongly suggest CoA: prominent ascending aorta contour, the change in aortic caliber at the coarctation site producing the "3" sign, and notching of the inferior margin of ribs 3–8 owing to erosion by large and developed collateral arteries.

Echocardiography is the definitive imaging modalities for diagnosing CoA and for identifying all associated cardiac defects; a sagittal view from the suprasternal notch should be used to visualize the posterior wedge-shaped shelf that characterizes true CoA. In neonates and infants, it is sometimes difficult to establish a proper diagnosis in the presence of PDA, and CoA may become evident once the duct closes. A typical Doppler flow pattern with persistent forward flow into diastole usually confirms a significant stenosis.

Key features, prior to any treatment, are the aortic arch morphology and the branching pattern of the head and neck vessels. If echocardiography is inconclusive, MR and CT are the preferred noninvasive techniques to evaluate the entire aorta, while cardiac catheterization is still the gold standard in case of complex CoA associated with other CHD: a peak-to-peak gradient >20 mmHg is indicative of significant CoA in the absence of well-developed collaterals.

Treatment. For sick neonates, PGE_1 infusion should be given to reopen the arterial duct; inotropic agents, diuretics, and, if necessary, mechanical ventilation should be started to treat CHF. All these measures aim at stabilizing the patient in preparation for surgery. In fact, the standard management of native CoA in neonates, infants, and young children is surgical repair [57]. Some different surgical techniques have been used: subclavian flap repair, patch aortoplasty, and, currently, resection with end to end anastomosis, via a left lateral thoracotomy or, in the presence of severely hypoplastic aortic arch, via a median sternotomy on cardiopulmonary bypass. For older children, adolescents, and adults with native CoA, in many specialized centers, balloon angioplasty (BA) with covered or non-covered stent implantation has become first choice treatment if anatomy is appropriate [57, 58] (Figs. 1.12 and 1.13). Procedure is generally performed under general anesthesia which reduces sympathetic drive and may result in a falsely low gradient across the CoA site.

Outcome. Surgical short-term complications include recurrent laryngeal or phrenic nerve damage, Horner syndrome, pleural effusion, and chylothorax. Short-term outcomes relate mostly to the clinical condition of the patient prior to surgery and the severity of associated cardiac lesions. For children and adolescents operated on, spinal cord injury with paraplegia is quite rare but is more common in patients with poor collateral circulation. Initially, long-term incidence of recurrent CoA after surgery approached 30%, whereas, nowadays, percentage has gone down to about 10% [59]. BA is mainly indicated in recoarctation in infants and young children providing excellent acute relief of obstruction but being associated with high rate of coarctation recurrence and big concerns regarding aneurysm formation and dissection. The use of covered stents has reduced significantly the incidence of dissection and aneurysm formation at the site of treated coarctation; furthermore, stents can be re-dilated later in life in case of recoarctation or residual stenosis.

Fig. 1.12 Angiography:
severe isthmic aortic
coarctation

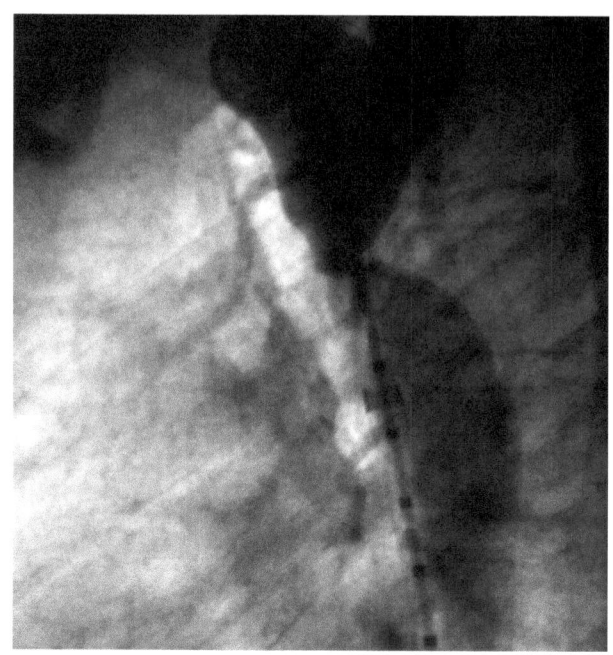

Fig. 1.13 Angiography
post-covered stent
implantation

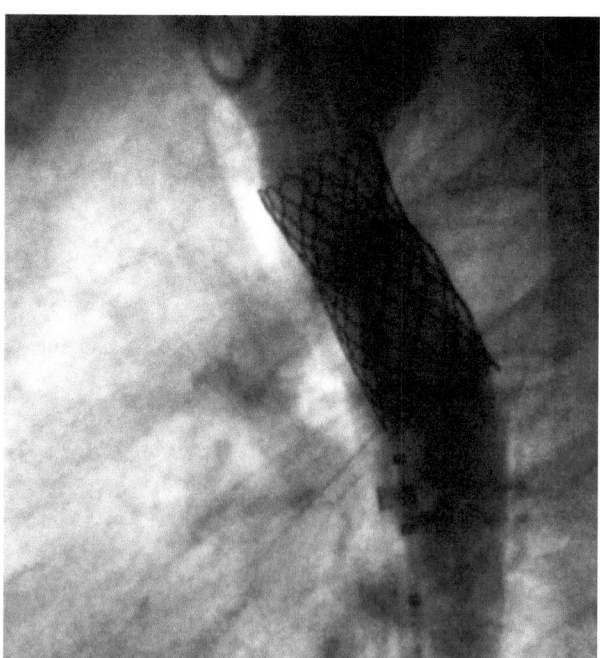

After BA with stenting, acute complications may include stent migration, the most important one occurring in 5% of cases; cerebrovascular accident, seen more frequently in older patients; and femoral artery injury resulting in leg ischemia or retroperitoneal bleeding [60]. Considering delayed complications, the incidence of aortic dissection or aneurysm formation following stenting is reported at approximately 10% of cases, most commonly at the site of the narrowest segment of CoA. The vast majority of aneurysms are small and can be managed conservatively [60, 61].

Any successful CoA treatment is usually effective in lowering systemic blood pressure, but during follow-up at least one-third of patients remain hypertensive demonstrating that CoA is not purely an isolated mechanical obstruction but a complex aortic vasculopathy involving many factors such as arterial stiffness and elasticity, endothelial function, and renin-angiotensin system. Hypertension is definitely the most important long-term concern, being a key determinant of late morbidity and mortality [62, 63]. The most relevant predictor of problematic hypertension long after repair is the age at treatment; the lowest rate is seen in those repaired under 1 year of age.

Interrupted Aortic Arch
Interrupted aortic arch (IAA) accounts for approximately 1.5% of all CHD, and 15% of IAA patients have DiGeorge syndrome. The anatomical spectrum varies from an extreme form of CoA to an absence of an arch segment. According to the site of interruption, three different types are described:

(a) Type A: The interruption is distal to the origin of left subclavian artery; it occurs in 30% of cases (Fig. 1.14).
(b) Type B: The interruption is between the left carotid and left subclavian arteries (Fig. 1.15); it occurs in 43% of cases. DiGeorge syndrome is reported in about 50% of patients.
(c) Type C: The interruption is between the innominate and left carotid arteries; it occurs in 17% of cases.

VSD is the most common associated anomaly seen in approximately 73% of these cases. A PDA is invariably present with IAA, and the descending aorta is a continuation of the ductus. Bicuspid aortic valve occurs in 60% of all cases, subaortic stenosis occurs in about 20%, and truncus arteriosus and AP window occur in about 10%.

Diagnosis. Neonates present with signs of CHF, variable degrees of cyanosis, and respiratory distress. Due to the frequent association of VSD, differential cyanosis is uncommon. Peripheral pulses may be weak and thready; a gallop rhythm is usually present. On ECG, RVH is often seen in uncomplicated cases. On x-ray, cardiomegaly, increased pulmonary vascular markings, and pulmonary venous

Fig. 1.14 Type A aortic
arch interruption (1)

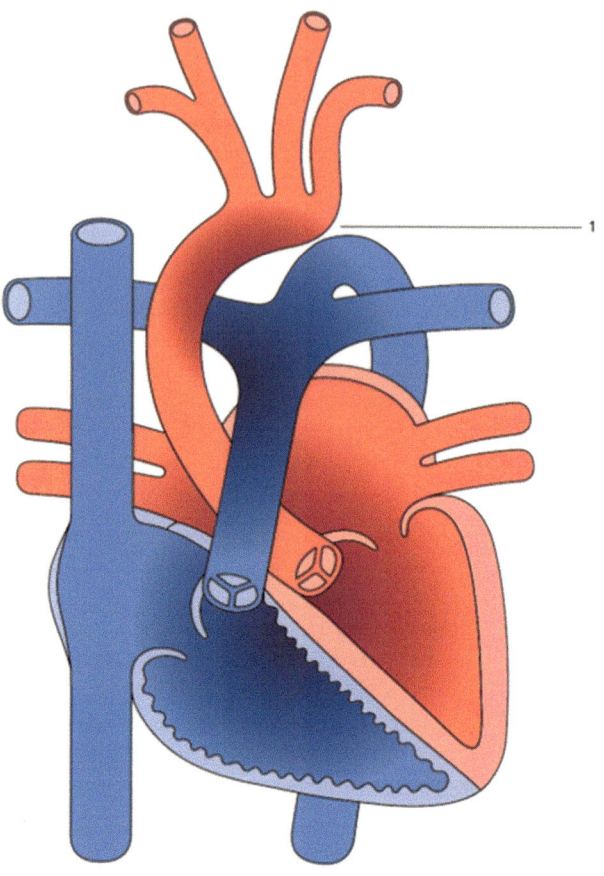

congestion are usually present; the upper mediastinum may be narrow in case of absence of thymus as in DiGeorge syndrome. Echocardiography is the preferred method for diagnosis and decision-making; it allows one to evaluate the type of interruption, the aortic valve, the cardiac function, and the associated CHD. Cardiac catheterization is rarely performed, in complex cases, just for diagnostic purposes.

Treatment. For sick neonates, PGE_1 infusion should be given to keep the arterial duct open; inotropic agents, diuretics, and, if necessary, mechanical ventilation should be started to treat CHF. All these measures aim at stabilizing the patient in preparation for surgery. In fact, the standard management of IAA and simple VSD is a single-step surgical repair [64]. If primary repair is not feasible, PA banding and interruption repair should be the initial operation followed by, at a later date, debanding and repair of other cardiac anomalies.

Outcome. Perioperative mortality can be as low as 10% for initial surgery [64]. Surgical short-term complications include recurrent laryngeal or phrenic nerve damage, ischemic cerebral accident, pleural effusion, and chylothorax. The long-term outcomes after conventional repair of IAA and VSD are acceptable; bicuspid

Fig. 1.15 Type B aortic
arch interruption (1)

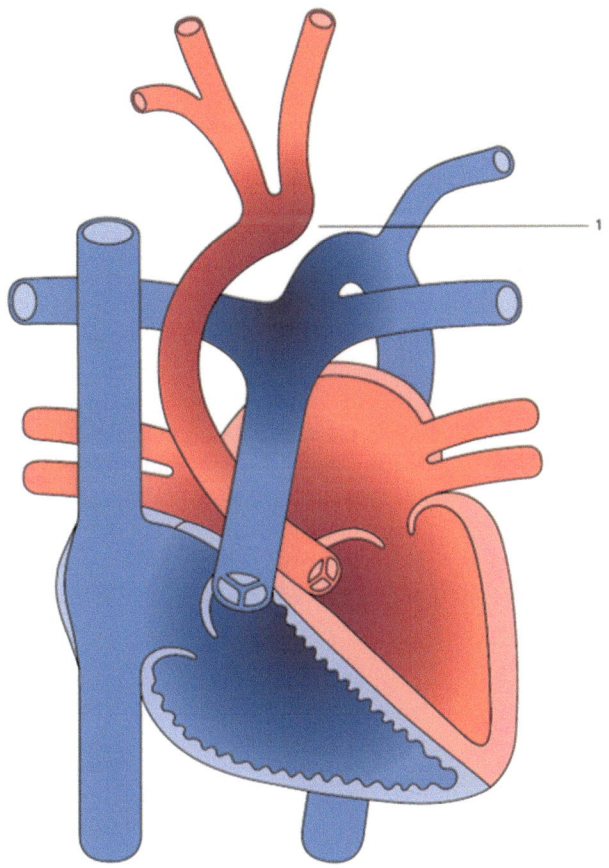

aortic valve is a significant risk factor for valve-related reinterventions [65].
Mortality rate is estimated in 3.6% at 2 years and about 39% at 21 years. Main
causes of reintervention are left ventricular outflow tract obstruction (LVOTO) and
recurrent aortic arch obstruction. Subjects with IAA demonstrate a significant burden of operative and transcatheter intervention and large magnitude deficits in exercise performance, health status, and health-related quality of life [66].

1.1.3   Right-Heart Congenital Heart Disease

1.1.3.1 Ebstein Anomaly
Ebstein anomaly (EA) accounts for <1% of all CHD with an equal distribution
between the sexes. It is a malformation which involves both the tricuspid valve (TV)
and the right ventricle (RV). Embryologically, TV leaflets arise from the myocardium through a process known as delamination which appears apically and pro-
ceeds to the atrioventricular junction. An incomplete and variable delamination,

involving the septal and posterior leaflet, results in an apically displaced and anteriorly rotated, toward the RVOT, zone of leaflet coaptation which can be considered as the "functional" TV orifice [67]. Due to the variable degree of delamination, leaflets can be very limited in excursion resulting in variable degree of regurgitation or, less frequently, stenosis. Also the anterior leaflet can have some myocardial attachments along its entire length and because the hinge point usually remains at the atrioventricular junction level, it shows a "sail-like" aspect which compensates for the abnormal septal and inferior leaflets. As a consequence of this apical and anterior displacement of the TV functional orifice, functionally RV is variably hypoplastic; the myocardium above the orifice becomes "atrialized" and, thus, thin and dysfunctional; the myocardium below the orifice typically possesses a more normal ventricular wall thickness but is still dysfunctional (Fig. 1.16). The RV impairment and the TV regurgitation decrease forward flow across the pulmonary valve reducing systemic cardiac output and increase right atrial dimensions and pressure thus favoring a right-to-left shunt through the interatrial communication; cyanosis depends upon the right-to-left shunting. Associated lesions include an ASD and less commonly a VSD or PDA; in complex forms of EA, pulmonary valve stenosis or atresia, tetralogy of Fallot, or left-sided abnormalities such as MV stenosis or regurgitation can be seen. Quite often, conduction system abnormalities coexist.

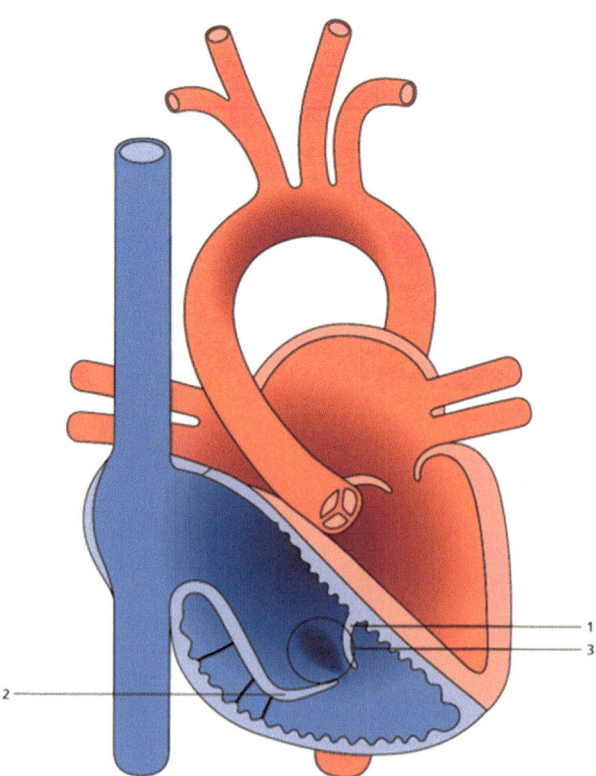

Fig. 1.16 Ebstein anomaly: (1) septal leaflet delamination abnormality. (2) Sail-like anterior leaflet. (3) Tricuspid valve regurgitation

Due to the large spectrum of anatomical features, clinical presentation and age at presentation can vary widely ranging from overt cardiac failure (dyspnea, poor feeding, and failure to thrive) or low pulmonary blood flow in neonates and infants with complex forms to almost normal findings in patients able to survive into adulthood. Approximately two-thirds of patients will present before 1 year of age and 10% will present prenatally [68]. A history of exertional dyspnea and palpitations is common in children, adolescents, and adults.

Diagnosis. Physical examination is extremely variable. Mild to severe cyanosis is usually observed as well as clubbing in older infants and children. Jugular venous distension is not common because the large RA and the atrialized RV dissipate the V wave; however it could be seen in case of severe TV regurgitation without interatrial communication. The heart examination may reveal split first and second heart sounds and/or third and fourth sounds resulting in a triple or quadruple rhythm; a soft holosystolic murmur is usually audible at the lower left sternal border. The lungs typically are normal on auscultation. Hepatomegaly is usually present.

Characteristic ECG findings of RA enlargement and RBBB are detected in most of the patients; 20–30% will display features of Wolff-Parkinson-White preexcitation with occasional episodes of supraventricular tachycardia (SVT). First-degree AV block occurs in about 40% of cases.

Due to the variability of the malformation, chest x-ray findings can range from normal to severe cardiomegaly (mainly involving the RA) with balloon-shaped heart and significantly reduced pulmonary vascular markings.

Echocardiography is the gold standard technique for morphologic and functional assessment of EA. One of the most diagnostic features is the apical displacement of the TV septal leaflet hinge point which is, in normal heart, slightly apical to mitral valve leaflet hinge point; the "displacement index" is measured in systole from the hinge point of anterior MV leaflet to the hinge point of tricuspid septal leaflet, where it begins to delaminate; if it is greater than 8 mm/m^2, a diagnosis of EA is made. Echo assessment should include TV regurgitation, RVOT obstruction, intracardiac shunts, and ventricular dimensions and function. Right heart morphology and function may alter LV geometry and subsequently function which can also be compromised by the presence of increased fibrosis within the LV myocardium since birth [69].

Cardiac MRI provides more accurate evaluation of ventricular size and function, whereas CT can help assess the coronary arteries in the adults. Cardiac catheterization can be useful only in selected and complex cases to evaluate intracardiac and intrapulmonary pressure before surgical intervention especially prior to a bidirectional cavopulmonary connection.

Treatment. Individual patient characteristics dictate how EA is managed. Patients with mild Ebstein require only regular observation. In severely cyanotic newborns, the RV is not able to generate enough pressure to open the pulmonary valve, and the R-L interatrial shunt is significant, resulting in functional pulmonary atresia and low pulmonary blood flow (PBF); PGE_1 should be given to keep the ductus arteriosus open as long as the PVR drops and antegrade flow across pulmonary valve increases. Subsequently patient's cyanosis will improve as a result of both TV regurgitation and R-L atrial shunt reduction.

Acute episodes of SVT may be treated effectively with adenosine, whereas beta blockers are commonly used as first-line preventive therapy for SVT of undetermined mechanism. In children with refractory arrhythmias, electrophysiology (EP) study and ablation should be considered; if preexcitation exists on baseline ECG, EP study and ablation should be performed before the first surgical intervention.

Only neonates with most severe forms of EA with significant TV regurgitation and/or severe RVOT obstruction will need palliative surgery consistent with a systemic-to-pulmonary arterial shunt (modified Blalock-Taussig shunt) which enables the patient to grow [70]. Indications for surgery in children, adolescents, and adults include worsening cyanosis, reduced exercise tolerance, progressive RV dilatation, and onset or progression of atrial arrhythmias. TV repair is preferred than replacement in patients less the 50 years of age; different surgical techniques have been reported, but currently, the Carpentier technique and the so-called cone reconstruction are the most effective. For patients older than 50, TV replacement with a bioprosthesis is the preferred procedure. In all patients undergoing surgery, intercardiac shunts are closed at the same time, whereas a bidirectional cavopulmonary shunt is performed in presence of markedly dysfunctional RV in order to reduce ventricle preload [71]. For patients experiencing recurrent atrial arrhythmias prior surgery, intraoperative ablation (maze procedure) is usually done. Cardiac transplantation is reserved only for the most severe, worst cases.

Outcome. Early mortality in neonates is related to right heart enlargement, severe tethering of all TV leaflets, pulmonary atresia, and LV dysfunction. Due to the medical management and surgical technique improvement over the last decades, mortality and morbidity for children with EA have been significantly reduced; consequently most children will live well into adulthood. Surgical mortality in adult patients is low, less than 3% in the current era [72]. The reoperation rate at 20 years postoperative is about 50%; the most recent procedure which has been developed for patients already operated for bioprosthesis is percutaneous valve-in-valve implantation; at the moment it is feasible in carefully selected cases [73]. Atrial arrhythmias (flutter and/or fibrillation) are the most frequent long-term complication occurring in up to one-third of operated patients [74]; even after maze procedure, recurrence rate is as high as 50% and may be the result of RA progressive enlargement secondary to worsening TV regurgitation and/or RV dysfunction. Recurrent hospitalizations are frequent with arrhythmias being, once again, the most common indications for readmission [74].

1.1.3.2 With Outflow Obstruction

Pulmonary Valve Stenosis

Pulmonary valve stenosis (PVS) with normal cardiac connections accounts for 8–12% of all CHDs. From an anatomical point of view, two forms are described: a tricuspid valve with thin leaflets, fusion of the cusps, and underdeveloped or absent commissures resulting in a dome-shaped valve, the so-called "doming," and narrow effective orifice; frequently this type of valve shows some degree of tethering to the sinotubular junction which can be mistaken for supravalvular pulmonary stenosis

Fig. 1.17 Congenital
pulmonary valve stenosis:
(1) dysplastic valve

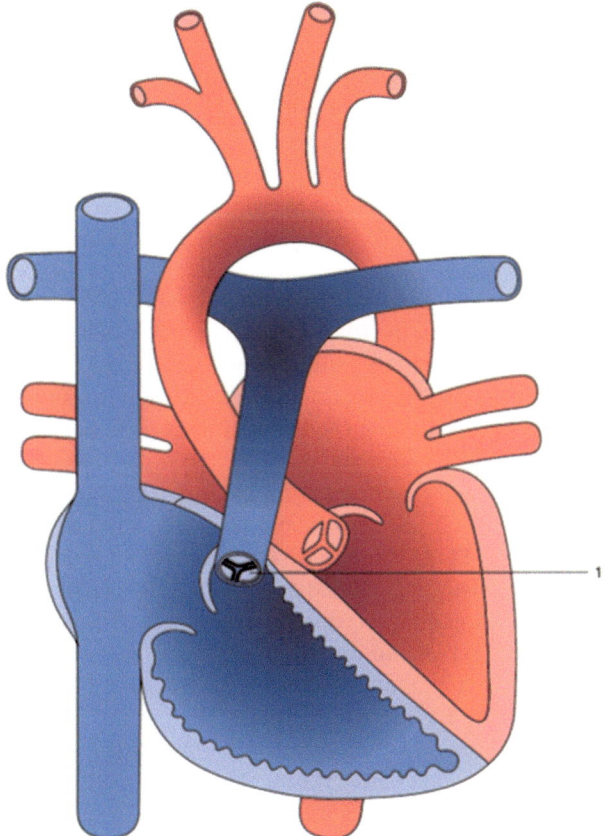

[75]; post-stenotic PA dilation is another common feature. The second form is the dysplastic one, characterized by thickened and irregular leaflets with variably hypoplastic annulus in the absence of cusp fusion (Fig. 1.17); it is typically associated with genetic syndromes such as Noonan, Williams, or Alagille syndrome.

Clinical presentation is determined by the severity of the stenosis varying from tachypnea and cyanosis in critical PVS with ductal-dependent PA circulation (due to RV hypertension, decreased output, and R-L shunt at the atrial level) to exertional dyspnea and easy fatigability in moderate to severe stenosis (due to RV inability to increase cardiac output to face the increasing demands of activity) or no symptoms as in mild obstruction; typically, these asymptomatic infants or children present with a systolic murmur at a routine pediatrician's visit.

Diagnosis. Clinical assessment is variable and correlates with severity and associated genetic syndromes. In newborns with critical stenosis, cyanosis is usually detected, and signs of CHF with hepatomegaly and peripheral vasoconstriction may be found. In children with at least moderate stenosis, a right ventricular tap and a systolic thrill may be present at the upper left sternal border; the S2 may split widely, and an ejection systolic murmur is best audible at the upper left sternal border, and it transmits well to the back too; the louder and longer the murmur, the more severe the stenosis is.

ECG usually shows right axis deviation and RVH, with strain pattern in case of severe stenosis; the degree of RVH correlates with the severity of the disease.

On chest x-ray of neonates with critical stenosis, lungs are oligemic, and varying degrees of cardiomegaly are present. In most of the children with moderate to severe PVS, cardiac silhouette is normal and will remain normal for a long time; as they get older, main PA enlargement may become prominent consistent with post-stenotic dilation.

TTE is the primary diagnostic modality, able to assess the features of the valve, the annulus size, the RV hypertrophy and dimensions, and the presence of interatrial shunt; Doppler study estimates pressure gradient across the stenotic valve; a gradient >70 mmHg is severe. Limited utility remains for CT and MRI for diagnostic purpose in this age group as well as cardiac catheterization whose role is strictly interventional.

Treatment. Newborns with critical PVS need emergency treatment to reduce mortality; PGE_1 infusion should be started as soon as possible in order to increase the size of PDA and thereby improve the pulmonary blood flow (PBF); once stabilized, neonates should undergo cardiac catheterization for percutaneous pulmonary valve balloon dilation which is the procedure of choice. Subsequently, PGE_1 may be discontinued keeping in mind that some neonates will still temporary require an additional source of PBF even after successful balloon dilation; this situation may occur when RV stiffness prevents appropriate diastolic ventricular filling or when infundibular muscular hypertrophy becomes more evident after the procedure, obstructing antegrade PV flow. This additional source can be either a PDA stent or a surgical mBTS.

If percutaneous balloon dilation is unsuccessful, surgical pulmonary valvotomy is urgently indicated in critically ill patients [76].

Infants, children, and adolescents with PVS are referred to PPV dilation when stenosis is diagnosed as severe or should become severe during a conservative follow-up. Surgical approach is required in case of resistant PVS which did not respond to previous balloon dilation. Dysplastic valves with annular hypoplasia are less likely to have a satisfying relief of obstruction.

Outcome. Short- and medium-term results for infants undergoing balloon dilation or surgical valvotomy are excellent [77]. As anesthesia, technology, and experience have improved, mortality and annular tear associated with percutaneous procedure are extremely low [78]; about 15% of all children undergoing percutaneous PV dilation will have residual subvalvular gradient of 10 mmHg or more which will typically regress by time. A significant immediate residual RV-to-PA gradient is considered one determinant of a suboptimal long-term outcome; infants with a smaller indexed pulmonary annulus are reported to have higher incidence of reintervention, ≤30%, due to restenosis [79]. Other causes for reintervention in the long term are as follows: congestive heart failure and RV dilation/dysfunction related to pulmonary valve regurgitation (PR). Operated patients have a lower transvalvular gradient during follow-up but greater valvar regurgitation. PR may be progressive;

approximately 25% of children with at least moderate PR initially increase to more than 50% with time. Estimated freedom from reintervention rate after surgery is 93.5% at 10 years and 87.7% at 20 years whereas, after percutaneous dilation, is 87.5% at 10 years and 84.4% at 20 years [80]. The most common reintervention consists of surgical PV replacement or transcatheter PV implantation.

Pulmonary Atresia with Intact Ventricular Septum

Pulmonary atresia with intact ventricular septum (PAIVS) is a rare form of cyanotic heart disease which accounts for fewer than 1% of all CHD and for approximately 3% of the critically ill newborns affected by CHD. Anatomical key features are as follows: complete obstruction at the PV level; intact interventricular septum; wide range of TV and RV abnormalities, ranging from severe hypoplasia to severe dilation; and possibility of communications between the RV cavity and epicardial coronary artery circulation (sinusoids) (Fig. 1.18).

Cyanosis is the typical neonatal presentation due to obligatory interatrial R-to-L shunting; the severity of cyanosis also depends on the amount of pulmonary blood flow (PBF), provided through the PDA, and the pulmonary vascular resistance.

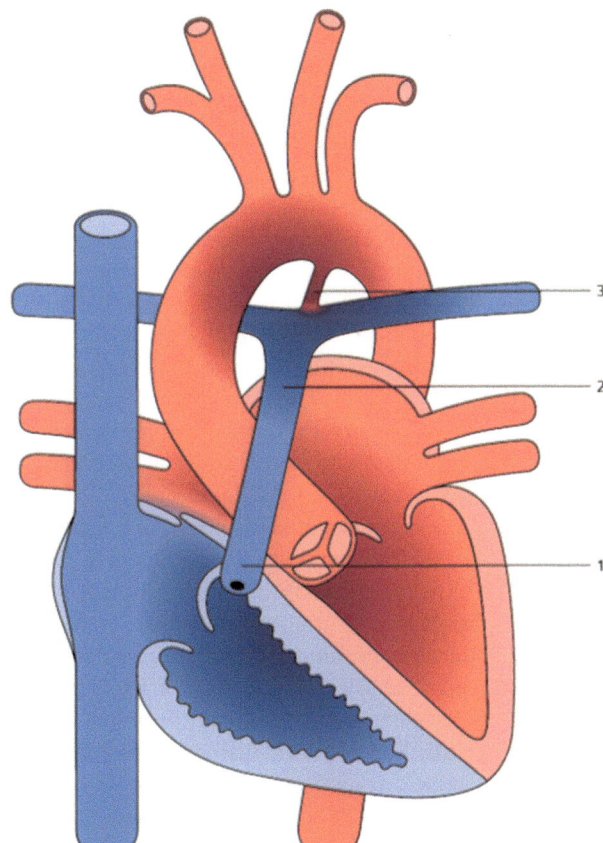

Fig. 1.18 Pulmonary atresia with intact septum: (1) Valvular atresia. (2) Main pulmonary artery. (3) PDA

Diagnosis. Variable degrees of cyanosis are detected; sometimes, in the presence of large PDA, neonates may have systemic oxygen saturation in the 90s, rendering the finding of cyanosis very subtle. Arterial pulses are generally well palpable. Auscultation reveals a single S2 with or without a murmur; generally the murmur is caused by TV regurgitation, rarely by coronary artery fistulae or markedly constricted ductus arteriosus.

On ECG, right atrial enlargement is common, occurring in about 70% of cases; the QRS axis is normal; LVH is usually present, whereas RV forces will depend on the degree of RV hypoplasia.

The cardiac silhouette on chest x-ray frontal projection can vary from normal to large, resulting from right atrial enlargement secondary to TV regurgitation; in case of severe regurgitation, cardiomegaly may resemble that observed in Ebstein anomaly. Pulmonary vascular markings are usually decreased with dark lung fields.

TTE is the definitive imaging modality for diagnosing and for addressing all the specific issues: a large PFO is present in most of the cases associated with R-L obligatory shunting. TV abnormalities are common and can vary from annular hypoplasia to Ebstein-like features or subvalvular leaflet tethering. Indeed, TV annular dimension is strongly correlated with the RV cavity size ranging from normal to severely hypoplastic, in case of small RV, or severely dilated in case of significant valvar regurgitation. Through the regurgitation jet, systolic RV pressure should be measured by Doppler and compared with systemic arterial blood pressure; most children with PAIVS have suprasystemic pressure secondary to complete obstruction at the PV level and the presence of a reasonably competent TV. Based on the presence or absence of the three portions, inlet, trabecular, and infundibular, RV cavity should be classified as tripartite, bipartite if only inlet and infundibular portions are present, or unipartite if the inlet portion is the only one developed [81]. RV systolic dysfunction is common at presentation due to extremely high afterload and not to a proper contractility impairment. PV atresia in most of the cases is functional rather than anatomical: in fact, three well-formed sinuses in the PA, thin valve leaflets, and normal or mildly hypoplastic annulus are usually found in this condition. Pulmonary arteries are commonly confluent and of normal size, whereas major aortopulmonary collateral arteries are quite unusual. Presence of right ventriculo-coronary communications, also known as RV-to-coronary fistulae or coronary sinusoids, is directly related to the degree of TV hypoplasia: the smaller the TV, the more likely the existence of sinusoids which may involve both the right and the left coronary system. Furthermore, variable degree of coronary artery stenosis can be detected within the coronary circulation at any level, both proximal and distal; if proximal significant obstruction is present, coronary perfusion depends mainly on RV cavity desaturated blood through the sinusoids; this is the typical feature of a condition known as RV-dependent coronary circulation which occurs, more likely, if the coronary stenosis is severe and proximal and varies from partially to totally dependent according to the extension of coronary system disease.

Cardiac catheterization with angiography is currently recommended in almost all the cases with PAIVS in order to assess the coronary circulation and, consequently, to evaluate the suitability for RV decompression.

Treatment. In the neonatal period, PGE$_1$ infusion should be started as soon as the diagnosis is suspected or confirmed to maintain the arterial duct open. Subsequently, the aims of treatment should be to decompress the RV if appropriate, to achieve an adequate PBF, and to have an unrestrictive flow across the ASD. Cardiac catheterization with RV angiography and aortogram is fundamental for decision-making: if RV dependence of a major portion of coronary circulation is confidently ruled out, RV decompression can be performed. Catheter-based radiofrequency perforation of pulmonary valve followed by valvar balloon dilation is nowadays the first-line procedure worldwide [82, 83]. Due to the frequently associated RV diastolic dysfunction secondary to the compliance impairment, hypertrophy, and/or hypoplasia, RV decompression quite often does not immediately result in adequate pulmonary and systemic blood flow and adequate oxygen saturation level (>75%). Therefore, an additional source of PBF may be required, consisting of either a surgical modified Blalock-Taussig shunt (mBTS) or transcatheter arterial duct stent implantation performed at the time of the initial catheterization or some days later in case of persisting inadequate systemic oxygen saturation once the arterial duct closes [84]. Modified BTS or PDA stent implantation is the procedure performed in all the neonates judged not suitable for RV decompression at the initial cardiac catheterization. A restrictive interatrial shunt is extremely rare in PAIVS and may require balloon atrial septostomy, at the time of cardiac catheterization, only in case of concomitant rudimentary RV and/or when RV decompression is contraindicated.

Outcome. After neonatal period, infants with PAIVS may follow two possible treatment strategies according to whether or not RV decompression has been performed:

(a) If unsuitable for decompression, patients will be managed along a univentricular pathway consisting of bidirectional cavopulmonary anastomosis (Glenn) at about 3–6 months of age, followed by total cavopulmonary anastomosis (Fontan) at about 2–5 years of age.

(b) If suitable for decompression, patients will follow different possible pathways:
   – Patients who continue to have hypoplasia of the RV and TV annulus will be directed to univentricular circulation.
   – Patients who show substantial growth of the RV cavity and TV annulus will be directed to biventricular circulation consisting of additional PBF source occlusion (if present) and ASD occlusion; all these procedures should be preceded by a complete cardiac catheterization including an ASD balloon occlusion test as well, in order to assess the RV capacity to handle all the systemic venous return.
   – Patients who show some growth of the RV cavity and TV annulus but not enough to support the entire PBF and to maintain adequate systemic oxygen saturation. These patients will be directed to a bidirectional cavopulmonary anastomosis with or without ASD closure. If the ASD is closed, patient will achieve a so-called one and a half ventricle circulation: the RV will accept the systemic venous return only from IVC while SVC blood reaches directly the pulmonary arteries via the cavopulmonary anastomosis [85]. If the ASD

cannot be closed because of the insufficient RV cavity growth, variable degrees of cyanosis will persist lifelong due to the right-to-left shunting across the defect. Regardless of ASD closure, in both anatomical situations, SVC will be exposed directly to the pulmonary vascular resistance via cavo-pulmonary anastomosis, whereas IVC will maintain normal or near-normal pressure regime avoiding long-term complications of venous hypertension such as protein losing enteropathy (PLE), ascites, and liver cirrhosis.

Later on, in adolescence and adulthood, the management of patients with PAIVS varies greatly depending on type of circulation achieved in early childhood. Those with coronary sinusoids and not suitable for decompression are at risk of developing chronic myocardial ischemia and infarction, ventricular dysfunction, and sudden death [86]; cardiac transplantation may become the only therapeutic option. Those who achieved a univentricular-Fontan circulation will be exposed to the risks commonly associated to this circulation: ventricular dysfunction, gastrointestinal complications such as cirrhosis and PLE, and pulmonary complications such as plastic bronchitis. Those who managed to reach biventricular or a one and a half ventricle circulation will likely experience pulmonary valve regurgitation as a result of trans-catheter or surgical RV decompression; therefore, percutaneous or surgical pulmonary valve replacement might become necessary, at some point, to stop RV dilation and to prevent long-term complications as much as possible.

Tetralogy of Fallot

Tetralogy of Fallot (TOF) occurs in 10% of all CHD and is the most common cyanotic defect seen in children beyond infancy. It involves the following four anatomic abnormalities of the heart: large malaligned VSD, anterior shift of the aorta over the VSD (overriding aorta), right ventricular outflow tract (RVOT) obstruction, and right ventricular hypertrophy (Fig. 1.19). All these anatomic findings are the result of one developmental anomaly: the anterocephalad deviation of the outlet septum which inserts, in the normal anatomy, into the central portion of the Y-shaped septo-marginal trabeculation of the RVOT. The obstruction is most frequently in the form of infundibular stenosis (45%) although it may be present at different levels at the same time: subvalvar, valvar, and supravalvar [87]. PA branches are usually small but confluent; stenosis at the origin of LPA is very common while systemic collateral arteries feeding into the lungs are occasionally detected, especially in severe forms of RVOT obstruction. The VSD is typically a perimembranous, unrestrictive defect which allows pressure equalization between RV and LV and, consequently, contributes in determining RVH. Approximately 25% have a right-sided aortic arch, and about 5% have coronary artery anomalies, some of which may change the surgical approach such as the anterior descending artery arising from the right coronary artery (RCA) and passing over the RVOT; this is the most common anomaly which prohibits any surgical incision in infundibular area. Atrioventricular septal defects occur in about 2% of the cases and should be considered in TOF patients with trisomy 21.

Fig. 1.19 Tetralogy of Fallot: (1) infundibular stenosis. (2) Malaligned VSD. (3) Overriding aorta. (4) RV hypertrophy

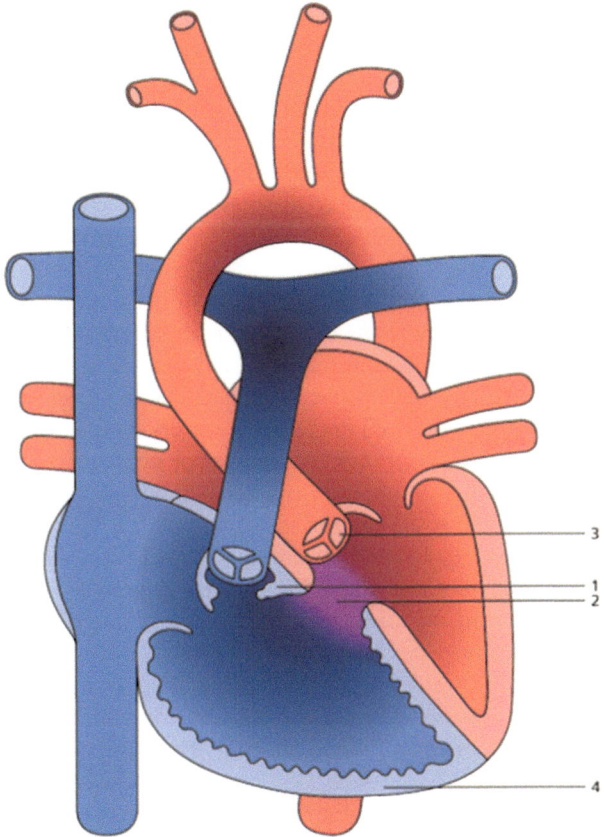

Within TOF, there is a wide spectrum of presentation: the degree of cyanosis depends on the degree of RVOT obstruction. This is quite variable, from a slight obstruction to the extreme variant of TOF with pulmonary atresia. With mild pulmonary stenosis, also known as "pink TOF," it behaves as a VSD with high PBF, normal oxygen saturation, and potential CHF symptoms early in life. Progression in RVOT obstruction may occur later on, as a result of hypertrophy of the RV and the septomarginal trabeculation, resulting in increasing cyanosis. Apart from pink TOF, all the other forms may experience the so-called hypoxic or hypercyanotic spells which occur in infants with a peak incidence between 2 and 4 months of age and manifest as a paroxysm of hyperpnoea, worsening cyanosis, irritability, and decreasing intensity of the heart murmur. They are often associated with prolonged crying or exercise, and they require immediate recognition and treatment because they can lead to serious complications such as limpness, convulsion, cerebrovascular accident, or even death. Some believe that spells may be explained by a catecholamine-induced spasm of the muscularized infundibulum resulting in acute worsening of RVOT obstruction, in acute increased amount of blood shunting R to L across the

VSD, and, eventually, in worsening cyanosis and acidosis. Some believe that SVR plays a primary role in the hypoxic spell etiology.

Another rare and unique clinical presentation is represented by TOF infants with absent pulmonary valve syndrome characterized by the presence of a rudimentary pulmonary valve apparatus and abnormal pulmonary artery development, resulting in mildly–moderately reduced PBF and markedly dilated pulmonary arteries which can cause compression of the main bronchi and gas exchange limitations.

Diagnosis. Variable degrees of cyanosis are detected at birth or shortly thereafter. Arterial pulses are generally well palpable. Auscultation reveals a normal S1, a single S2, and a long, loud ejection systolic murmur at the mid and upper left sternal border radiating to the back; the more severe the RVOT obstruction, the softer and shorter the systolic murmur. Furthermore, during hypoxic spell, murmur may disappear as less blood flows across the RVOT and more flows through the large VSD. On ECG, right QRS axis deviation is common in the cyanotic forms; the axis is normal in pink TOF, whereas it is superior or leftward in TOF with AVSD. RVH is common, but the strain pattern is unusual. Combined ventricular hypertrophy may be found in the acyanotic forms.

In cyanotic forms, the cardiac silhouette on chest x-ray frontal projection is characteristic: a concave main PA segment (secondary to reduced PBF) with an upturned apex (secondary to RVH), the so-called "boot-shaped" heart. In acyanotic forms, x-ray findings are almost indistinguishable from those of a small to moderate VSD.

TTE is the definitive diagnostic imaging modality for addressing all the four components that classify the disease, evaluating the total PBF including PDA and aortopulmonary collateral arteries, and ruling out any associated anomalies such as AVSD, right aortic arch, coronary anomalies, and pulmonary or systemic venous return abnormalities. Further investigations and imaging techniques such as CT, MR, or cardiac catheterization are rarely requested after an accurate and complete echocardiographic evaluation.

Treatment. PGE$_1$ infusion should be started in all TOF cases with arterial duct-dependent pulmonary circulation or in case of nonconfluent pulmonary arteries (PAs) with one branch supplied by the PDA; infusion should be maintained until a more definitive intervention can be performed either percutaneously or surgically. After neonatal period, it is important to recognize and treat hypoxic spells: the infant should be picked up and held in a knee-chest position in order to raise SVR and increase PBF. Supplemental oxygen is usually provided, but it has little demonstrable effect on arterial saturation. When noninvasive treatment fails, analgesic therapy, such as morphine sulfate, should be given subcutaneously or intramuscularly or intravenously if an access is obtained. Fluid volume can increase RV preload, whereas beta blocker, propranolol, can lower heart rate, improve RV filling, and stop catecholamine surge. Acidosis should be promptly treated with intravenous sodium bicarbonate in order to prevent PVR rise. If the spell does not respond to these measures, intubation and mechanical ventilation should be considered as well as intravenous peripheral vasoconstrictor, such as norepinephrine, to raise SVR and promote PBF.

Oral propranolol is often used to prevent hypoxic spells while waiting for an optimal time for surgery. Recurrent spells are an indication for intervention.

Surgical management includes both palliative and repair procedures:

(a) Palliative procedures. In order to achieve an adequate PBF and enable the infant to grow properly till the age of repair, a Gore-Tex interposition shunt, modified Blalock-Taussig shunt (mBTS), placed between the subclavian artery and the ipsilateral pulmonary artery, is the procedure of choice. Indications for mBTS vary from institution to institution, but it usually is performed in children with hypoplastic PAs.

(b) Repair procedure. It consists of patch closure of the VSD and relief of RVOT obstruction with patch augmentation under cardiopulmonary bypass and circulatory arrest; if the stenosis involves PV annulus, transannular patch augmentation is performed at the expanse of creation of free pulmonary regurgitation (PR). Over time, surgical strategy for VSD closure has shifted from a transventricular approach to a transatrial plus transpulmonary approach with the aim of reducing ventriculotomy scar with its potential arrhythmogenic effect. Patients with extreme hypoplasia or atresia of RVOT/PV, or those with left coronary artery crossing the infundibulum, are not good candidates for patch augmentation, but they will benefit from RV-to-PA valved conduit implantation. Optimal timing of repair is still under debate; although several strategies have been developed, almost all the institutions perform repair by 12 months of age [88, 89]. A worldwide accepted strategy is to delay the repair until the patient is older than 3–4 months of age unless cyanosis dictates palliative shunt implantation; this way seems to reduce, as much as possible, the need of transannular patch and hence of consequent PR [90]. Many other institutions have been promoting an early TOF repair in neonatal period to avoid RVH, to lower the risk of hypoxic spells, and to improve PA growth and development [91].

Over the last few decades, interventional cardiac catheterization has become a valid option for some selected patients, as premature TOF neonates, as an effective initial palliation: procedure consists of stent implantation in the RVOT [92].

Outcome. mBTS has a surgical mortality rate of about 1%. Generally, for surgical repair, mortality rate is about 2%. After repair, the majority of patients have normal oxygen saturation and no residual shunt. Symptom-free survival in children after TOF repair is excellent with 30-year survival rates approaching 90%; however, survival is less than expected for the general population at all times [93]. The most common late complication is chronic PR, whereas residual RVOT obstruction and PA stenosis are less frequent but significant late sequelae [94]. Chronic PR is the major contributor to long-term morbidity and mortality: it leads to progressive RV dilation and dysfunction, arrhythmias, and functional tricuspid valve regurgitation. PV replacement with a biological valve is the treatment of choice for patients with severe PR and RV dysfunction and/or symptoms related to arrhythmias, both atrial and ventricular. Surgical replacement has been for a long time the only technique available; nowadays percutaneous pulmonary valve implantation (PPVI) is a valid and effective alternative either in native RVOT, in selected patients, or in dysfunctioning RV-PA conduit [95]. Cardiac MR [96] and cardiopulmonary exercise test provide a lot of information used in clinical decision-making to establish the right timing for PV replacement. Atrial flutter and fibrillation are the most frequent arrhythmias encountered in the late follow-up, whereas prevalence of ventricular arrhythmias increases with age and is associated with LV dysfunction [97]. Atrial arrhythmias can be treated with a surgical ablation, maze procedure, at the time of PV replacement, whereas sustained ventricular tachycardia (VT) or aborted sudden cardiac death (SCD) should be addressed with ICD implantation for secondary prevention. SCD due to ventricular arrhythmias is the most common cause of death after TOF repair with a risk of about 3–6% over the 30-year follow-up period. Progressive aortic valve regurgitation along with aortic root dilation may be seen in 15–18% of patients after repair as a long-term complication as well [98].

Tetralogy of Fallot and Pulmonary Atresia with Ventricular Septal Defect

TOF and pulmonary atresia with VSD occurs in approximately 15–20% of all tetralogy cases. Chromosome 22q11 deletion and infants of diabetic mothers have a strong association with this pathology. Intracardiac anatomy resembles that of TOF in all features except for the presence of pulmonary atresia which is the extreme form of RVOT obstruction and may be at the infundibular and/or at valvar level. Typical of this CHD is the disposition of the pulmonary arteries and their relationship to additional sources of PBF; the pulmonary supply is most commonly mediated through a PDA (70%) and less commonly through major aortopulmonary collateral arteries (MAPCAs) (30%). PDA is usually small and long and arises from the aortic arch with an acute angle and courses downward. PAs anomalies can widely vary in terms of degree of hypoplasia, nonconfluence, and abnormal distribution:

- In general, the more hypoplastic are central PAs, the more developed is the MAPCA circulation pulmonary supply.
- Central PAs are nonconfluent in about 15% of patients. Usually, in the presence of PDA, central PAs are confluent in 70% of cases. If the PAs are nonconfluent, the PDA may supply just one of the pulmonary branches, whereas the contralateral lung will be supplied by MAPCAs.
- Incomplete distribution of one or both PAs to all lung segments occurs in about 80% of patients with nonconfluent PAs compared to 50% with confluent PAs.

Also MAPCAs can widely vary in terms of origin, caliber, course, and pattern of anastomosis with the pulmonary circulation. Some of them derive from bronchial arteries which originate from ascending aorta and make an intrapulmonary anastomosis, being the sole suppliers to the target lung segments. Other collaterals originate from aortic vessels, such as subclavian, intercostal or internal mammary arteries, and usually anastomose with the central PAs. Another type of MAPCAs, the most common one occurring in about two-thirds of patients, is represented by collaterals that arise from descending aorta and usually anastomose with PAs at the hilum level, resulting in so-called dual blood supply for that specific corresponding lung segment [99]; these vessels are often stenotic at some point of their course or tend to become stenotic over time.

Cyanosis is the common clinical presentation which may become evident early after birth or later on, according to the patency of arterial duct and how extensive the collateral artery supply is. In case of increased PBF, infant may present with signs of CHF within the first weeks of life.

Diagnosis. Some degree of cyanosis is obligatory, ranging from mild to severe, and may be detected at birth or thereafter. Arterial pulses are generally well palpable. Auscultation reveals a normal S1 and a single S2; a systolic or a continuous murmur may be audible in the presence of PDA or collaterals. ECG usually shows RVH and right QRS axis deviation. On chest x-ray, quite often the heart appears as a "boot-shaped" silhouette whose size varies according to the amount of PBF: the higher is the PBF, the larger will be the cardiac size. A combination of areas of increased and decreased pulmonary vascular marking is characteristic of patients with MAPCAs. TTE is very useful and accurate for addressing all the anatomic components that classify the disease, providing many details about RVOT variable anatomy which ranges from well-developed tract to an imperforate pulmonary valve to a complete muscular atresia without a demonstrable infundibulum, the total PBF including PDA and aortopulmonary collateral arteries, and the presence of associated anomalies such as AVSD, right aortic arch, coronary anomalies, and pulmonary or systemic venous return abnormalities. Although MAPCAs can be detected on echocardiogram, further imaging modalities are usually required in order to better define the PBF and to plan treatment strategy. CT and three-dimensional CT or MR are able to clearly delineate the origin and distribution of systemic-to-pulmonary collaterals and the anatomy of native PAs in most of the patients with some limitations such as in case of severe central PA hypoplasia. Therefore, cardiac catheterization still remains the most accurate technique used to assess all the sources of PBF and their arborization and to measure hemodynamics within native PAs and MAPCAs.

Treatment. PGE_1 infusion should be started in all cases with duct-dependent pulmonary circulation or nonconfluent PAs with one branch supplied by the PDA; infusion should be maintained until a more definitive intervention can be performed either surgically or percutaneously. According to the anatomy and hemodynamics, surgical management may differ as follows:

(a) Single-stage repair. Complete, primary surgical repair is feasible when adequate size central PAs exist and the central PA connects without obstruction to sufficient areas of both lungs; it consists of closing the VSD and creating a continuity between RV and central PA via a patch or conduit implantation.

(b) Staged repair. When criteria for single-stage repair are not met, surgical strategy should both promote maximal central PA growth and improve the PA distribution in order to supply as many lung segments as possible. To promote central PA growth, different techniques have been used: mBTS has been performed extensively but with the disadvantage of iatrogenic stenosis of the PA at the level of the anastomosis; for very hypoplastic but confluent central PAs, a "central shunt" is a valid option which consists of anastomosis of the small main PA to the side of the ascending aorta but with the disadvantage of risk of excessive PBF and CHF [100] and RVOT reconstruction with a patch, leaving the VSD open or partially closed with fenestrated patch.

To improve PA arborization, for patients with multiple MAPCAs, so-called unifocalization procedure is performed: It consists of connecting those collateral arteries, being the sole suppliers of some lung segments, to native PAs in order to achieve a single source of perfusion.

Alternative percutaneous interventional procedures exist and have been performed routinely in some centers and in some selected patients: PDA stenting to palliate neonates or infants pending later surgical repair, RVOT perforation, and stenting to create a continuity between the RV and the main PA, delaying surgical intervention for weeks or even months [101].

Outcome. Surgical repair can be performed, even at neonatal age, with a relatively low mortality rate albeit higher than that associated with repair of TOF and pulmonary stenosis. In terms of morbidity, early postoperative period can be complicated by the onset of RV restrictive physiology secondary to RV compliance impairment and consequent low cardiac output state; this condition may be worsened by arrhythmias, such as junctional ectopic tachycardia, and severe PR resulting from transannular patch implantation.

Long-term outcome for repaired patients is similar, in many cases, to that observed for patients with TOF and PS. Children who had RV-PA conduit implantation commonly required recurrent conduit changes throughout childhood due to body growth and throughout adolescence and adulthood due to conduit dysfunction (stenosis and/or regurgitation); at present, if the original conduit is larger than 16 mm and can be dilated and stented to that size or above, PPVI can be done successfully and has become the percutaneous procedure most performed in TOF patients with pulmonary atresia. Mid- and long-term outcome of patients who have undergone unifocalization is affected by many factors: the type of RVOT reconstruction, the number of lung segments recruited, the development of native PAs, the presence of collateral and/or PA stenosis in combination of pulmonary regurgitation, and the degree of RV dysfunction. Interventional cardiac catheterization plays a major role in treating pulmonary vascular bed stenosis with balloon dilation and stent implantation and in closing residual VSD with device. Another group of patients who requires careful and regular follow-up includes both survivors of early attempts at palliation in the early era of congenital surgery and unoperated adult patients; cyanosis can be improved by stenting the shunt connections or stenotic MAPCAs [102].

1.1.4   CHD with Anomalous Origin of Great Arteries

1.1.4.1 Transposition of the Great Arteries

Transposition of great arteries (TGA) accounts for 2–5% of all CHD with a prevalence of about 0.2–0.3 of 1000 births; it is more common in males than in females with a ratio of 2–3:1. It derives from truncal ridge and infundibulum normal spiraling rotation failure during fetal life which results in discordant ventriculo-arterial connection: aorta arises from the morphologically RV and is located anteriorly and to the right of PA (D-transposition), whereas the PA arises from morphologically LV (Fig. 1.20).

Consequently pulmonary and systemic circulations flow in parallel instead of in series, having oxygenated blood pumped by the LV into the lungs via the PA and back to the LV and deoxygenated blood pumped by the RV to the body via the aorta and back to the RV. This hemodynamic condition is incompatible with life unless a communication exists between the two circulations which allows a mixing between

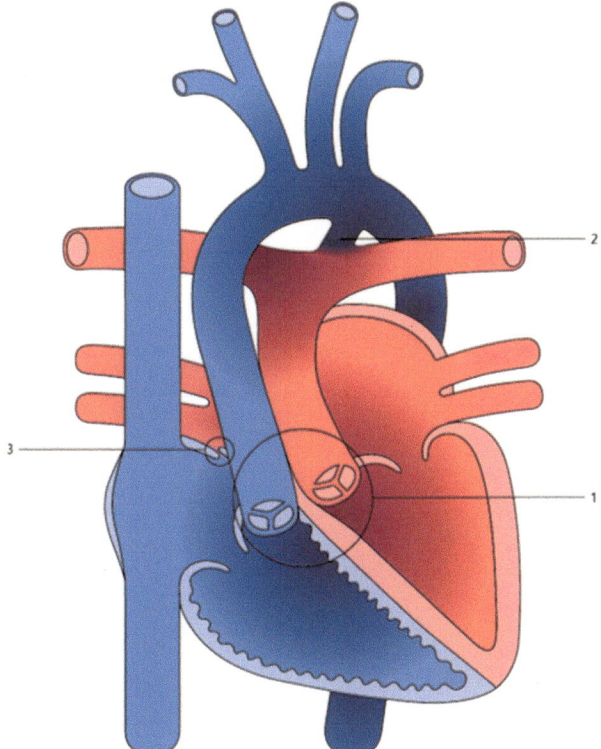

Fig. 1.20 Transposition of the great arteries: (1) discordant ventricular-arterial connection. (2) PDA. (3) PFO

oxygenated and deoxygenated blood. Effective systemic blood flow is the amount of oxygenated blood coming from the lungs which reaches systemic circulation through the anatomic shunts; effective PBF is the amount of deoxygenated blood coming from the body which reaches the pulmonary circulation through the anatomic shunts.

During neonatal period, PDA and mainly PFO usually maintain an adequate mixing because they ensure the effective systemic/pulmonary blood flow going respectively into the aorta and the PA; as the PDA starts to close and PFO by itself is restrictive in size, infant develops severe cyanosis.

Approximately one-half of patients with TGA have an intact interventricular septum (IVS). VSD is present in 30–40% of D-transposition cases and may be located anywhere within the septum (Fig. 1.21).

Associated lesions with TGA-VSD are left ventricular outflow tract (LVOT) obstruction in 30% of cases, at valvar (Fig. 1.22) and subvalvar level, coarctation of the aorta, interrupted aortic arch, overriding and straddling of the atrioventricular valve, and coronary anomalies.

Coronary arteries usually arise from the two facing sinuses which are opposed directly to the pulmonary valve; their origin, course, and branching pattern may vary significantly affecting surgical mortality at the time of the repair, the so-called

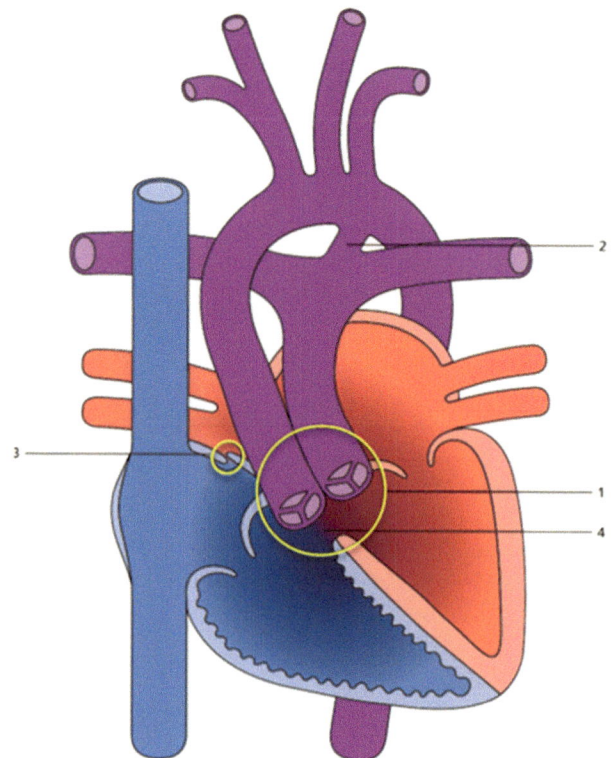

Fig. 1.21 Transposition of the great arteries: (1) Discordant ventriculo-arterial connection. (2) PDA. (3) PFO. (4) Subaortic VSD

Fig. 1.22 Transposition of the great arteries: (1) discordant ventriculo-arterial connection. (2) PDA. (3) PFO. (4) Ventricular septal defect. (5) Pulmonary valve stenosis

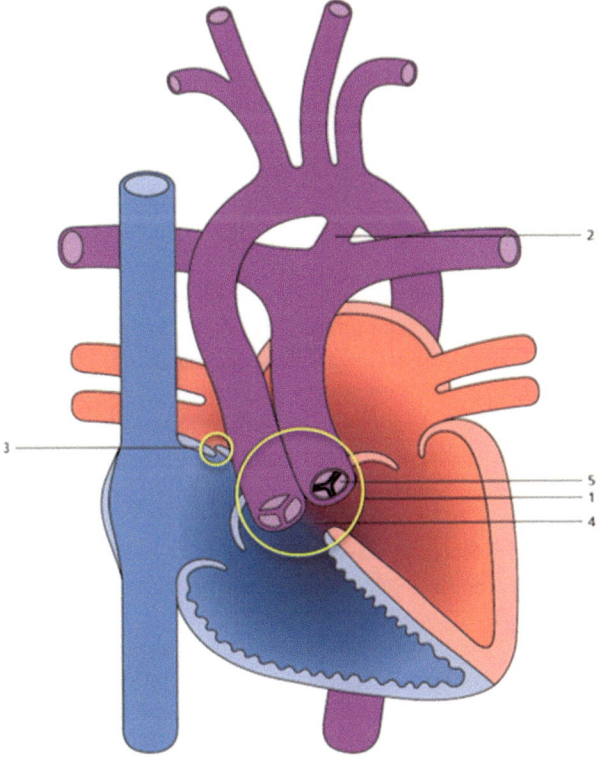

arterial switch operation (ASO). Yacoub surgical classification, currently used worldwide, describes all the coronary anomalies encountered, including the origin of left coronary from the right facing sinus, a single coronary artery, and intramural course [103].

Unoperated children with TGA-IVS have a tendency to develop POVD within months to years, whereas babies with TGA and large VSD without pulmonary stenosis may develop POVD earlier, within 6–12 months.

Diagnosis. Cyanosis from birth is always present as well as arterial hypoxemia with or without acidosis; hypoxemia does not respond to oxygen. Neonatal reversed differential cyanosis is a typical finding, resulting from blood circulations in parallel: arterial oxygen saturation is higher in the postductal extremities than in the preductal ones due to the amount of oxygenated blood which reaches the descending aorta from the PA through the PDA. Signs of CHF, with tachypnea, dyspnea, and failure to thrive, develop during the newborn period as PVR decreases. On auscultation S2 is single and loud. No murmur is audible in infants with TGA-IVS, whereas a systolic ejection murmur will be detected in TGA-VSD due to increased blood flow across the LVOT and pulmonary valve.

On ECG, RVH is usually present and persists thereafter. In case of associated large VSD or PDA or POVD, combined ventricular hypertrophy may be seen.

The cardiac silhouette on chest x-ray frontal projection is characteristic: a narrow superior mediastinum, secondary to anterior position of the aorta which obscures PA, the so-called egg on a string. Vascular markings and cardiac size depend on the amount of PBF and tend to increase in the presence of large VSD and/or PDA.

TTE is the modality of choice for addressing all the components that classify the disease and to achieve all the information required for planning the management: the origin and course of the great arteries which run parallel, in their proximal portion, in parasternal long axis view; both arterial valves can be seen in parasternal short-axis view as double circles; PA is identified by observing bifurcation of the artery; presence and size of PFO/ASD and PDA, being the sites of blood mixing; any associated anomalies such as VSD, PS, LVOT obstruction, and CoA; and the origins and courses of coronary arteries by using parasternal and apical views.

Treatment. Oxygen is given in case of severe hypoxia in order to lower PVR and increase PBF. Metabolic acidosis should be corrected, and, depending on the degree of mixing, PGE1 infusion should be started to maintain ductal patency. All infants with TGA-IVS and restrictive atrial communication should undergo emergency percutaneous balloon atrial septostomy (BAS), the Rashkind procedure: a balloon-tipped catheter is advanced into the LA through the PFO and then, after having inflated the balloon, is abruptly withdrawn to the RA in order to enlarge the inter-atrial communication; if effective, the oxygen saturation will rise to 10% or more due to the improvement of intracardiac mixing [104]. After successful BAS, neonates can wait for surgical repair even without prostaglandin infusion if oxygen saturation does not drop too much, below 70%, as the PDA closes. For TGA-IVS patients, ASO is the procedure of choice since the late 1980s and is usually performed by the first 3–4 weeks of life before PVR drops to normal level, and, consequently, morphologic LV systolic pressure decreases making the LV "deconditioned"; in fact, morphological LV should be able to support systemic circulation after surgery. It consists of anatomic correction by transecting the great arteries above the level of sinotubular junction, relocating the aorta over the morphological LV and the PA over the morphological RV; moving PA bifurcation anteriorly to the ascending aorta, according to the so-called Lecompte maneuver; and, finally, transferring the coronary artery buttons to the "neoaorta"; the latter is a critical part of the operation especially in case of coronary pattern abnormalities.

Prior the ASO introduction, before the early 1980s, physiological correction used to be performed by switching the right- and left-sided blood at the atrial level, using either the Mustard or the Senning technique. Atrial switch consists of creating intra-atrial baffles to redirect the blood, using, respectively, prosthetic material in Mustard operation or right atrial and atrial septal tissue in Senning operation. These techniques are still performed in rare cases such as "double-switch" operation (combined with arterial switch or Rastelli operation), palliative atrial switch, or isolated ventricular inversion.

For patients with TGA-VSD and/or CoA, associated lesions are usually repaired at the same time as ASO. For patients with significant pulmonary valve stenosis which contraindicates ASO, Rastelli or Nikaidoh operation is used. In Rastelli technique, the pulmonary and systemic venous blood are switched at the ventricular level by creating an intraventricular tunnel between the VSD and the aortic valve which connects LV to the aorta and by placing a conduit between the RV and main PA.

In Nikaidoh technique, there is reconstruction of both ventricular outflow tracts by patch augmentation, but there are variations on it which are currently used as well.

Outcome. Survival without surgery is unlikely. The early surgical mortality rate for ASO is between 2–5%, whereas the overall 5-year survival exceeds 90% [105]. PA stenosis is the most frequent complication after ASO: possible causes include scarring and retraction of the tissue used to fill the coronary artery button sites, tension at the anastomotic site in case of inadequate mobilization of the distal PAs, and abnormal growth of the suture lines. Balloon dilation and stent implantation are usually effective to treat stenosis. Dilation of the aortic root and consequent neoaortic valve regurgitation are common, especially in patients who had VSD closure, but not significant or progressive. Coronary artery complications, stenosis or occlusion, have been reported in 5–7% after ASO and have been associated with ventricular dysfunction and sudden death [106]; usually these lesions can be treated percutaneously, during cardiac catheterization. Cardiac catheterization used to be performed, later in childhood, even in asymptomatic patients after ASO, in order to assess coronary artery circulation.

Following the Rastelli repair, often the RV-to-PA conduit will become stenotic and/or regurgitant with the need of replacement during adolescence or adulthood; if the original conduit is larger than 16 mm and can be dilated and stented to that size or above, PPVI can be done effectively. Subaortic stenosis may develop at the level of LV to aortic valve tunnel and may require reintervention. After atrial switch operation, some mid- and long-term complications may occur: sinus node dysfunction and atrial arrhythmias (mainly intra-atrial reentry tachycardia) are the most frequent and progressive; by 20 years, only 40% of patients remain in sinus rhythm [107]; pacemaker implantation is required for symptomatic sinus node dysfunction and arrhythmias. Because the morphological RV remains the systemic ventricle, progressive ventricular dysfunction is usually observed in long-term follow-up; symptoms are relatively uncommon until the systemic RV failure is advanced. Intra-atrial baffle leakage and/or obstruction occurs in about 10% of patients and may be addressed by interventional techniques or surgical revision. Sudden death may occur in up to 10%–12% of these patients, mainly related to arrhythmias.

1.1.4.2 Congenitally Corrected Transposition of the Great Arteries

Congenitally corrected transposition of the great arteries (ccTGA) accounts for about 0.05% of all CHD. There is an increased incidence among families who have had a previous child with ccTGA with a recurrence risk in siblings approximately 2–5%. It is characterized by discordant atrioventricular (A-V) and ventriculo-arterial (V-A) connections, resulting in functionally corrected circulation because the oxygenated blood comes into the LA, goes into the morphologically RV, and then flows out into the aorta, whereas deoxygenated blood comes into the RA, goes into the morphologically LV, and then flows out into the pulmonary artery (Fig. 1.23). This abnormal configuration is secondary to impaired cardiac looping during embryologic development. In 90% of ccTGA patients [108], there are associated

Fig. 1.23 Congenitally corrected transposition of the great arteries: (1) morphologically RV. (2) Morphologically LV. (3) Morphologically LA. (4) Morphologically RA

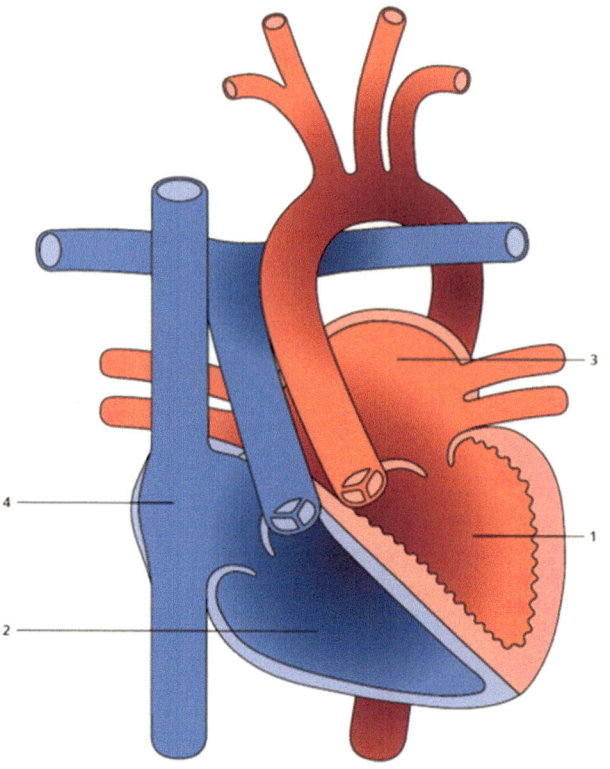

CHDs as follows: a VSD in 60–80%, mainly perimembranous; LVOT obstruction/PVS in 30–50%; tricuspid valve anomalies, in about 90% of autopsy cases, which can vary from mild valvar dysplasia to Ebstein-like features with variable degree of regurgitation; and heart position abnormalities such as dextrocardia (heart placed mainly in right-sided chest) in about 30% of cases. Because the pulmonary valve is wedged between the atrial septum and the mitral valve, there is a malalignment between the interatrial and interventricular septum causing an abnormal arrangement of the conduction system; instead of the normal position, at the apex of triangle of Koch, AV node is located just beneath the opening of right atrial appendage, at the lateral margin of the area of PV-to-MV continuity. This anatomic condition predisposes to AV conduction disturbance which can occur in fetal life as well. A complete AV block is present in 10% of ccTGA neonates at birth, whereas the risk of AV block occurrence is about 2–3%/year.

Coronary arteries usually arise from aortic sinuses adjacent to the PA and show an epicardial distribution which follows their respective ventricle; coronary anomalies can occur as well.

Clinical presentation is widely variable according to the underlying anatomy: patients are usually asymptomatic when ccTGA is not associated with other defects and the disease is found incidentally later on in life. In case of VSD and PVS, variable degree of cyanosis may be detected. Signs of CHF may appear during first weeks of life in case of large VSD or severe bradycardia. Exertional dyspnea and reduced exercise tolerance may develop with worsening tricuspid valve, the systemic AV valve, regurgitation.

Diagnosis. Cyanosis is detected in case of associated VSD and PVS. Bradycardia, tachycardia, or irregular rhythm may be the reason for cardiology referral. S2 is loud and single at the upper left sternal border. A pansystolic murmur can be audible at the lower sternal border in case of VSD or tricuspid regurgitation; an ejection systolic murmur at the upper sternal border is typical of LVOT obstruction/PVS.

In usual atrial arrangement and levocardia, ECG usually shows Q waves in the right precordial leads (V1) and absent Q wave in the left precordial leads (V5–V6); this is the result of abnormal initial ventricular depolarization which occurs from right to left in a superior and anterior direction, according to the abnormal ventricular arrangement [109]. On chest x-ray, a straight left upper cardiac border is a characteristic finding in case of normal atrial arrangement and levocardia; other cardiac position abnormalities are easily detected. Cardiomegaly and increased vascular markings are associated with large VSD, whereas pulmonary venous congestion and left atrial enlargement are seen in significant systemic, tricuspid valve regurgitation.

TTE is extremely useful and accurate for addressing all the anatomic components, following a segmental approach, and for taking many details about the associated lesions. The aorta is no longer in fibrous continuity with the AV valve and is usually anterior and to the left of the PA. TV anatomy and function require careful examination.

CT and MRI can provide a complete, noninvasive evaluation of the cardiac morphology and hemodynamics but require anesthesia for children.

Treatment. In neonates with severe PVS or severe coarctation or aortic arch interruption, PGE1 infusion should be given to keep arterial duct patency until surgical intervention. Infants born with complete AV block may require a pacemaker soon after birth.

Repair strategies for ccTGA associated with other CHDs are multiple and include the "physiological"-classic repair, single or 1.5-ventricle repair, and the "double-switch" operation, so-called "anatomic" repair.

The "physiological" biventricular repair aims at restoring normal circulatory patterns and hemodynamics by closing VSD, relieving LVOT obstruction, repairing or replacing the TV, or, when needed, LV-to-PA conduit implantation; the key point is that the patient remains with a systemic morphologically RV which tends, over time, to deteriorate in function along with TV regurgitation worsening. In patients with straddling AV valves or unbalanced ventricles, a univentricular-Fontan circulation is the final target. Double-switch operation is an alternative biventricular repair which aims at restoring the normal anatomy leaving the morphologically LV as the systemic ventricle; it consists of an atrial switch (Mustard or Senning) combined with an arterial switch or Rastelli procedure [110].

Outcome. Infants with significant TV regurgitation and progressive AV block are at higher risk of morbidity and mortality. Most patients with ccTGA do well during childhood and adolescence and survive into adulthood; outcome determinants are systemic RV function, TV regurgitation, and progressive conduction disturbances. In adulthood, most ccTGA patients start to experience morbidity and mortality in their 30s and 40s; those with associated lesions are at higher risk of developing RV dysfunction and CHF than those without associated defects [111].

Surgical mortality rates have improved significantly over the last decades, and a gradual shift from physiological to anatomic repair has been observed worldwide; systemic RV function and TV function are still the most important outcome determinants in long-term prognosis. Regardless of type of operation, 10-year survival has been estimated between 70 and 75% [112].

1.1.4.3 Double Outlet Right Ventricle

Double outlet right ventricle (DORV) accounts for 1–2% of CHD with an incidence of about 0.1/1000 births. It could be associated with chromosome 22q11 deletion, as the other conotruncal anomalies, with polymalformative syndromes and a heterotaxy syndrome, the right isomerism.

DORV is not a single entity but refers to that group of CHD in which both outflow tracts arise entirely or predominantly from the RV and which physiologically may behave like VSD, TGA, TOF, or single ventricle. Associated anomalies include ASD, VSD, AVSD, AV valve abnormalities, PDA, PVS, CoA, and coronary anomalies. Different DORV classifications exist, based on great artery relationship or the position of the VSD in relation to the great arteries. The great vessels can lay side by side, or aorta rightward and anterior to PA, or aorta rightward and posterior to PA, or aorta leftward and anterior to the PA. VSD position can vary: subaortic, closer to the aortic valve (Fig. 1.24); subpulmonary, closer to the pulmonary valve, the so-called Taussig-Bing anomaly; doubly committed, equally committed to both arterial valves; and, then, noncommitted, far from both arterial valves. The most frequent position is subaortic, 58–68%, followed by subpulmonary one in about 60% of cases [113].

Because more than 60% of infants with DORV with subaortic VSD have some degree of pulmonary stenosis, they will present, clinically, like infants with TOF: mild stenosis will not protect from high PBF and, consequently, from CHF; severe stenosis will determine low PBF and severe cyanosis. Neonates and infants with DORV and subpulmonary VSD will present like those with TGA and VSD, therefore with variable degree of cyanosis and possibly CHF. In this setting, there is a frequent association with subaortic obstruction and aortic coarctation which should be suspected in case of cardiogenic shock at presentation, as the PDA closes.

Diagnosis. As mentioned before, variable degree of cyanosis may be detected in both forms of DORV. S2 is loud. An ejection systolic murmur may be audible at the upper sternal border. ECG shows right axis deviation, RVH. LVH may be seen during infancy in Taussig-Bing anomaly, whereas first-degree AV block is more common in Fallot-type DORV.

Chest x-ray shows normal heart size with an upturned apex in the Fallot type, whereas cardiomegaly and increased vascular markings are characteristic of TGA-type DORV.

Fig. 1.24 Double outlet RV: (1) normally related great arteries. (2) Subaortic VSD

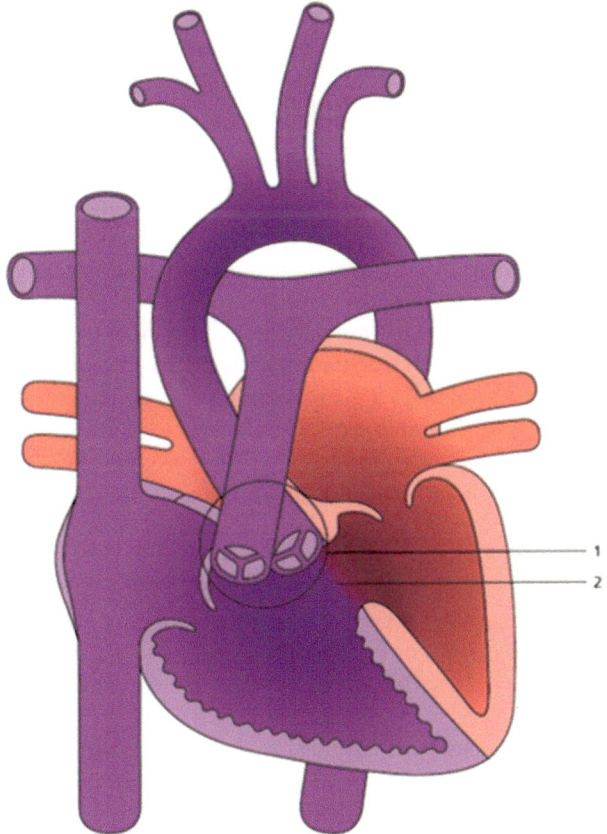

TTE is diagnostic in almost all cases and should be based on accurate sequential, segmental approach for addressing all the components that classify the disease and to achieve all the information required for planning the management: VSD position, great artery relationship, associated anomalies, coronary artery origins, and proximal course should be investigated.

Treatment. In neonates with Fallot-type DORV, the PBF is often well balanced, so they do not require any medical treatment. In case of Taussig-Bing anomaly, severe cyanosis should be treated with PGE1 infusion; if cyanosis does not meliorate despite the presence of PDA, a Rashkind balloon atrial septostomy may be necessary to improve blood mixing and oxygen saturation. Diuretics may be helpful to treat CHF.

Fallot-type DORV surgical management is similar to that for TOF patients: repair can be performed either in neonatal period or within the first 4–6 months of life by VSD closure with patch, directing LV into the aorta, and by relieving RVOT obstruction with infundibular and/or transannular patch or with RV-to-PA conduit implantation in case of coronary anomaly at the level of infundibulum. Some neonates with severe PS may require an mBTS as a first surgical procedure, followed by complete repair and takedown of the shunt later on.

TGA-type DORV surgical management is similar to that for TGA patients: repair can be performed within the first 3–4 weeks of life by VSD closure with patch along with an arterial switch operation. Coa, if present, can be treated at the same time of the repair.

Outcome. Within the DORV group, the Fallot type is the anatomic variation with the lowest surgical mortality; best overall survival, about 96% at 15 years [114]; lowest ongoing complication rate; and best freedom from reoperation, estimated about 87% at 15 years. Pulmonary valve regurgitation and/or stenosis and RV-PA conduit dysfunction are the most common complications during long-term follow-up. TGA-type DORV patients have a 15-year survival rate of approximately 90% with an estimated 15-year freedom from reoperation of 72% [114]. Survival is lower for those who underwent CoA repair as well. Cardiac catheterization used to be performed, later in childhood, even in asymptomatic patients after ASO, in order to assess coronary artery circulation.

1.1.4.4 Truncus Arteriosus

Truncus arteriosus (TA) occurs in 1–4% of all CHDs. Of the other conotruncal anomalies (TOF, TGA, and DORV), TA may be associated with chromosome 22q11 deletion typical of DiGeorge syndrome, in about 35% of the cases [115], and with another polymalformative syndrome such as CHARGE association which comprises coloboma, heart disease, choanal atresia, retardation of growth, genitourinary abnormalities, and esophageal atresia. It consists of a single great artery arising from the cardiac ventricles through a single arterial valve which is most often placed over a large VSD, in 70–90% of cases; rarely, the common trunk arises entirely from the RV. TA gives rise to the pulmonary, systemic, and coronary circulation. It is the result of abnormal embryological great artery septation and is frequently associated with a large variety of other CHDs which includes partial or total anomalous pulmonary venous drainage, CoA, or type B aortic arch interruption. Coronary anomalies are detected in more than half of the patients. The truncal valve is most commonly tricommissural, followed by bicommissural and then by quadricommissural; valvar leaflets can be thickened and redundant with stenosis, regurgitation, or both [116]. Four types of TA are described according to Collett and Edwards classification, based on the origin of PAs from the common arterial trunk.

- Type I: The main PA arises from the common arterial trunk and the divides into the RPA and LPA (Fig. 1.25).
- Type II: Both PAs arise independently from the posterior aspect of the arterial trunk.
- Type III: Both PAs arise independently from the lateral aspect of the arterial trunk.
- Type IV: No PAs but arteries, supplying the lungs, arise from the anterolateral aspect of the descending aorta.

Fig. 1.25 Truncus arteriosus type I: (1) common arterial trunk. (2) Common arterial valve. (3) VSD. (4) Pulmonary arteries

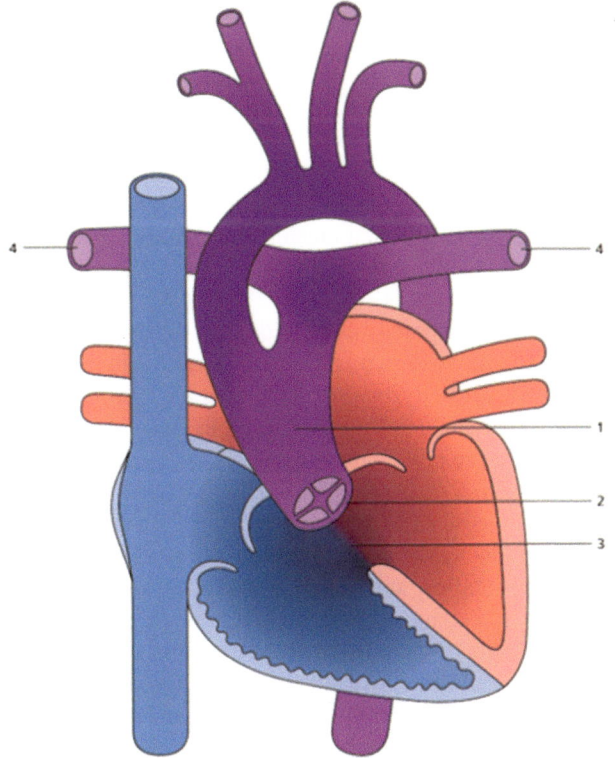

Clinical presentation is dependent on the amount of PBF: in case of mild obstruction to PBF, patients will present with signs of CHF, tachypnea, failure to thrive, and mild degree of cyanosis; situation can be worsened by truncal valve dysfunction and/or by the physiological decrease of PVR within 6–8 weeks of age. Poor development is often associated with DiGeorge syndrome. If not repaired, the condition will lead to POVD as early as 6 months of age, leading to poor results with late surgical correction. Later presentation is often associated with pulmonary hypertension and possible Eisenmenger syndrome. In case of significant impediment to PBF, patients will present with at least moderate cyanosis and hypoxemia and less signs of CHF.

Diagnosis. Variable degrees of cyanosis are usually present. Peripheral pulses are bounding with a wide pulse pressure. On auscultation, S2 is single and loud; a pansystolic murmur may be detected at the left sternal border, whereas a diastolic decrescendo murmur is audible in presence of truncal valve regurgitation. In case of TA type IV, a continuous murmur may be heard over either side of the chest or at the interscapular area. ECG may show RVH or LVH or combined ventricular hypertrophy in more than 70% of the patients. Chest x-ray may reveal cardiomegaly and increased pulmonary vascular markings according to the amount of PBF. A right aortic arch is seen in 25–30% of cases. TTE is diagnostic in almost all cases and should be based on accurate sequential, segmental approach for addressing all the components that classify the disease and to achieve all the information required for planning the management: VSD dimension, truncal valve anatomy and function, coronary artery origins, PA origin and dimension, aortic arch, and any associated CHD.

If TTE is inadequate for preoperative assessment, CT and MR are very helpful especially for extracardiac anatomy but require general anesthesia.

Treatment. Medical management should stabilize neonates or infants in preparation for surgical repair. In case of CHF, anticongestive treatment should be commenced.

Surgical repair is usually carried out within the first 6 months of life by VSD patch closure, directing the LV blood to the truncal valve, and by PA separation from the arterial trunk and connection to RV with the interposition, in Rastelli procedure, of a RV-to-PA conduit; in this way, the truncal valve will become the "neo-aortic" valve [117].

Outcome. Currently, surgical repair, even at an early age, is performed with low mortality rate and excellent chance of survival with good quality of life well into adulthood. Severe truncal valve regurgitation, type B interrupted aortic arch, coronary anomalies, and genetic anomalies are considered significant risk factors for perioperative morbidity and mortality. In general reoperation later on in life is required for truncal valve replacement and/or RV-to-PA conduit replacement; both can be performed with low morbidity and mortality rates. Some of the mid- and long-term complications, such as residual shunts at atrial, ventricular, or pulmonary levels, or discrete pulmonary branches stenosis or RV-to-PA conduit dysfunction, may be addressed with transcatheter interventions. Unoperated patients who have developed Eisenmenger syndrome have the poorest long-term prognosis [118].

1.1.5   The "Functional-Univentricular Heart"

Hearts with functional single ventricle are rare, comprising 1–2% of all CHDs. This group includes a large variety of CHD with single atrioventricular connection (tricuspid atresia, mitral valve atresia, double-inlet LV) and/or severe hypoplasia of one ventricle and its own atrioventricular valve (hypoplastic left heart syndrome, unbalanced complete AVSD) (Fig. 1.26). Although, from anatomic and physiological aspects, these lesions can vary widely, they can be considered collectively taking into account the management pathway, the so-called single ventricle pathway.

Clinical presentation may differ a lot, according to the underlying anatomy: neonates with well-balanced circulation may show mild cyanosis and normal growth with no signs of CHF; if one of the outflow tracts is significantly obstructed, neonates may present with variable degrees of cyanosis and low PBF or low cardiac output state, requiring emergency care; if both outflow tracts are unobstructed, neonates may present with signs of CHF.

Diagnosis. Physical findings depend on the amount of PBF. With high PBF, mild cyanosis and CHF signs are present; single S2 and a systolic murmur are audible

Fig. 1.26 Functional univentricular heart: (1) aortic valve atresia. (2) LV hypoplasia. (3) Ascending aorta hypoplasia. (4) PDA. (5) ASD

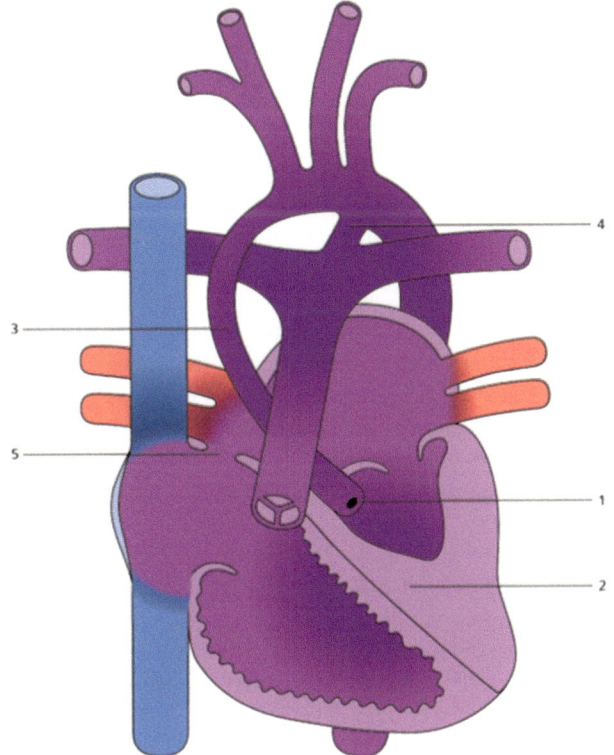

along the upper sternal border. With low PBF, moderate to severe cyanosis is present; S2 is single and loud; an ejection systolic murmur may be audible at the upper sternal border. On ECG, ventricular hypertrophy pattern may be seen in most or all precordial leads. Chest x-ray may reveal cardiomegaly and increased pulmonary vascular markings according to the amount of PBF.

TTE is the modality of choice for assessing all the anatomic details, considering the complexity of this group of CHD. It should be performed using a through sequential, segmental approach, including atrial and visceral situs, A-V and V-A connections, cardiac valves, outflow tracts, and great artery anatomy and their relationship.

Treatment. Affected neonates often require PGE1 infusion for pulmonary or systemic outflow tract obstruction. Surgical management consists of a staged approach: in the neonatal period, a palliative procedure may be necessary to increase the PBF via an mBTS or to reduce PBF via a PA banding or to optimize the systemic cardiac output via a Damus-Kaye-Stansel or Norwood procedure. Subsequently patients will be managed along a univentricular pathway consisting of bidirectional cavopulmonary anastomosis and Glenn procedure, followed later on by total cavopulmonary anastomosis (TCPC) and Fontan operation. Glenn procedure consists of superior vena cava-ipsilateral pulmonary artery anastomosis and is routinely performed at about 3–6 months of age [119]. The TCPC or Fontan operation aims to separate completely systemic and pulmonary venous circulations by directing inferior vena cava deoxygenated blood into the PA via an intracardiac or extracardiac conduit. The original procedure described by Kreutzer and Fontan was a right atrial to main PA anastomosis; then, over time, different modifications had been used; currently it is performed using an extracardiac conduit between the IVC and ipsilateral PA, at about 18 months to 5 years of age [120]. Because of its preload dependency, any Fontan circulation requires the following elements to work properly: good ventricular function, both systolic and diastolic, and low PVR and normal pulmonary vascular bed, both arterial and venous. If any concern arises about one of these elements, a fenestration can be created in the Fontan conduit at the time of the operation, in order to allow systemic venous blood to enter into the atrium and to lower systemic venous pressure at the expense of some degree of oxygen desaturation and hypoxemia. Fenestration was thought to reduce Fontan pressure and the duration of pleural drainage and to maintain a reasonable cardiac output in the immediate postoperative period [121].

Outcome. Interstage morbidity and mortality are mainly related to the onset of some complications such as ventricular dysfunction, AV valve regurgitation, PA stenosis, and PVR rise. To note that after Glenn procedure and takedown systemic-to-pulmonary shunt, coronary circulation is no longer exposed to a diastolic runoff caused by the shunt. Conversely, if some degree of PA hypoplasia persists after the Glenn, it will be challenging to treat because venous flow is a less potent stimulator of arterial growth than pulsatile arterial flow.

Patients with TCPC are at risk for multiple long-term complications which involve multiple apparatus; cardiac, pulmonary, hepatic, gastrointestinal, and neurological problems may occur starting from 5 to 10 years after the operation. Intraatrial arrhythmias [122], especially for people who had atrio-pulmonary anastomosis, such as atrial flutter, atrial tachycardia, or atrial fibrillation, are difficult to treat either medically or interventionally and tend to have high rate of recurrency. Sinus node dysfunction is common, occurring in about 45% of patients after 5–7 years; it may require pacemaker implantation. Liver dysfunction due to chronically elevated central venous pressure can lead to fibrosis, cirrhosis (30%), and hepatic tumors (2.9%) mainly hepatocellular carcinoma [123]. The occurrence of plastic bronchitis and protein losing enteropathy, whose etiology is still partially unknown, may be the alarming feature of a failing Fontan circulation. Moderately reduced exercise tolerance is observed in the majority of these patients due to poor conditioning, elevated systemic vascular resistance, lack of a subpulmonary ventricle, and sinus node dysfunction. Heart failure and sudden cardiac death are the leading causes of mortality; the incidence of heart failure increases with age. At some point, heart transplantation may become the only effective option in Fontan patients with untreatable arrhythmias and/or protein losing enteropathy and/or overt cardiac failure; survival after transplantation is similar to that observed in patients without complex CHD [124].

1.1.6   Miscellanea

1.1.6.1 Partial Anomalous Pulmonary Venous Connection

Partial anomalous pulmonary venous connection (PAPVC) occurs in <1% of all CHD and is found commonly in Noonan and Turner syndromes, up to 18%. There is a frequent association with left isomerism, the polysplenia form of heterotaxy. In PAPVC, one or more, but not all, pulmonary veins drain into the systemic venous circulation instead of entering the left atrium. Multiple combinations are possible; the right pulmonary veins (RPVs) are involved twice as often as the left pulmonary veins (LPVs). The following forms are the most frequent:

- RPVs may drain into the SVC (Fig. 1.27), at any level even in the azygos vein, or directly into RA; there is a common association with sinus venosus defect ASD.

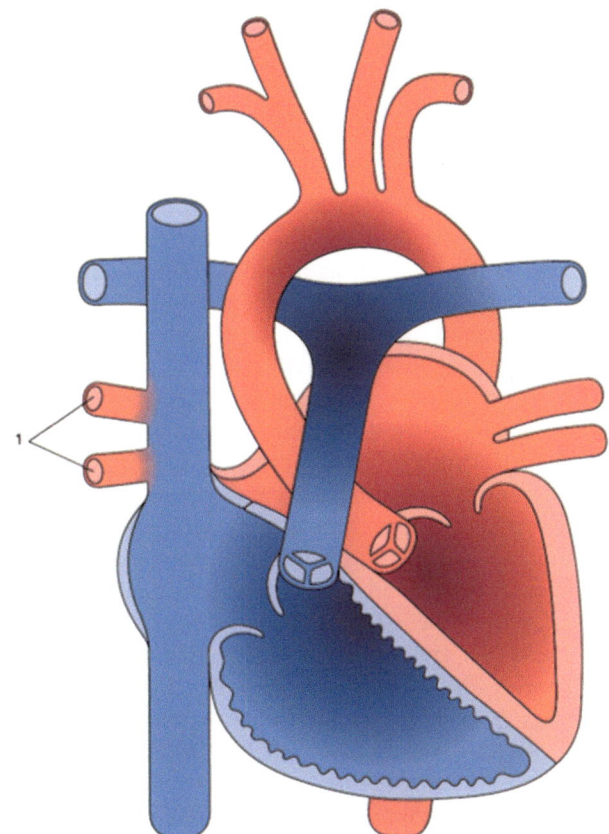

Fig. 1.27 Partial anomalous pulmonary venous connection. (1) Two right pulmonary veins into SVC

- RPVs may drain into the IVC at any level; it is typical of the so-called scimitar syndrome in which the affected part of the right lung has the characteristics of a sequestration: hypoplastic, with abnormal bronchi and abnormal arterial supply which comes directly from the descending aorta. The right PA is usually hypoplastic as well and the atrial septum is typically intact.
- Left upper pulmonary vein may drain into the left innominate vein via an anomalous vertical vein; an ASD is typically present.

Clinical presentation of PAPVC is quite similar to that of an ASD: being an acyanotic defect, symptoms depend on the amount of L-to-R shunting. If a single vein drains anomalously, it carries less than 25% of the pulmonary venous return, resulting in a hemodynamically insignificant shunt; however, patients may become symptomatic later on in life due to LV diastolic dysfunction or worsening LA capacitance. When all but one of the pulmonary veins are involved, patients may present in infancy or early childhood with dyspnea on exertion, repeated respiratory tract infection, and asthma. Rarely older patients present with PH and PAPVC should be considered in the differential diagnosis. Two forms of scimitar syndrome exist with two different presentations: the infantile form and the adult one. Infants may present with some degree of cyanosis, recurrent pneumonia, PH, poor feeding, and failure to thrive. In adults, symptoms and PH are quite rare, and often the syndrome is discovered incidentally when a chest x-ray shows dextrocardia and/or lung hypoplasia.

Diagnosis. When associated with ASD, S2 is split widely and fixed; without ASD, S2 is normal. A 2–3 ejection systolic murmur may be audible at the upper left sternal border as well as a mid-diastolic tricuspid rumble. ECG may reveal RA enlargement, incomplete RBBB, and RVH. On chest x-ray, RA, RV, and PA dilation may be seen in case of large L-to-R shunt, along with increased pulmonary vascular markings. Occasionally, a dilated SVC, a crescent-shaped vertical shadow in the right lower lung (the "scimitar sign"), or a widened superior mediastinum may suggest the site of the anomalous connection. In scimitar syndrome, lung hypoplasia and dextrocardia are easily detected. On TTE, the diagnosis of PAPVC requires a high index of suspicion: dilation of RA and RV in the absence of a large ASD should raise the suspicion as well as a large coronary sinus in the absence of a left SVC. In scimitar syndrome, subcostal views may be helpful to detect the anomalous connection to IVC and, sometimes, the aortopulmonary collateral supplying the affected lung; usually the RPA is small in caliber. If TTE is not conclusive for the diagnosis, CT and MR are excellent imaging modalities. Cardiac catheterization is required whenever PH is suspected or, in older adults, to rule out coronary artery disease.

Treatment. Symptomatic infants or children may require diuretics in case of high PBF. Definitive therapy is surgery that is recommended with a significant L-to-R shunt (> 2:1) or when more than one vein is involved or in case of recurrent pneumonia. In asymptomatic children, repair is delayed until early school age. The surgical approach may vary greatly, according to the anomalous anatomy: in case of RPVs into SVC with ASD, repair is performed by rerouting the anomalous veins into the LA via a patch through the ASD. For scimitar syndrome, resection of the abnormal lung may be necessary [125]; interventional cardiac catheterization may play a role in closing aortopulmonary collateral artery with device. Nowadays, surgical mortality rate is very low. The major long-term concerns are pulmonary vein stenosis, at the level of surgical reimplantation or within the baffles created for rerouting the anomalous vein. After scimitar syndrome repair, a 13-year freedom from pulmonary venous drainage obstruction is approximately 85%, regardless of the surgical technique used [126].

1.1.6.2 Total Anomalous Pulmonary Venous Connection

Total anomalous pulmonary venous connection (TAPVC) is a cyanotic disease which accounts for 1% of all CHDs. Occurrence is typically sporadic. It could be associated with both forms of heterotaxy. There is a marked male preponderance for the infracardiac type with a 4:1 ratio. It is the result of an abnormal incorporation of the common pulmonary vein into the posterior LA which may lead to persistency of fetal connections to the fetal venous systems. In TAPVC all the pulmonary veins drain directly or indirectly into the systemic venous circulation. A R-to-L shunt at the atrial level is necessary for life, to allow blood to enter into left-sided circulation to maintain systemic cardiac output. Based on the anatomic site of the connection, TAPVC can be classified into the following four types: supracardiac 49%, cardiac 16%, infracardiac 26%, and mixed 9% [127].

- Supracardiac: The pulmonary venous confluence drains superiorly into the left cardinal system via a vertical vein which is not a persistent left SVC because its position is more posterior; vertical vein usually runs anterior to the LPA and then enters the left innominate vein; rarely it courses between LPA and the left mainstem bronchus and may become obstructed.
- Cardiac: The pulmonary venous confluence drains into the coronary sinus or directly into RA; obstruction is uncommon (Fig. 1.28).

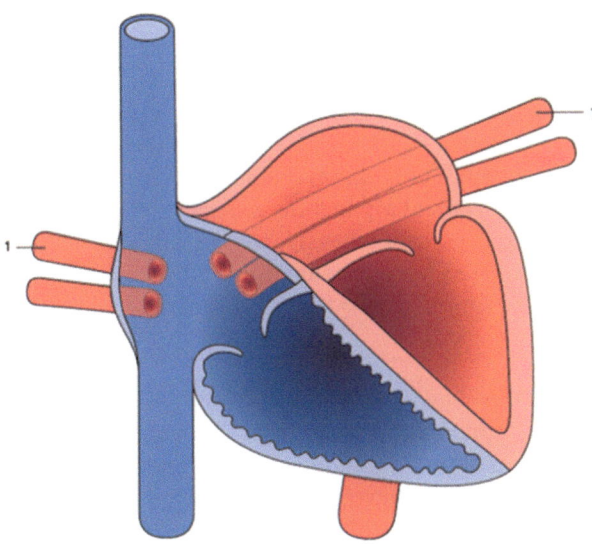

Fig. 1.28 Cardiac total anomalous pulmonary venous connection. (1) Pulmonary veins

- Infracardiac/infradiaphragmatic: The pulmonary venous confluence, via a vertical vein, courses through the esophageal hiatus anterior to the esophagus and then enters into the portal vein or, more rarely, the ductus venosus or hepatic vein or IVC. Obstruction is typical of this form and can occur at different levels: at the esophageal hiatus, at the hepatic sinusoids, or at the ductus venosus as the duct closes postnatally.
- Mixed: The veins drain to at least two different levels; most frequently three veins drain together into the coronary sinus, while the left upper vein drains into the left innominate vein.

For all the forms described, obstruction can rarely occur at the atrial level, should the ASD/PFO become restrictive.

Clinical presentation depends on whether the pulmonary venous return is obstructed. Neonates with unobstructed TAPVC are usually asymptomatic at birth with minimal degree of cyanosis; as the PVR decreases during the first weeks of life, PBF increases and patients gradually develop symptoms of pulmonary overcirculation: tachypnea, feeding difficulties, recurrent respiratory infections, and failure to thrive. Without treatment, 75–85% of cases will die by 1 year of age.

Neonates with obstructed TAPC typically present early after birth and develop symptoms within the first few days: moderate to severe cyanosis, tachypnea with retraction, and signs of respiratory distress. Cyanosis worsens with feeding in the infracardiac type due to the compression of the pulmonary vein confluence by the food-filled esophagus.

Diagnosis

- Unobstructed TAPVC: Hyperactive RV impulse is present. S2 is widely split and fixed; a 2–3/6 ejection systolic murmur is usually audible along with a mid-diastolic tricuspid rumble. ECG shows RA dilation and RVH. On chest x-ray, cardiomegaly is present with increased vascular markings. In supracardiac form, the "snowman" sign, due to enlarged superior mediastinum (vertical vein, dilated innominate vein, and dilated SVC), may be seen but rarely before 4 months of age.
- Obstructed TAPVC: Moderate to severe cyanosis is present. A loud and single S2, indicative of severe PH, along with a gallop rhythm is audible. Typically, heart murmur is absent. Pulmonary crackles and hepatomegaly are present. ECG is not particularly helpful and shows RVH but not RA dilation. On chest x-ray there is no cardiomegaly, and the lung parenchyma is markedly abnormal with pulmonary venous congestion and edema; in severe obstruction, diffuse ground glass appearance becomes evident and could be misdiagnosed as respiratory distress syndrome.

TTE is the modality of choice for assessing all the anatomic details and should be performed using a thorough sequential, segmental approach. The intracardiac anatomy, the pulmonary veins, the pulmonary venous confluence, the entire route of drainage, and the level of the obstruction should be identified quite clearly.

Treatment. In older infants with unobstructed TAPVC and presenting with signs of pulmonary overcirculation, diuretics may be helpful until surgical correction. Because obstruction can develop late, close follow-up is mandatory. Surgical repair is the definitive therapy and is usually carried out shortly after the diagnosis.

Infants with obstructed TAPVC are critically ill and require aggressive medical stabilization, mechanical ventilation, and inotropic support prior to surgical repair which should be performed as soon as possible after the diagnosis as an emergency procedure. Surgical techniques depend on the anatomy of TAPVC and aim at rerouting the pulmonary venous drainage back to the LA via an unobstructed course.

Outcome. Surgical mortality rate is about 5% [128]. Immediate postoperative period can be tough especially in case of significant residual PH which can affect early prognosis and survival. Mid and long term are mainly related to residual or progressive pulmonary venous obstruction which can occur in 10% of cases; some risk factors for significant postoperative venous obstruction have been identified and include hypoplastic or stenotic pulmonary veins and the absence of a common venous confluence at the time of operation. Atrial arrhythmias may occur along with sinus node dysfunction.

1.1.6.3 Anomalous Origin of Left Coronary Artery from the Pulmonary Artery

Anomalous origin of left coronary artery from the pulmonary artery (ALCAPA) occurs in about 0.2% of all CHD with an incidence of 1/300,000 infants. It can cause myocardial ischemia, infarction, and congestive heart failure within the first few months of life and carries a risk of sudden cardiac death in all age groups. The anomalous coronary artery usually arises from the main PA (Fig. 1.29); because coronary perfusion depends on the diastolic pressure gradient existing between the PA and the myocardium supplied by that left coronary artery (LCA), when diastolic PA pressure decreases, LV myocardial ischemia and/or infarction can occur. These critical events may happen as PVR decreases after birth, before coronary collaterals from the right coronary artery (RCA) are well developed. Gradually, over time, after collaterals have enlarged, there will be high flow in the enlarged RCA and in the coronary collaterals supplying the LCA and significant retrograde flow into the PA.

The timing of presentation depends on the development of coronary collateral circulation supplying the LCA from the RCA. Symptoms usually appear at 2–3 months of life and consist of recurrent acute episodes of distress (anginal pain) and CHF such as feeding difficulties and failure to thrive.

Occasionally, children, adolescents and even adults may present with exercise intolerance, fatigue, palpitations, chest pain, or arrhythmias. Late presentation is associated with significant collateral coronary circulation that has been preserving LV function.

Diagnosis. Tachypnea, diaphoresis, tachycardia, and poor peripheral perfusion are commonly present. On auscultation gallop rhythm may be audible, whereas significant murmur is usually absent. ECG usually shows an anterolateral myocardium infarction pattern consisting of deep (>3 mm) and wide (>30 ms) Q waves, inverted T waves, and ST segment elevation in leads I, aVL, and V3–V6. On chest

Fig. 1.29 Anomalous
origin of left coronary
artery from the pulmonary
artery. (1) LCA from the
PA. (2) RCA from the
aorta

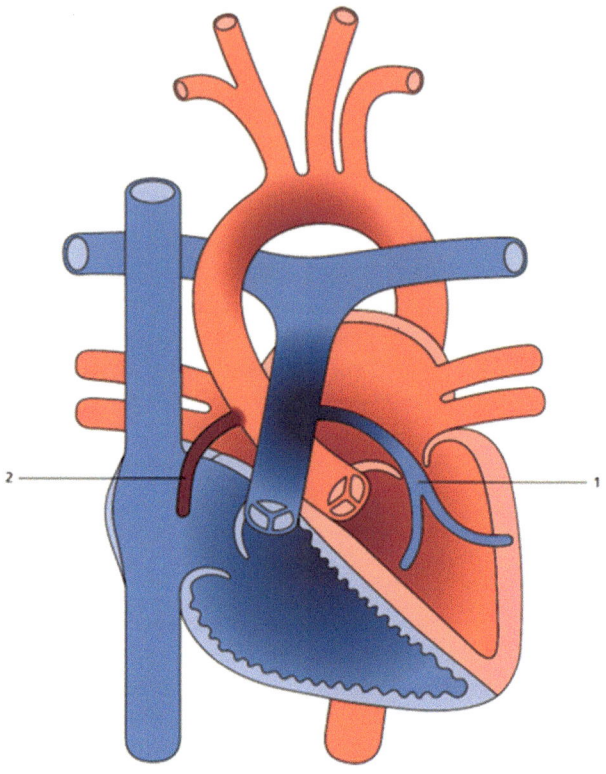

x-ray, cardiomegaly and pulmonary edema are common. TTE shows a markedly dilated LV with poor systolic function with variable degree of MV regurgitation due to papillary muscle ischemia. The coronary artery origins should be fully interrogated, in parasternal short-axis view, by 2D imaging and then by color Doppler flow in order to study the flow direction within the coronaries as well [129]. The endocardium and MV papillary muscles may appear echo-bright, indicating prior infarction. Cardiac catheterization has been the gold standard for diagnosing ALCAPA; however, over the last decade, CT but mainly MR has often replaced cardiac catheterization as the preferred diagnostic modality.

Treatment. All the medical treatments are a bridge to surgical treatment; inotropic support and/or diuretics may be helpful to stabilize the patient. Surgical correction is the definitive treatment and is usually carried out shortly after the diagnosis. Surgical technique may vary; the most common approach consists of translocation of the anomalous artery from PA to the aorta. Another procedure termed the Takeuchi repair allows in situ rerouting of the LCA by creating an intrapulmonary baffle; unfortunately it may result in supravalvar pulmonary stenosis later on.

Also in adolescents and adults, surgical techniques are multiple: reimplantation of LCA from PA to the aorta, coronary arterial bypass grafting from the aorta to the left anterior descending artery with closure of the anomalous coronary from inside the PA, and closure of the anomalous coronary from inside the PA only. Regardless of the technique used, the aim is to remove the L-to-R shunt from the LCA to the PA in order to stop any coronary steal.

Outcome. Although LV function may remain significantly impaired immediately after surgery, usually, in most of the cases, it gradually improves, often going back to normal value. Also functional outcomes in the long-term follow-up are very good for children operated on, despite the severe initial LV dysfunction at presentation. An important issue is the residual, significant MV regurgitation which could be seen in about one-third of the patients.

In patients operated on in adolescence or in adulthood, the RCA tends to decrease to normal size, and the collaterals appear to involute within 3 or more years after surgery. LV function may not recover as much as in infants or children. LV function and LV myocardial damage are the most relevant determining factors in the long-term survivals.

1.1.7 Heterotaxy

Heterotaxy does not define a single specific condition but includes many cardiac and systemic anomalies characterized by an abnormal arrangement across the left-right axis of the body of the internal thoracic and abdominal organs secondary to an embryological failure in differentiation. The key feature of heterotaxy is the mirror-image duplication of normally unilateral structures; some patients appear to have bilateral right-sidedness, so-called right isomerism, and others bilateral left-sidedness, so-called left isomerism. This abnormality becomes evident in the lungs, each of which may show either three lobes and a short bronchus (right isomerism) or two lobes and a long undivided bronchus (left isomerism). At cardiac level, atrial appendages may exhibit isomerism of the pectinate muscles, and a strong association is seen between bronchial morphology, lungs, and atrial appendages. Within the atrium, it is the appendages that are the most constant components; their shape and the particular morphology of their junction with the rest of the atrium permit them to be distinguished as morphologically right or left. Furthermore, a strong association, up to 85%, exists between pulmonary, bronchial, and atrial isomerism and abdominal visceral arrangement; right atrial isomerism is usually associated with absence of the spleen, so-called asplenia syndrome, whereas left atrial isomerism is commonly associated with multiple spleens, so-called polysplenia syndrome. CHDs are usually present in heterotaxy, and they can vary from mild to severe complexity; some CHDs can be seen in both forms of isomerism, such as AVSD, although more prevalent in the right one, about two-thirds of cases, compared to half in left isomerism. Other CHDs occur much more commonly in right isomerism such as pulmonary stenosis, TGA, and TAPVC.

Two extracardiac conditions are frequently seen in patients with heterotaxy: impaired immune system secondary to asplenia or malfunctioning spleen or dysfunctional cilia and bowel obstruction secondary to gut malrotation.

Because of the complexity of heterotaxy, patients should be evaluated following a sequential, segmental approach to properly describe systemic and cardiac anatomy: evaluation should address the thoracoabdominal situs, cardiac position, atrial situs, A-V and V-A connections, cardiac looping, great artery relationship, and systemic and pulmonary vein connections.

Focusing on atrial and abdominal situs, the following arrangements are described: solitus, inversus, right-sided isomerism, and left-sided isomerism.

References

1. Hoffman JI, Kaplan S. The incidence of congenital heart disease. J Am Coll Cardiol. 2002;39(12):1890–900.
2. Park MK. Pediatric cardiology for practitioners. 4th ed. St Louis: Mosby; 2002.
3. Anderson RH, Baker EJ, Penny D, Redington AN, Rigby ML, Wernovsky J. Paediatric cardiology. 3rd ed. Philadelphia: Elsevier; 2009.
4. Triedman JK, Newburger JW. Trends in congenital heart disease. The next decade. Circulation. 2016;133:2716–33.
5. Anderson RH, Brown NA, Webb S. Development and structure of the atrial septum. Heart. 2002;88:104–10.
6. John Sutton MG, Tajik AJ, McGoon DC. Atrial setal defect in patients ages 60 years or older: operative results and long-term postoperative follow-up. Circulation. 1981;64:402–9.
7. Schneider B, Zienkiewicz T, Jansen V, et al. Diagnosis of patent foramen ovale by transesophageal echocardiography and correlation with autopsy findings. Am J Cardiol. 1996;77:1202–9.
8. Furlan AJ, Reisman M, Massaro J, Mauri L, Albers GW, Felberg R, Herrmann H, Kar S, Landzberg M, Raizner A, Wechsler L, CLOSURE I Investigators. Closure or medical therapy for cryptogenic stroke with patent foramen ovale. N Engl J Med. 2012;366:991–9.
9. Butera G, Romagnoli E, Carminati M, Chessa M, Piazza L, et al. Treatment of isolated secundum atrial septal defects: impact of age and defect morphology in 1013 consecutive patients. Am Heart J. 2008;156:706–12.
10. Hoffman JI, Kaplan S, Liberthson RR. Prevalence of congenital heart disease. Am Heart J. 2004;147:425–39.
11. Roos-Hesselink JW, Meijboom FJ, Spitaels SE, et al. Excellent survival and low incidence of arrhythmias, stroke and heart failure long-term after surgical ASD closure at young age. A prospective follow-up study of 21-33 years. Eur Heart J. 2003;24:190–7.
12. Rhodes LA, Keane JP, et al. Long follow up (up to 43 years) of ventricular septal defect with audible aortic regurgitation. Am J Cardiol. 1990;66:340–5.
13. Simpson JM, Miller O. Three-dimensional echocardiography in congenital heart disease. Arch Cardiovasc Dis. 2011;104:45–56.
14. Nygren A, Sunnegard J, Berggren H. Preoperative evaluation and surgery in isolated ventricular septal defects: a 21 years perspective. Heart. 2005;83:198–204.
15. Carminati M, Butera G, Chessa M, Drago M, Negura D, Piazza L. Transcatheter closure of congenital ventricular septal defects with Amplatzer occluders. Am J Cardiol. 2005;96:52L–8L.
16. Roos-Hesselink JW, Meijboom FJ, Spitaels SE, Van Domburg R, Van Rijen EH, Utens EM, Bogers AJ, Simoons ML. Outcome of patients after surgical closure of ventricular septal defect at a young age: longitudinal follow-up of 22-34 years. Eur Heart J. 2004;25:1057–62.
17. Butera G, Carminati M, Chessa M, Piazza L, Micheletti A, Negura DG, Abella R, Giamberti A, Frigiola A. Transcatheter closure of perimembranous ventricular septal defects. Early and long term results. J Am Coll Cardiol. 2007;50:1189–95.

18. Carminati M, Butera G, Chessa M, De Giovanni J, Fisher G, Gewillig M, Peuster M, Piechaud JF, Santoro G, Sievert H, Spadoni I, Walsh K. Transcatheter closure of congenital ventricular septal defects: results of the European Registry. Eur Heart J. 2007;28:2361–8.
19. Holzer R, De Giovanni J, Walsh K, Tometzki A, Goh T, Hakim F, Zabal C, de Lezo JS, Cao QL, Hijazi ZM. Transcatheter closure of perimembranous ventricular septal defects using the Amplatzer membranous ventricular septal defect device occluder: immediate and midterm results of an international registry. Catheter Cardiovasc Interv. 2006;68:620–8.
20. Hlavacek AM, Crawford FA Jr, Chessa KS, Shirali GS. Real-time three-dimensional echocardiography is useful in the evaluation of patients with atrioventricular septal defects. Echocardiography. 2006;23:225–31.
21. Dimopoulos K, Inuzuka R, Goletto S, et al. Improved survival among patients with Eisenmenger syndrome receiving advanced therapy for pulmonary arterial hypertension. Circulation. 2010;121:20–5.
22. Najm HK, Coles JG, Endo M, et al. Complete atrioventricular septal defects: results of repair, risk factors and freedom from reoperation. Circulation. 1997;96(9 Suppl):II-311–5.
23. Patel SS, Burns TL, Kochilas L. Early outcomes and prognostic factors for left atrioventricular valve reoperation after primary atrioventricular septal defect repair. Paediatr Cardiol. 2012;33:129–40.
24. Bergin ML, Warnes CA, Tajik AJ, Danielson GK. Partial atrioventricular canal defect: long-term follow-up after initial repair in patients > or = 40 years old. J Am Coll Cardiol. 1995;25:1189–94.
25. Benson LN, Cowan KN. The arterial duct: its presence and patency. In: Anderson RH, Baker EJ, Macartney FJ, et al., editors. Paediatric cardiology. 2nd ed. London: Churchill Livingstone; 2002. p. 1404–59.
26. Schwartz MC, Nykanen D, Winner LH, et al. Trancatheter patent ductus arteriosus occlusion in small infants. Congenit Heart Dis. 2016;11(6):647–55.
27. Backes CH, Cheatham SL, Deyo GM, et al. Percutaneous patent ductus arteriosus (PDA) closure in very preterm infants: feasibility and complications. J Am Heart Assoc. 2016;5(2):e002923.
28. Jaspal D, Chessa M, Piazza L, Negura D, Micheletti A, Bussadori C, Butera G, Carminati M. Initial experience with the new Amplatzer duct occluder II. J Invasive Cardiol. 2009;21:401–5.
29. Pedra CA, Sanches SA, Fontes VF. Percutaneous occlusion of the patent ductus arteriosus with the Amplatzer device for atrial septal defect. J Invasive Cardiol. 2003;15:413–7.
30. Boudjemline Y. The new Occlutech(®) patent ductus arteriosus occluder: single centre experience. Arch Cardiovasc Dis. 2016;109(6–7):384–9.
31. Barnes ME, Mitchell ME, Tweddell JS. Aortopulmonary window. Semin Thorac Cardiovasc Surg Pediatr Card Surg Annu. 2011;14(1):67–74.
32. Kosmač B, Eicken A, Kühn A, Heinrich M, Ewert P. Percutaneous device closure of an aortopulmonary window in a small infant. Int J Cardiol. 2013;168(3):e102–3.
33. Alsoufi B, Schlosser B, McCracken C, et al. Current outcomes of surgical management of aortopulmonary window and associated cardiac lesions. Circulation. 2016;133(19):1907–10.
34. Avari M, Nair S, Kozlowska Z, Nashef S. Cor triatriatum sinistrum: presentation of syncope and atrial tachycardia. BMJ Case Rep. 2017;14:2017.
35. Said SM, Ibrahimiye AN, Punn R, Hanley FL. Hemoptysis as a rare presentation of cor triatriatum sinister. J Thorac Cardiovasc Surg. 2015;150(5):e73–5.
36. Naimo PS, Konstantinov IE. Cor triatriatum sinister: is it less sinister in older patients? J Thorac Cardiovasc Surg. 2015;150(5):e77–8.
37. Saxena P, Burkhart HM, Schaff HV, et al. Surgical repair of cor triatriatum sinister: the Mayo Clinic 50-year experience. Ann Thorac Surg. 2014;97(5):1659–63.
38. Ruckman RN, Van Praagh R. Anatomic types of congenital mitral stenosis: report of 49 autopsy cases with considerations of diagnosis and surgical implications. Am J Cardiol. 1978;42(4):592–601.

39. Fuller S, Spray TL. How I manage mitral stenosis in the neonate and infant. Semin Thorac Cardiovasc Surg Pediatr Card Surg Annu. 2009;12:87–93.
40. McElhinney DB, Sherwood MC, Keane JF, et al. Current management of severe congenital mitral stenosis: outcomes of transcatheter and surgical therapy in 108 infants and children. Circulation. 2005;112(5):707–14.
41. Kojori F, Chen R, Caldarone CA, et al. Outcomes of mitral valve replacement in children: a competing-risks analysis. J Thorac Cardiovasc Surg. 2004;128(5):703–9.
42. Caldarone CA, Raghuveer G, Hills CB, et al. Long-term survival after mitral valve replacement in children aged <5 years: a multi-institutional study. Circulation. 2001;104(12 Suppl 1):I143–7.
43. Gunther T, Mazzitelli D, Schreiber C, et al. Mitral valve replacement in children under 6 years of age. Eur J Cardiothorac Surg. 2000;17(4):426–30.
44. Perloff JK, Child JS. Clinical and epidemiologic issues in mitral valve prolapse: overview and perspective. Am Heart J. 1987;113(5):1324–32.
45. Hayek E, Gring CN, Griffin BP. Mitral valve prolapse. Lancet. 2005;365(9458):507–18.
46. Webb JG, Harnek J, Munt BI, et al. Percutaneous transvenous mitral annuloplasty: initial human experience with device implantation in the coronary sinus. Circulation. 2006;113(6):851–5.
47. Weinsaft JW, Devereux RB, Preiss LR, et al. Aortic dissection in patients with genetically mediated aneurysms: incidence and predictors in the GenTAC registry. J Am Coll Cardiol. 2016;67(23):2744–54.
48. Fernandes SM, Sanders SP, Khairy P, et al. Morphology of bicuspid aortic valve in children and adolescents. J Am Coll Cardiol. 2004;44:1648–51.
49. Maskatia SA, Ing FF, Justino H, et al. Twenty-five year experience with balloon aortic valvuloplasty for congenital aortic stenosis. Am J Cardiol. 2011;108:1024–8.
50. Ross DN. Replacement of aortic and mitral valves with a pulmonary autograft. Lancet. 1967;2:956–8.
51. McCrindle BW. Independent predictors of immediate results of percutaneous balloon aortic valvotomy in children. Valvuloplasty and Angioplasty of Congenital Anomalies (VACA) Registry Investigators. Am J Cardiol. 1996;77(4):286–93.
52. Geva A, Mc Mahon CJ, Gauvreau K, et al. Risk factors for reoperation after repair of discrete subaortic stenosis in children. J Am Coll Cardiol. 2007;50(15):1498–504.
53. Scott DJ, Campbell DN, Clarke DL, et al. Twenty-year surgical experience with congenital supravalvar aortic stenosis. Ann Thorac Surg. 2009;87(5):1501–7.
54. McBride KL, Zender GA, Fitzgerald-Butt SM, et al. Linkage analysis of left ventricular outflow tract malformations (aortic valve stenosis, coarctation of the aorta, and hypoplastic left heart syndrome). Eur J Hum Genet. 2009;17:811–9.
55. Niwa K, Perloff JK, Bhuta SM, Laks H, et al. Structural abnormalities of great arterial walls in congenital heart disease: light and electron microscopic analyses. Circulation. 2001;103:393–400.
56. Baumgartner H, Bonhoeffer P, DeGroot N, et al. ESC guidelines for the management of grown-up congenital heart disease. Eur Heart J. 2010;31:2915–57.
57. Matsui H, Adachi I, Uemura H, Gardiner H, Ho SY. Anatomy of coarctation, hypoplastic and interrupted aortic arch: relevance to interventional/surgical treatment. Expert Rev Cardiovasc Ther. 2007;5:871–80.
58. Egan M, Holzer RJ. Comparing balloon angioplasty, stenting and surgery in the treatment of aortic coarctation. Expert Rev Cardiovasc Ther. 2009;7:1401–12.
59. Thomson JDR, Mulpur A, Guerrero R, et al. Outcome after extended arch repair for aortic coarctation. Heart. 2006;92:90–4.
60. Holzer R, Qureshi S, Ghasemi A, et al. Stenting of aortic coarctation: acute, intermediate and long-term results of a prospective multi-institutional registry—Congenital Cardiovascular Interventional Study Consortium (CCISC). Catheter Cardiovasc Interv. 2010;76:553–63.

61. Forbes TJ, Moore P, Pedra CA, Zahn EM, et al. Intermediate follow-up following intravascular stenting for treatment of coarctation of the aorta. Catheter Cardiovasc Interv. 2007;70:569–77.

62. Hager A, Kanz S, Kaemmerer H, et al. Coarctation Long-term Assessment (COALA): significance of arterial hypertension in a cohort of 404 patients up to 27 years after surgical repair of isolated coarctation of the aorta, even in the absence of restenosis and prosthetic material. J Thorac Cardiovasc Surg. 2007;134:738–45.

63. Eicken A, Pensl U, Sebening W, Hager A, et al. The fate of systemic blood pressure in patients after effectively stented coarctation. Eur Heart J. 2006;27:1100–5.

64. Brown JW, Ruzmetov M, Okada Y, et al. Otcomes in patients with interrupted aortic arch and associated anomalies: a 20-year experience. Eur J Cardiothorac Surg. 2006;29(5):666–73.

65. Sugimoto A, Ota N, Miyakoshi C, et al. Mid- to long-term aortic valve-related outcomes after conventional repair for patients with interrupted aortic arch or coarctation of the aorta, combined with ventricular septal defect: the impact of bicuspid aortic valve. Eur J Cardiothorac Surg. 2014;46(6):952–60.

66. O'Byme ML, Mercer-Rosa L, Zhao H, et al. Morbidity in children and adolescents after surgical correction of interrupted aortic arch. Pediatr Cardiol. 2014;35(3):386–92.

67. Anderson KR, Zuberbuhler JR, Anderson RH, et al. Morphologic spectrum of Ebstein's anomaly of the heart: a review. Mayo Clinic Proc. 1979;54(3):174–80.

68. Sharland GK, Chita SK, Allan LD. Tricuspid valve dysplasia or displacement in intrauterine life. J Am Coll Cardiol. 1991;17(4):944–9.

69. Celermajer DS, Dodd SM, Greenwald SE, et al. Morbid anatomy in neonates with Ebstein's anomaly of the tricuspid valve: pathophysiologic and clinical implications. J Am Coll Cardiol. 1992;19(5):1049–53.

70. Starnes VA, Pitlick PT, Bernstein D, et al. Ebstein's anomaly appearing in the neonate. A new surgical approach. J Thorac Cardiovasc Surg. 1991;101(6):1082–7.

71. Quinonez LG, Dearani JA, Puga FJ, et al. Results of the 1.5-ventricle repair for Ebstein anomaly and the failing right ventricle. J Thorac Cardiovasc Surg. 2007;133(5):1303–10.

72. Brown ML, Dearani JA, Danielson GK, et al. The outcomes of operations for 539 patients with Ebstein anomaly. J Thorac Cardiovasc Surg. 2008;135(5):1120–36.

73. Roberts PA, Boudjemline Y, Cheatham JP, et al. Percutaneous tricuspid valve replacement in congenital and acquired heart disease. J Am Coll Cardiol. 2011;58(2):117–22.

74. Brown ML, Dearani JA, Danielson GK, et al. Functional status after operation for Ebstein anomaly: the Mayo Clinic experience. J Am Coll Cardiol. 2008;52(6):460–6.

75. Stamm C, Anderson RH, Ho SY. Clinical anatomy of the normal pulmonary root compared with that in isolated pulmonary valvular stenosis. J Am Coll Cardiol. 1998;31(6):1420–5.

76. Coles JG, Freedom RM, Olley PM, et al. Surgical management of critical pulmonary stenosis in the neonate. Ann Thorac Surg. 1984;38(5):458–65.

77. Holzer RJ, Gauvreau K, Kreutzer J, et al. Safety and efficacy of balloon pulmonary valvuloplasty: a multicentre experience. Catheter Cardiovasc Interv. 2012;80:663–72.

78. McCrindle BW. Independent predictors of long-term results after balloon pulmonary valvuloplasty. Circulation. 1994;89:1751–9.

79. Karagoz T, Asoh K, Hickey E, et al. Balloon dilation of pulmonary valve stenosis in infents less than 3 kg: a 20-year experience. Catheter Cardiovasc Interv. 2009;74:753–61.

80. Voet A, Rega F, Van de Bruaene A, et al. Long term outcome after treatment of isolated pulmonary valve stenosis. Int J Cardiol. 2012;156:11–5.

81. Bull C, de Leval MR, Mercanti C, et al. Pulmonary atresia and intact ventricular septum: a revised classification. Circulation. 1982;66:266–80.

82. Justo RN, Nykanen DG, Williams WG, et al. Transcatheter perforation of the right ventricular outflow tract as initial therapy for pulmonary valve atresia and intact ventricular septum in the newborn. Catheter Cardiovasc Diagn. 1997;40:408–13.

83. Humpl T, Soderberg B, McCrindle BW, et al. Percutaneous balloon valvotomy in pulmonary atresia with intact ventricular septum: impact on patient care. Circulation. 2003;108:826–32.

84. Gewillig M, Boshoff DE, Dens J, et al. Stenting the neonatal arterial duct in duct-dependent pulmonary circulation; new techniques, better results. J Am Coll Cardiol. 2004;43:107–12.
85. Kreutzer C, Mayorquim RC, Kreutzer GO, et al. Experience with one and a half ventricle repair. J Thorac Cardiovasc Surg. 1999;117:662–8.
86. Patel A, Farrell P, Harris M, et al. Acquired ventricular septal aneurysm in a patient with pulmonary atresia with intact ventricular septum. Cardiol Young. 2012;22:227–9.
87. Anderson RH, Jacobs ML. The anatomy of tetralogy of Fallot with pulmonary stenosis. Cardiol Young. 2008;18(Suppl 3):12–21.
88. Kirsch RE, Glatz AC, Gaynor JW, et al. Results of elective repair at 6 months or younger in 277 patients with tetralogy of Fallot: a 14-year experience at a single center. J Thorac Cardiovasc Surg. 2014;147(2):713–7.
89. He GW, Liu XC, Kong XR, et al. The current strategy of repair of tetralogy of Fallot in children and adults. Cardiol Young. 2008;18(6):608–14.
90. Morales DL, Zafar F, Fraser CD Jr. Tetralogy of Fallot repair: the right ventricle infundibulum sparing (RVIS) strategy. Semin Thorac Cardiovasc Surg Pediatr Card Surg Annu. 2009:54–8.
91. Norwood WI, Rosenthal A, Castaneda AR. Tetralogy of Fallot with acquired pulmonary atresia and hypoplasia of pulmonary arteries. Report of surgical management in infancy. J Thorac Cardiovasc Surg. 1976;72(3):454–7.
92. Cools B, Boshoff D, Heying R, et al. Transventricular balloon dilation and stenting of the RVOT in small infants with tetralogy of Fallot with pulmonary atresia. Catheter Cardiovasc Interv. 2013;82(2):260–5.
93. Nolleret G, Fischlein T, Bouterwek S, et al. Long-term survival in patients with repair of tetralogy of Fallot: 36-year follow up of 490 survivors of the first year after surgical repair. J Am Coll Cardiol. 1997;30(5):1374–83.
94. Anderson RH. Paediatric cardiology. 3rd ed. Philadelphia, PA: Churchill Livingstone/Elsevier; 2010.
95. Burchill LJ, Wald RM, Harris L, Colman JM, Silversides CK. Pulmonary valve replacement in adults with repaired tetralogy of Fallot. Surg Pediatr Card Surg Ann. 2011;14:92–7.
96. Geva T. Repaired tetralogy of Fallot: the roles of cardiovascular magnetic resonance in evaluating pathophysiology and for pulmonary valve replacement decision support. J Cardiovasc Magn Reson. 2011;13:9.
97. Khairy P, Aboulhosn J, Gurvitz MZ, et al. Arrhythmia burden in adults with surgically repaired tetralogy of Fallot: a multi-institutional study. Circulation. 2010;122(9):868–75.
98. Niwa K, Siu SC, Webb GD, et al. Progressive aortic root dilatation in adults late after repair of tetralogy of Fallot. Circulation. 2002;106:1374–8.
99. Rossi RN, Hislop A, Anderson RH, et al. Systemic-to-pulmonary blood supply in tetralogy of Fallot with pulmonary atresia. Cardiol Young. 2002;12(4):373–88.
100. Al Abib HF, Jacobs JP, Mavroudis C, et al. Contemporary patterns of management of tetralogy of Fallot: data from the Society of Thoracic Surgeons Database. Ann Thorac Surg. 2010;90(3):813–9.
101. Dohlen G, Chaturvedi RR, Benson LN, et al. Stenting of the right ventricular outflow tract in the symptomatic infant with tetralogy of Fallot. Heart. 2009;95(2):142–7.
102. Redington AN, Somerville J. Stenting of aortopulmonary collaterals in complex pulmonary atresia. Circulation. 1996;94(10):2479–84.
103. Yacoub MH, Radley-Smith R. Anatomy of the coronary arteries in transposition of the great arteries and methods for their transfer in anatomical correction. Thorax. 1978;33(4):418–24.
104. Rashkind WJ, Miller WW. Creation of an atrial septal defect without thoracotomy: a palliative approach to complete transposition of the great arteries. JAMA. 1966;196:991–2.
105. Kempny A, Wustmann K, Borgia F, et al. Outcome in adult patients after arterial switch operation for transposition of the great arteries. Int J Cardiol. 2013;167(6):2588–93.
106. Mayer JE Jr, Sanders SP, Jonas RA, et al. Coronary artery pattern and outcome of arterial switch operation for transposition of the great arteries. Circulation. 1990;82(5 Suppl):IV139–45.
107. Gelatt M, Hamilton RM, McCrindle BW, et al. Arrhythmia and mortality after the Mustard procedure: a 30-year single-center experience. J Am Coll Cardiol. 1997;29:194–201.

108. Presbitero P, Somerville J, Rabajoli F, et al. Corrected transposition of the great arteries without associated defects in adult patients: clinical profile and follow up. Br Heart J. 1995;74:57–9.
109. Anderson RC, Lillehei CW, Lester RG. Corrected transposition of the great vessels of the heart. Pediatrics. 1957;20:626–46.
110. Sano T, Riesenfeld T, Karl T, et al. Intermediate-term outcome after intracardiac repair of associated cardiac defects in patients with atrioventricular and ventriculoarterial discordance. Circulation. 1995;92:272–8.
111. Graham TP Jr, Bernard YD, Mellen BG, et al. Long-term outcome in congenitally corrected transposition of the great arteries: a multi-institutional study. J Am Coll Cardiol. 2000;36:255–61.
112. Horer J, Schreiber C, Krane S, et al. Outcome after surgical repair/palliation of congenitally corrected transposition of the great arteries. J Thorac Cardiovasc Surg. 2008;56:391–7.
113. Sondheimer HM, Fredom RH, Olley PM. Double-outlet right ventricle: clinical spectrum and prognosis. Am J Cardiol. 1977;39:709–14.
114. Brown JW, Ruzmetov M, Okada Y, et al. Surgical results in patients with double-outlet right ventricle: a 20-year experience. Ann Thorac Surg. 2001;72:1630–5.
115. Radford DJ, Perkins L, Lachman R, et al. Spectrum of DiGeorge syndrome in patients with truncus arteriosus : expanded DiGeorge syndrome. Pediatr Cardiol. 1988;9:95–101.
116. Elzein C, Ilbawi M, Kumar S, et al. Severe truncal valve stenosis. J Card Surg. 2005;20:589–93.
117. McGoon DC, Rastelli GC, Ongley PA. An operation for the correction of truncus arteriosus. JAMA. 1968;205:69–73.
118. Niwa K, Perloff JK, Kaplan S, et al. Eisenmenger syndrome in adults: ventricular septal defect, truncus arteriosus, univentricular heart. J Am Coll Cardiol. 1999;34:223–32.
119. Young WG Jr, Sealy WC, Houck WS Jr, et al. Superior vena cava-right pulmonary artery anastomosis in cyanotic heart disease. Ann Surg. 1963;157:894–901.
120. McElhinney DB, Petrossian E, Reddy VM, et al. Extracardiac conduit Fontan procedure without cardiopulmonary bypass. Ann Thorac Surg. 1998;66:1826–8.
121. Laks H. The partial Fontan procedure. A new concept and its clinical application. Circulation. 1990;82:1866–7.
122. Stephenson EA, Lu M, Berul CI, et al. Arrhythmias in a contemporary Fontan cohort: prevalence and clinical associations in a multicenter cross-sectional study. J Am Coll Cardiol. 2010;56:890–6.
123. Baek JS, Bae EJ, Ko JS, et al. Late hepatic complications after Fontan operation: non-invasive markers of hepatic fibrosis and risk factors. Heart. 2010;96:1750–5.
124. Kanter KR, Mahle WT, Vincent RN, et al. Heart transplantation in children with a Fontan procedure. Ann Thorac Surg. 2011;91:823–9; discussion 829–30.
125. Brown JW, Ruzmetov M, Minnich DJ, et al. Surgical management of scimitar syndrome: an alternative approach. J Thorac Cardiovasc Surg. 2003;125(2):238–45.
126. Najm HK, Williams WG, Coles JG, et al. Scimitar syndrome: twenty years' experience and results of repair. J Thorac Cardiovasc Surg. 1996;112:1161–9.
127. Seale AN, Uemura H, Webber SA, et al. Total anomalous pulmonary venous connection: morphology and outcome from an international population-based study. Circulation. 2010;122(25):2718–26.
128. Hancock Friesen CL, Zurakowski D, Thiagarajan RR, et al. Total anomalous pulmonary venous connection: an analysis of current management strategies in a single institution. Ann Thorac Surg. 2005;79:596–606.
129. Frommelt PC, Berger S, Pelech AN, et al. Prospective identification of anomalous origin of left coronary artery from the right sinus of valsalva using transthoracic echocardiography: importance of color Doppler flow mapping. Pediatr Cardiol. 2001;22:327–32.

Routine and Emergency Bedside Equipment Setup

Samantha Scolari

Abstract

Designing a specific care approach for children with congenital heart disease (Cardiologia Pediatrica, McGraw-Hill, Milan, 1988) requires considerable hands-on knowledge and skills while also drawing on specific cardiology, paediatrics, intensive care, anatomy, physiology and pathophysiology elements.

As no similarities exist with other patient types, thorough clinical observation should be the starting point. This, combined with comprehensive knowledge of the anatomy, physiology and clinical condition of an individual patient, will be the key to drafting a customised patient care pathway, in which an experienced nurse (From novice to expert: excellence and power in clinical nursing practice, Italian edition: L'eccellenza nella pratica clinica dell'infermiere, McGraw-Hill, Milan, 2003) does make a difference.

2.1 Children and Their Specificities

A child's organism [1] evolves continuously and steadily, unlike that of an adult: as the body grows in size, its external appearance changes, and, most importantly, all the bodily functions develop along with growth, gradually evolving into adulthood. For this reason, children cannot be viewed as "small adults"; rather, they should be considered as individuals who evolve and develop through a number of stages, each of which is seamlessly connected to the previous and following phases yet retains specific features.

The development of a child is a complex phenomenon, starting with conception and continuing into adulthood, whereby changes involve not only the skeleton,

S. Scolari
University Hospital S. Orsola Malpighi, Bologna, Italy

© Springer International Publishing AG, part of Springer Nature 2019
S. F. Flocco et al. (eds.), *Congenital Heart Disease*,
https://doi.org/10.1007/978-3-319-78423-6_2

muscles, organs and functions but, more generally, also intellectual, communication and motor skills. This is a genetically determined process, which is affected by the family and the social environment the child lives in.

Specific care concerns in the case of paediatric heart patients require a diverse and thorough knowledge from the nursing staff, to cater to the needs of all patient types: paediatric patients (neonatology, paediatrics, obstetrics), heart or cardiac surgery patients (cardiology, surgery, paediatric cardiology/cardiac surgery) and acute patients (intensive resuscitation, pharmacology, anaesthesiology). In addition, transversal skills and knowledge are required to provide qualified patient care across all patient types (psychology, systemic counselling, palliative care). This knowledge background allows the nursing staff providing care to acute paediatric heart patients to prioritise their efforts.

2.2   ACHD/GUCH and Their Specificities

Grown-ups with congenital heart defects are subjects [2] who were born with a cardiovascular anomaly and who underwent surgical palliation when growing up that modified their anatomy and, consequently, physiology, hence enabling them to reach adulthood.

These subjects might seek care for other conditions or physiological situations such as pregnancy, just like any other adult; however, they exhibit multiple problems that are intrinsically related to their physiological and anatomical status and which affect their haemodynamic balance.

Given their specific condition, integrating these patients into "universal" diagnosis and treatment courses requires close supervision by an experienced paediatric cardiologist and nurse, who might support and assist their fellow healthcare professionals, providing adequate counselling as needed.

2.3   A Comparison Between Children and Adults

The physiological specificities [3] of the growing body of a child imply that symptoms in paediatric patients present differently than in adults (Table 2.1). Newborn children exhibit evolving haemodynamic features that are mainly related to the beginning of pulmonary ventilation and to a patent ductus arteriosus, which obliterates spontaneously over a few days. This might involve, for instance, physiologically lower saturation levels. The organs of a child, such as the liver, the kidneys and the brain, are more prone to adapt to extreme conditions. Children are highly reactive, expressing the considerable vital potential of a growing body. When assessing signs and symptoms, one should always consider that the child might suffer from associated congenital anomalies that have not been diagnosed yet. Children can express their discomfort using very reliable indicators when they are unwell: a flaccid newborn baby [4] who is lacking appetite cannot be defined as "lazy", and an irritable infant who cannot find comfort and consolation when being fed or cuddled

Table 2.1 Specificities of paediatric patients having an effect on the symptoms and treatment course as compared to adult subjects

Children	Adults
Evolving haemodynamic status	Stable haemodynamic status
Full organ adaptability	Reduced organ adaptability
Greater response capacity	Lower response capacity
Possible still undiagnosed associated anomalies	Associated conditions, if any (e.g. allergies), are usually known
Reliable but mainly non-specific ways for reporting discomfort	Possible interference of the patient's emotions on the symptoms
Natural dependency on parents and limited ability of deferring needs	Rational capabilities for managing discomfort

is unquestionably indicating that something is not right, and such a behaviour cannot be viewed as a "tantrum". Finally, as children naturally depend on their reference parent, they are extremely sensitive to their parent's mood, and the parenting style might affect the child's response capacity.

All these things considered, therefore, we can state that children are not small adults in any respect.

2.4   Setup of Patient Care Stations in General and Intensive Care Units

Patient care stations in a paediatric cardiology/cardiac surgery unit include the following:

- Patient bed.
- Equipment for vital signs monitoring.
- Equipment for peripheral or central venous/arterial catheterisation.
- Equipment for airway management and oxygen therapy (as needed).
- Pre-diluted and patient-specific emergency medications.
- Medical emergency trolley for urgency/emergency management.
- Equipment for urinary catheterisation.
- Supplies for surgical drain insertion.

These "patient units" differ between a *general (ward)* and an *intensive care* scenario.

Ward patients, in fact, exhibit sufficient haemodynamic stability to enable vital sign monitoring as needed, non-intensive clinical observation supported by surveillance from a caregiver as well as oral, intravenous or oxygen therapy as needed and planned by the physician, based on the patient's clinical status.

Conversely, intensive care patients are haemodynamically unstable and, as such, require continuous vital signs monitoring, dedicated observation of their clinical status, continuous IV medication administration and respiratory support by intubation, as needed.

Table 2.2 Patient bed

Routine	Emergency
The bed should be appropriate to the patient's size and weight, and ensure proper comfort; the headboard and side rails should be easily removable, and a rigid board should be available that can be placed under the patient, should resuscitation be necessary	The bed should be appropriate to the patient's size and weight, and ensure proper comfort based on the patient's conditions and clinical stability; the headboard and side rails should already be adjusted to the required patient care; the bed should be equipped with a pressure-relief mattress and an integrated rigid board, along with the electronic systems usually required in an intensive care setting

Incubator, neonatal care station, paediatric surgical bed, extendable paediatric surgical bed, adult surgical bed

Table 2.3 Equipment for vital signs monitoring

Routine	Emergency
Vital signs monitoring is usually performed as needed; based on the type of care, a bedside or portable multifunction monitor can be used to enable: • Heart rate monitoring via electrodes attached to the patient's chest • Respiratory monitoring, either using the same electrodes or manually, by counting the number of breaths and assessing the breathing pattern • Saturation measurement by pulse oximetry • Non-invasive and occasional blood pressure measurement • Peripheral or axillary/tympanic temperature measurement	Vital signs are usually monitored continuously, and the following parameters are displayed: • Heart rate and tracing • Respiratory rate • Oxygen saturation • Invasive or non-invasive blood pressure • Peripheral or core temperature along with other parameters, as appropriate • Cardiac output • Capnometry • FiO_2 • Central venous pressure • Pulmonary blood pressure

Multifunction monitor, portable pulse oximeter, monitoring systems with dedicated slots for all required parameters

Having made this distinction, we can move on to analyse bedside equipment setup, differentiating between a *routine* situation, involving general care patients who exhibit a stable haemodynamic and clinical status, and a clinically unstable situation that might deteriorate into haemodynamic instability and into *emergency/urgency*, as is the case for an intensive care patient (Tables 2.2, 2.3, 2.4, 2.5, 2.6, 2.7, 2.8, and 2.9).

2.5   Managing an Urgency/Emergency Situation

Urgency is defined as a severe impairment of a patient's health conditions, which is not immediately *life-threatening* [1]. In this scenario, it is crucial to restore the balance of all vital functions so as to prevent the situation from deteriorating into an emergency.

Table 2.4 Equipment for peripheral or central venous/arterial catheterisation

Routine	Emergency
Ward patients usually take their therapy orally; however, the need for parenteral medication administration may arise. Patients who received previous intensive care possibly have a central, percutaneous or peripheral venous line already in place, and if adequate care of the vascular access is maintained, they may continue to receive therapy during their hospital stay as well. Should a sudden deterioration of the clinical state of an otherwise stable patient require placing a vascular access, moving the patient to a different room is usually preferred, whenever possible. By doing this, the patient's bed and room are maintained as a safe place where they can feel protected. The procedure is performed in a different room, for instance, a treatment room, and support is provided by the caregiver to limit the patient's fear, using team distraction techniques. Where needed, an anaesthetist may provide pharmacological pain management and sedation, as appropriate Should action be taken urgently, the procedure can be performed bedside using the medical emergency trolley, which contains all the required supplies for emergency venous access placement	Generally, intensive care patients already have a central/percutaneous venous or arterial line in place, as required by their current therapy. Should replacing an access line become necessary, for example, in the case of catheter malfunction, the required supplies are available in the drawer units by the patient care station. Additional supplies can be found in the emergency trolley or in the drawer units/cabinets in the open space of the intensive care unit, containing all the necessary spare materials to cope with various patient needs. Given the patient's unstable conditions, vascular access line placement is usually performed bedside, with anaesthesiological support to provide pain management and limit fear, as the caregiver is very unlikely to attend in such a situation

Single- or multi-lumen central venous catheters in a variety of sizes, single-lumen arterial catheters, umbilical catheters, peripheral venous lines in a variety of sizes, PICC or midline catheters in a variety of sizes, supplies required to insert a central or peripheral line, supplies required to set up an infusion line

In an emergency scenario, vital function impairment is life-threatening for the patient and requires prompt initiation of resuscitation to try to keep the patient from dying.

2.5.1 How Are Children Different from Adults?

Both urgency and emergency are serious situations, but the time to take action shortens considerably from the first to the second scenario.

The success rate of resuscitation is inversely proportional to *time*.

Children exhibit considerable adaptability to situations where the haemodynamic balance and the acid-base homeostasis are altered.

This, however, constitutes a hazard to their lives every time the *non-specific signs* [3] from their bodies are overlooked or are not interpreted correctly by their caregivers.

Young patients can maintain a fragile balance for quite a long time. However, if appropriate action is not taken to eliminate the cause of such decompensation, the situation might deteriorate rapidly into a condition that sometimes leaves very little time to act.

Table 2.5 Equipment for airway management and oxygen therapy (as needed)

Routine	Emergency
Bedside oxygen therapy management in an ordinary inpatient scenario involves the choice of the oxygen delivery mode, therapy prescription and treatment administration. Possible options include nasal prongs, a facemask, a Venturi mask, a non-rebreather mask, an oxygen hood or CPAP, as per the patient's needs and tolerance to the selected administration mode Usually, just the necessary equipment for emergency respiratory support is set up by the patient care station, including an appropriately sized non-self-inflating bag (0.5 L, 1 L or 2 L), facemask and Guedel airway Suitably sized naso-oropharyngeal and tracheobronchial aspiration tubes should also be available bedside	Patients may undergo oxygen therapy as explained in the routine scenario or might require oxygen administration by mechanical ventilation through orotracheal or nasotracheal intubation In this case, the patient care station is equipped with a non-self-inflating bag, a facemask and a Guedel airway, just as in a routine scenario. In addition, a self-inflating bag is made available to ventilate the patient using a different FiO_2, together with the necessary equipment for reintubation (if need be), weaning and extubation. Endotracheal tubes are supplied in the exact size, along with the next larger and the next smaller size. Available equipment also includes a suitably sized Magill forceps, a handpiece (as needed) or a reinforced (also semi-rigid) tube in the case of an adult patient, lubricant, tape for tube fixation and a laryngoscope with conveniently sized straight and curve blades Weaning requires an angled perforated connector and a tube holder. Nasal prongs, a facemask, an oxygen hood or free-flow oxygen are required after extubation. Aspiration tubes and bronchoalveolar lavage supplies shall be provided for sterile secretion aspiration

Oxygen therapy management: nasal cannulas; conventional oxygen facemask; Venturi mask; non-rebreather mask; oxygen hood; CPAP using a facemask, a hood or nasal prongs
Airway management: non-self-inflating bag; facemask, Guedel airways; oxygen supply source
Intubation management: cuffed/uncuffed endotracheal tubes; tubes for normal or difficult intubation (semi-rigid) or reinforced endotracheal tubes; handpiece; Magill forceps; lubricant spray; laryngoscope and straight or curved blades; tracheobronchial aspiration tubes, self- or non-self-inflating bag; oxygen supply source; tape for tube fixation and external tube holder; anaesthetic medications
Weaning management: intubation supplies + angled or straight perforated connector; non-self-inflating bag connected to an oxygen supply source; anaesthetic medications

Table 2.6 Pre-diluted and patient-specific emergency medications

Routine	Emergency
Usually, bedside pre-diluted emergency medicines based on each patient's weight are not required in a general case scenario. Such medications are available in the emergency trolley and can be used as needed Concentrations are standardised by patient weight categories, hence making pharmacological management in an urgency somewhat easier	For an intensive care patient, conversely, urgent pre-diluted medications should be prepared daily, based on the patient's weight, body size, type and pharmacological requirements, hence making them more readily available in a critical scenario. In such a context, an emergency trolley is useful but no longer necessary, as a conventional medical cart or a specially prepared cabinet at each care station already contains the required supplies to respond to an emergency and stabilise the patient A multifunction semi-automated or manual external defibrillator with pacing capability should be made available in the emergency trolley

The sets of pre-diluted medications and their respective concentrations are agreed upon by each unit with their teams

Table 2.7 Medical emergency trolley for urgency/emergency management

Routine	Emergency
The emergency trolley becomes a paramount and essential component in an ordinary inpatient scenario, as it is impossible to set up a care station featuring all the required supplies to deal with an emergency	In an intensive care scenario, conversely, patient care stations are equipped with all the supplies required to respond to an emergency for a specific patient, as far as possible; in such a context, the emergency trolley becomes an important reference for managing emergency arrhythmias through the multifunction defibrillator

Each unit can decide how to set up the emergency trolley, by coding suitable procedures and drafting specific operational instructions, as needed

Table 2.8 Equipment for urinary catheterisation

Routine	Emergency
Ward patients do not usually require diuresis supervision via catheterisation. The required supplies can be found as needed in specific drawer units/cabinets that are set up in the ward, as the procedure is not urgent	Usually, diuresis balance monitoring through urinary catheterisation is routine for intensive care patients. Repositioning a urinary catheter may be required following removal, or as the clinical conditions of the patients vary, or in an emergency scenario, after the patient has been stabilised In such an event, the necessary equipment can be found in designated drawer units/cabinets within the intensive care unit, as setting up these supplies bedside for each patient would be unnecessary

Latex or silicone urinary catheters in a variety of sizes; urinary catheterisation set; drainage system chosen for diuresis control

However, children have an outstanding ability to *recover*, even when the situation was desperate just shortly before.

A child's organism is very responsive to balance restoration and exhibits early signs of improved and more stable conditions.

Conversely, adults have a more limited adaptability to alterations of the haemodynamic and acid-base balance; they can express their discomfort, providing their caregivers with meaningful hints, and usually go from feeling well to being unwell without many intermediate steps.

This being said about the differences between children and adults, a further distinction should be made concerning the *etiopathogenesis* of cardiopulmonary arrest.

In adults, cardiac arrest occurs as a consequence of a shockable rhythm in approximately 85% of cases.

Malignant arrhythmias occur only rarely in children, and cardiac arrest never happens suddenly (except for paediatric cardiac patients) but rather as the final event following a series of respiratory or haemodynamic alterations, which—if left untreated—gradually lead to respiratory arrest, to bradycardia and, eventually, to cardiac arrest (Table 2.10).

Table 2.9 Supplies for surgical drain insertion

Routine	Emergency
General care patients do not usually have surgical drains, as this occurs only rarely and in specific cases (postoperative chylothorax or wound drainage) In the first case, patients experience a postoperative complication, usually a few days after surgery, which makes it necessary to insert or keep a thoracic drainage tube to prevent chyle build-up. It may take a shorter or longer time for the accidentally injured thoracic duct to heal, and patients are moved to the general care unit, as they no longer require an intensive monitoring The second case involves patients who underwent haemodynamic procedures requiring surgical isolation of a vessel or placement of a final PM or ICD device. A surgical drainage tube is usually inserted in the implantation pocket, with a low vacuum, gravity, negative pressure or continuous suction collection system and is removed after a few days, if no complications arise For both patient types, should the drain become dislodged or occluded, the tube shall be reinserted under aseptic conditions and subject to prior patient sedation	Intensive care patients are more likely to have drainage tubes in place, especially after cardiac surgery, and/or following haemodynamic procedures (as set out in the column at the side), or as a consequence of cardiac/pulmonary complications The type and amount of leaking fluid are assessed to consider whether fluid supplementation is indicated Drain removal and insertion can be performed in the intensive care unit, as the environment, monitoring conditions and life support capabilities allow for such a procedure In this case, the required supplies are found in specific drawer units/cabinets

Insertion: trocar catheters; set for sterile field preparation; operator attire (gown, surgical mask with face shield, sterile gloves, footwear); drain collection system (low vacuum, gravity, negative pressure, continuous suction); surgical set for drain insertion; medications required for local and/or general anaesthesia

Removal: supplies for sterile field preparation; operator attire; scalpel; sterile pads; disinfectant; plaster

Table 2.10 Specificities of the operational approach in children and in adults

Children	Adults
• Parameter monitoring: Peripheral and rectal temperature, respiratory rate detection method	• The breathing pattern is more important than the respiratory rate. No peripheral and/or rectal temperature measurement
• Access sites: Umbilical vein, central venous line (first choice), saphenous peripheral access	• Access sites: Multiple peripheral lines (cephalic, brachial vein), no access via the umbilical vein, central venous line (second choice)
• Specific urgent medications: Prostaglandins	• Standard doses
• Greatest dosing accuracy because of differing units of measurement	
• Materials and sites: Nasotracheal/orotracheal intubation with an uncuffed, non-reinforced tube is preferred	• Materials and sites: Orotracheal intubation with a cuffed, reinforced tube is preferred
• Defibrillator: Special pads and shock power based on patient's weight	• Standard pads, standard shock

Given all of the above, the priority lies in *promptly identifying* the alteration of vital functions and in critically observing the patient's vital signs and clinical status.

Specific skills and knowledge in the field of paediatrics are required, along with a critical capacity of observing the patient and a good diagnostic acumen, taking nothing for granted.

Children often send out non-specific signals that parents sometimes intercept first, which they cannot explain and which they report to the healthcare professionals.

It is up to the latter to interpret such information, discriminating between useful indications and mere data.

When I started working in the Paediatric Cardiology Unit, I was most impressed with my colleagues' ability to read between the lines and grasp what children were trying to say.

Children communicate their world using *different languages* than the traditional ones; therefore, everybody working in the paediatric field should learn to speak those languages, in order to ensure good interaction with children and their parents.

The very same priorities apply to adult patients, and usually good communication and interaction with these subjects makes work easier for the operators.

2.5.2   Operational Implications (Table 2.11)

2.5.3   Priorities and Cooperation

Prompt recognition of the signs and symptoms indicating an alteration of the vital functions is the key to taking all the necessary measures to compensate for (or to eliminate) the risk factors, in order to prevent progressive balance deterioration.

Table 2.11 Operational implications in urgency and emergency

Urgency	Emergency
Alteration of vital functions, with no immediate threat to life	Immediate threat to life
Operational implications	
• Observation, assessment and early interpretation of signs and symptoms • *Interdisciplinarity* • Importance of waiting, as needed, when it comes to surgical procedures, so as to assess the best timing for intervention • Early assessment of deterioration into an emergency • Greater difficulty in managing instability • Nurses as mediators of the child's and parents' needs • Receiving the child and their parents in relation to the child's condition • Monitoring the child and measuring the parameters in the best moment • Ongoing assessment and adjustment of all actions taken	• Preparedness • *Interdisciplinarity* • Immediate need for non-surgical and surgical procedures to support vital functions • Knowledge and proper implementation of the procedures • Ability and flexibility in adjusting procedures to different age groups and conditions • Nurses as a mediators of the parents' needs • Receiving the child, first, and then the parent(s) • Vital functions monitoring and support • Stabilisation of the patient's conditions • Intensive care provision

Prevention is paramount and involves promptly restoring ventilation, oxygen saturation, blood volume and acid-base homeostasis, so as to break the chain of events that might lead to cardiac/respiratory failure and eventually to cardiac arrest, in some cases.

The problem should be identified and focused on; then, after *assessing* the situation, one or multiple *actions* should be taken to solve it.

Having a clear idea of the series of required assessments and actions makes it possible to respond effectively and efficiently. The urgency algorithm provided in the European Resuscitation Council guidelines educates and instructs on the proper, standardised behaviour.

Managing an emergency requires great emotional effort of the operators; knowing exactly what to do helps keeping one's mind focused and temporarily distracts from the huge emotional load of such an event.

2.5.4 Managing an Emergency Situation

The three following elements are paramount during an emergency.

2.5.4.1 The Division of Roles

A leader is appointed within the working group, who will serve as operations coordinator. He/she should be aware of the role they were assigned and should act so as to "direct" the other operators working with them.

The less people will be giving orders, the less confusion and tension there will be.

2.5.4.2 The Coordination Between Operators

During an emergency, an operator will be dealing with respiration; others will be dealing with the heart, the medications and the vascular accesses; and someone will take care of alerting the relevant advanced medical service providers (anaesthetist, cardiologist, heart surgeon, etc.).

The team leader should coordinate all efforts and divide roles as clearly as possible, so that each operator is fully engaged in a step of the treatment process, without hampering the work of their fellow operators.

This optimises both the timing and the results, prevents confusion from arising and allows the members of the team to act as if they were one single person with many hands.

This approach enables all the operators working in an urgency/emergency situation to act in a coordinated way.

2.5.4.3 The Management of Physical Space

Properly managing and organising the space where the team will be working is equally important, especially when it comes to paediatric patients, and this goes without saying if we consider a child's body size and compare it to that of an adult.

Proper physical demarcation of the space is paramount: the space around the head is required to provide ventilation; the space around the torso to allow for patient monitoring, CPR and defibrillation (where needed); and the space around the vascular access for preparing and delivering the required medications.

Defining the roles and dividing the space enable each operator to focus entirely on their relevant link of the chain of survival, without hindering others.

Conclusions

By their very nature, paediatric patients and ACHD/GUCH have specific features that make them rather fragile whenever physiological compensation mechanisms are altered.

Furthermore, children have an outstanding ability to recover even in severe impairment situations. An accurate observation of any change in their health conditions allows taking timely actions, hence posing fewer risks to little patients.

In the case of grown-ups with congenital heart disease, a multidisciplinary [5] treatment approach under the supervision of a paediatric cardiologist and an experienced nurse ensures the best possible results in terms of patient health recovery.

Patient care stations must be equipped with all the required devices and supplies to ensure an effective and efficient medical response whenever the patient's health conditions are altered, both in an emergency and in an urgency situation.

Lastly, proper management of an emergency/urgency situation partly contributes to improving patient outcomes.

References

1. Irc-Simeup. PALS pediatric advanced life support. Milan: Masson; 2004.
2. Carano N, Squarcia U. Cardiologia Pediatrica. Milan: McGraw-Hill; 1988.
3. European Resuscitation Council. European pediatric immediate life support [ERC's 2010 Guidelines].
4. Hogg T. Secrets of the baby whisperer, Italian edition: Il linguaggio segreto dei neonati. Milan: Mondadori; 2002.
5. Scolari S. Il case manager in Cardiologia e Cardiochirurgia Pediatrica. Possibilità applicative ed impatto organizzativo. Dissertation, Master in Management infermieristico. Alma Mater Studiorum Università di Bologna, academic year 2006/2007.

Vital Signs: Parameters, Frequency, and Pediatric and Cardiac Early Warning Scores

3

Veronica Mattioli

Abstract

- Vital parameters are indicative of the person's general conditions and are listed below: respiratory rate, heart rate, blood pressure, temperature, and neurocognitive state.
- Respiratory rate increases in any condition of respiratory fatigue due to airway obstruction, difficulty in gas exchange, or increased metabolic demands.
- In addition to respiratory dynamics, it is important to evaluate oxygen saturation, a useful parameter of the tissue oxygenation state at a peripheral level.
- Heart rate, blood pressure, refill time, and cyanosis evaluation indicate any condition of circulatory failure that, if not promptly corrected, can lead to multiorgan damage.
- Temperature can be detected in various sites including core, near-core, and peripheral: this parameter is a sign of effective or poor peripheral perfusion.
- Finally, neurocognitive impairment may be both respiratory and circulatory failure.
- Multiparameter scales can be used to evaluate vital parameters, such as PEWS and C-CHEWS.

V. Mattioli
Paediatric and Developing Age Cardiology and Heart Surgery Unit, Department Cardio-Vascular and Thoracic, University Hospital of Bologna Policlinico S. Orsola-Malpighi, Bologna, Italy

© Springer International Publishing AG, part of Springer Nature 2019
S. F. Flocco et al. (eds.), *Congenital Heart Disease*,
https://doi.org/10.1007/978-3-319-78423-6_3

3.1   Introduction

The measurement and interpretation of vital parameters are an important moment of the medical investigation; the detection of vital parameters is relatively simple and easy to learn, but interpreting measurements and integrating them in health-care and in the medical assessment require knowledge, problem-solving skills, critical thinking, and experience [1]. Measurement accuracy is of paramount importance: a wrong value or its wrong interpretation can have very serious consequences.

The general aspect is the observation of the child at distance, even before starting examining the subject, spontaneous movements, the way the child talks, skin complexion, his/her way of breathing, quality of crying, and the child's attitude toward receiving comfort from parents and/or operators. The approach with a child is age related. Usually, children under 6 months are not frightened by strangers; it is sufficient to avoid harsh or annoying stimulations. From 6 months to 3 years, the child's attitude is related to the behavior and the degree of tranquility of parents; over 3 years the child generally has a more comprehensive and cooperative attitude, although in a stressful situation he/she can regress.

Hereinafter, vital signs will be analyzed one by one (Table 3.1).

Vital parameters are indicative of the person's general conditions and are listed below:

1. *Respiratory rate*
2. *Heart rate*
3. *Blood pressure*
4. *Temperature*

As a vital sign, despite not being traditionally defined a vital parameter, we can include the patient's *neurocognitive state*.

Table 3.1 Pediatric vital parameters [2, 3]

Age	HR awake (bpm)	HR asleep (bpm)	RR (breaths per minute)	SAP (mmHg)	DAP (mmHg)	SatO$_2$
Newborn baby (0–30 days)	100–180	80–160	40–60	60–90	20–60	95–100%
Nursing infant (1–12 months)	100–160	75–160	30–60	87–105	53–66	
Early childhood (1–2 years)	80–110	60–90	24–40	95–105	53–66	
Late childhood (3–6 years)	70–100	60–90	22–34	96–110	55–69	
School age (7–12 years)	65–110	60–90	18–30	97–112	57–71	
Adolescent (13–15 years)	60–90	50–90	12–16	112–128	66–80	

Dap Diastolic Arterial Pressure; *Sap* Systolic (Or Systems) Arterial Pressure

3.1.1 Respiratory Rate

Three main questions must be answered in order to detect a possible respiratory failure in children:

- Has breathing workload increased?
- Is breathing effective?
- Are there signs of breathing ineffectiveness borne by other organs? [4]

3.1.1.1 Signs of Increased Breathing Workload

- Increase/decrease in respiratory rate (a decrease in respiratory rate is often a severe sign of respiratory exhaustion, index of imminent respiratory arrest)
- Assessment of ventilatory dynamics (abdominal or thoracic excursions)
- Presence of thoracic or jugular retractions
- Nasal flaring
- Onset of expiratory groan to increase intrathoracic pressure and prevent alveoli from collapsing during expiration: tirage (inspiratory effort with jugular retraction), cornage, and stridor (inspiratory sounds) [4]

Breathing effectiveness is measured with:

- Thorax auscultation.
- Observation of thoracic movements or in the newborn baby/nursing infant, of abdominal excursions. Reduced thorax expansion is a sign of breathing ineffectiveness. Newborn babies and nursing infants breath using abdominal muscles: thorax breathing starts at around 2–3 years of age and is complete at approximately 6–7 years of age [4].

3.1.1.2 The Effects of Respiratory Failure on Other Organs (Indirect Signs)

Are evaluated considering:

- Increased or decreased heart rate: usually, in respiratory failure, it is increased, whereas a prolonged hypoxia causes bradycardia.
- Skin complexion (pale in hypoxia, whereas cyanosis is a late sign).
- The child's mental state: a hypoxic child is initially agitated and very difficult to comfort; as the hypoxic state persists, or following CO_2 accumulation, the child gradually becomes lethargic until losing consciousness. In nursing infants, a mental status impairment may be difficult to recognize.
- The presence of apneas (breathing pauses lasting>15 s) is a severe sign of risk of respiratory arrest.
- The arterial transcutaneous oxygen saturation gives indirect information on ventilation efficiency at tissue level [4].

Breathing assessment is an important aspect during a patient examination, particularly in the child who fails to report a possible state of respiratory distress. The breathing characteristics that should be considered are frequency of respiratory acts, breathing mode and respiratory dynamics, and assessment of skin complexion and of peripheral perfusion.

Respiratory rate is the number of breaths per minute; each breath consists of an inspiratory phase and an expiratory phase. Alterations of respiratory rate are as follows:

- Bradypnea: abnormal decrease in breaths per minute, in children this can be a serious sign of respiratory exhaustion and hypoxia [4]
- Tachypnea: considerable increase in the respiratory rate than usual, it is indicative of a greater request in ventilation needs and, therefore, of an increased breathing workload [4]
- Apnea: absence of breathing or pause in breathing exceeding 15 s, continues apnea is a synonym of respiratory arrest and is not compatible with life [5].

Breathing nature should be assessed in addition to the respiratory rate, in particular, its depth and the effort required to maintain an effective breathing.

- Dyspnea: increased respiratory effort, subjective feeling of difficulty in breathing. It is associated with the activation of accessory respiratory muscles and is the expression of airway obstruction or reduced expandability of lung parenchyma. Dyspneic newborn babies and nursing infants typically present nasal flaring together with intercostal and jugular retractions and thoracoabdominal strain gauge (a greater diaphragmatic activation results in the lowering of the abdominal viscera with abdominal globosity and a simultaneous flattening of the chest) [1].
- Polypnea: is an increase in lung volumes, with increased breathing rate (*tachypnea*) or increased intensity of breathing acts (*hyperpnea*) [1].
- Orthopnea: is a form of dyspnea accentuated in the supine position and forces patients to a sitting position; this is typical of patients with heart failure [1].
- Hyperpnea: increased breathing depth, it occurs in several cases including fever, acidosis, anxiety, and pulmonary diseases of different origin [5].
- Grunting: is a forced expiration when the glottis is partially closed that occurs in case of hypoxia, atelectasis, pneumonia, or pulmonary edema [1].

3.1.1.3 Transcutaneous Oxygen Saturation (SatO$_2$) Monitoring

Saturation monitoring by pulse oximetry is a useful parameter of the state of tissue oxygenation at a peripheral level; however, we should bear in mind that measurements are unreliable when there is peripheral vasoconstriction such as in conditions of shock, severe anemia, or hypothermia [4]. See the following reference values:

Normal values 95–100%
Mild hypoxia 91–94%
Moderate hypoxia 86–90%
Severe hypoxia: inferior to 86%

Measurement can be carried out on hands, feet, ear lobe, and frontal lip. According to the site, pulse oximetry needs a different device, and in some cases, the site determines also one of the possible diagnostic discriminants; for example, in ductus-dependent *aortic coarctation* (Botallo's duct still patent), saturation at upper limbs can be higher than that measured at lower limbs that are affected by blood mixing carried by the ductal flow (blood not yet oxygenated).

Recognition of a Potential Circulatory Failure
The recognition of signs of circulatory failure is extremely important in critically ill children, because the deterioration of cardiovascular functions produces an inadequate perfusion of organs and tissues; this results in a reduced supply of oxygen and nutrients with local hypoxia, metabolic acidosis, and anaerobic induction [4].

If such failure is not promptly corrected, cell death occurs, with multiorgan damage. Early recognition of a state of shock allows doctors to quickly start the right treatment, preventing a worsening of the acidosis condition and the related organ damage [4]. For a proper management of circulatory failure, doctors should evaluate heart rate, assessment of peripheral pulses compared with central pulses, capillary refill time, and high blood pressure.

3.1.2 Heart Rate, Refill Time, and Cyanosis

Pulse characteristics include frequency, pace, and quality. The rate refers to the number of beats per minute, pace refers to the regularity of pulsations, and quality refers to the power of the palpated pulse.

Heart rate: It is the number of beats per minute and corresponds to the number of cardiac contractions in a minute. When the heart rate exceeds normal values, we talk about *tachycardia*; when the value is below the normal range, we speak of *bradycardia* (*for values see* Table 3.1).

Character: It is represented by the power or amplitude of the pulse, that is, by the power that the wave of blood flow pressure exerts against the artery elastic wall. It is defined *full* when a strong pulse is perceived and *weak* when the pulse is feeble and reduced below the fingertips palpating the wrist.

Pace: It expresses the ratio between the single pulse beats. It can be *regular* when the intervals between individual pulses remain constant (rhythmic) and *irregular* when the intervals between individual pulses are not constant (arrhythmic).

The pulse detection sites are carotid, temporal, brachial, ulnar, apical, radial, femoral, popliteal, and posterior tibial.

3.1.2.1 Signs of Cardiocirculatory Failure
- Tachycardia: may be physiological as the compensation result for the alteration of another parameter, such as in fever, in hypoxia, due to increased metabolic demands for hemodynamic imbalance, in anemia, in electrolyte or acid-base

imbalance, in hypotension, in shock (hypovolemic, hemorrhagic, septic, cardiogenic, hypoxic), in lung hyper-flow, and in low systemic capacity [4]. In any case, the cause must be identified and a solution found to prevent cardiocirculatory collapse. Even in case of arrhythmia, it is necessary to understand its origin to decide for the most appropriate treatment.

- Bradycardia: negative prognostic signs occur when there is hypoxemia, hypothermia, hypoglycemia, metabolic and acid-base disorders, bradyarrhythmias, vagal reflexes, apneas, and central nervous system disorders (all pathologies triggering intracranial hypertension) [4]. It is probably related to a patient's problem, and a prompt solution prevents cardiac arrest.
- Central and peripheral pulses: the reduction or absence of these pulses indicates a sign of peripheral hypoperfusion and severe shock. [4] Peripheral pulses are the first ones to disappear, followed by reduced renal perfusion and abdominal organs perfusion, and gradually central pulses disappear generating a state of shock. In addition to the radial pulse, the femoral pulse is particularly important in children: if it is perceived with difficulty and delayed with respect to the radial pulse, an *aortic coarctation* may occur. The perception of a strongly beating pulse may suggest an increase in cardiac output due to anemia, anxiety, physical activity, or medical conditions such as a patent arteriosus duct or aortic valve failure. Conversely, a weak pulse is present in heart failure and aortic stenosis.
- *Capillary refill time*: is assessed by exerting pressure for 5 s at the presternal site; skin complexion should return rosy in 2 s. If prolonged by >2 s, it is a sign of inadequate peripheral perfusion. The assessment must be related to the patient's anatomy and physiology in a known heart patient. A reduction in skin perfusion is an early sign of shock. In addition to a longer refill time, poor perfusion indices are pallor, peripheral cyanosis, cutaneous marbling, and the presence of cold extremities [4].
- Blood pressure: in children, serious circulatory deficiency can be present even when blood pressure is normal; hypotension is often a late, preterminal sign of circulation failure [4]. Hypertension can be related to pain, agitation, aortic coarctation, and postsurgical hemodynamic adjustments. Hypotension may be a sign of shock or a drug-mediated effect.

If a child is in a state of shock, the assessment of central and peripheral pulses and the refill time is faster and more effective than taking blood pressure. Blood pressure should be checked over time to monitor the response to resuscitation therapy.

3.1.2.2 Effects of Circulatory Failure on Other Organs (Indirect Signs)

- Respiratory rate and breathing nature: a high respiratory rate without signs of respiratory distress can be a sign of metabolic acidosis due to circulatory failure.
- Skin and temperature: a cold, marbled, pale, hypothermic skin indicates a defect in perfusion. Pallor and sweating may occur rarely in newborn babies and small children as an expression of myocardial ischemia. On the contrary, sweating

during meals is more common, and it can be the expression of latent heart failure (e.g., in the presence of a large interventricular defect).
- Neurological status: a deficient circulation, with cerebral hypoperfusion, can cause a status of agitation or lethargy till unconsciousness.
- *Diuresis*: the decreased excretion of urine is one of the signs of hypoperfusion. Normal diuresis in a child is 1–2 mL/kg/h. A lower diuresis, in the absence of renal disease, is a sign of poor perfusion [4].

3.1.2.3 Cyanosis

Cyanosis means a characteristic dark-purple color of the lips, nail bed, skin, and mucous membranes due to oxygen desaturation in the blood. It is therefore necessary to observe the color of the skin and mucous membranes of the mouth, lips, and nail beds (in black children observe only mucous membranes). Generally, cyanosis is secondary to:

- Circulation defects that bypass right to left shunt pulmonary circulation or congestive heart failure with stasis and increased hemoglobin peripheral desaturation
- Pulmonary alterations resulting in poor ventilation failure or a block in oxygen diffusivity from pulmonary alveoli to capillaries

A reduced peripheral circulation triggers acrocyanosis, so, for example, in sepsis, in cold-dependent vasoconstriction, it is also important to remember that acrocyanosis is a normal event in the newborn baby in the first hours of his/her life; it is in fact defined as innocent cyanosis (which is why the saturation probe, usually, should be put at the wrist and not at the extremities) [1].

In the heart child, cyanosis is usually due to venous blood flowing directly into the systemic circulation without passing through the lungs: this implies the lack of blood oxygenation. In some heart diseases, cyanosis may be present from birth (tetralogy of Fallot, transposition of great vessels, tricuspid atresia) or appear later in the first 6 months of life (some cases of tetralogy of Fallot, pulmonary stenosis with VSD, other heart diseases at the closure of the Botallo's duct). In this latter case, low blood oxygenation can be sufficient to the energy demand of the small body of a resting newborn baby, but growth and increased organic demands are bound to lead to the clinical manifestations of chronic hypoxia (polypnea, reduced tolerance to efforts, reduced weight gain) or acute hypoxia (hypoxic crisis). Chronic hypoxia related to cyanosis triggers an increase in arteriovenous circulation at the level of the distal phalanges of hands and feet (drumstick fingers, hippocratic nails) and the stimulation of anaerobic metabolism with increased lactic acid and more or less severe acidosis [1].

3.1.3 Blood Pressure

It can be defined as the pressure exerted by blood against the elastic walls of arteries. Systolic blood pressure (SBP) is the pressure inside arteries when blood is ejected by the heart. Diastolic blood pressure (DBP) is the pressure in the arterial circulation during the relaxation phase of the cardiac muscle.

Table 3.2 Width of armbands for measuring BP [6]

Age	Armband width (cm)
Newborn baby	4
Infant	6
Child	9
Young adult	10
Adult	13

Pressure values for different age groups are given in Table 3.1.

In children, a state of shock can be present even when blood pressure is normal: hypotension is often a late and preterminal sign of circulation failure. When blood pressure drops in children in a state of shock, cardiac arrest is imminent [4].

Blood pressure can be measured in both arms and legs. There are armbands of different width according to the different sizes of pediatric patients (they must cover 2/3 of an arm's length and more than half of its circumference): if an armband is too small, pressure values could be wrongly high; on the other hand, if it is too large, values will be slightly reduced.

Reasonable dimensions for armbands (Table 3.2):

Blood pressure varies according to the child's age; it progressively increases in the first 6 months of life, remains stable up to 6 years, and increases again during puberty. Physical exercise, coughing, excitement, and effort can increase systolic blood pressure in children also 40–50 mmHg above usual values. We talk about hypertension when blood pressure is stable above the values considered normal for the child's age. Kidney diseases, pathologies of the central nervous system, increased calcium concentration in the plasma, and *aortic coarctation* (BP is high in the upper limbs and low in the lower limbs) are some of the causes. Hypotension is associated with anemia, dehydration, severe infections, and *aortic or mitral stenosis* [1].

3.1.4 Temperature

Temperature can be detected in various sites: core, near-core, and peripheral.

Core body temperature is detected in the pulmonary artery, the tympanic membrane, the distal part of the esophagus, and the nasopharynx; it obviously involves invasive techniques and the use of electronic sensors [7].

In the *pulmonary artery* (or alternatively in a large artery), detection is carried out through the Swan-Ganz catheter or the pulse-induced contour cardiac output (PiCCO). Swan-Ganz is considered the gold standard as it measures temperature right in the bloodstream. *In the esophagus, the nose, and the pharynx and in the tympanic membrane* (different is the measurement of temperature in the ear), temperature is measured with an electronic sensor by means of a specific probe [7, 8].

When these sites are not available, other detection sites, so-called *near-core*, are used; these are the rectum, the bladder, and the oral cavity, peripheral sites that do not reflect the direct core temperature but the reflected one [7, 8].

In the *rectum*, measurement can be influenced by the presence of feces and bacteria, which produce heat; therefore, rectal temperature is often higher than core temperature [7]. Measurement can be done with an electronic sensor or by means of a thermometer (strongly not recommended due to the risk of rupture, perforation, vagal stimulation).

Temperature in the *bladder*, measured with an appropriate bladder catheter equipped with a sensor, totally depends on the urine flow: the higher the flow, the more accurate the value and the closer to that of the pulmonary artery and vice versa [7].

The oral site is strongly not recommended by many authors.

Peripheral body temperature detection sites are the armpit and skin surface; they are noninvasive and involve the measurement by means of electronic or chemical thermometers and electronic skin sensors. *Armpit* temperature can be also measured with an electronic skin sensor, alternating the right and left armpit for preventing pressure sores.

Measurements in newborn babies and children are preferably to be done in the tympanic (with an infrared thermometer) and armpit sites.

Usually, in pediatrics peripheral temperature is measured at the foot (sole or fingers) and is related to skin complexion. Low peripheral temperature is usually associated with cold, pale skin or with peripheral cyanosis, skin marbling, and extension of the refill time. A normal peripheral temperature ranges between 30° and 34°. It is a sign of effective or poor peripheral perfusion and can be a sign of inadequate systemic flow. Armpit temperature ranges between 36° and 37°; core temperatures deviate by approximately half degree compared to armpit temperature, also one degree in case of bladder temperature.

In newborn babies, especially if preterm, there is a temperature control problem due to immaturity of the thalamic thermoregulation system. They are strongly influenced by ambient temperatures.

Usually, there is a reduction of the peripheral temperature simultaneously with the disappearance of peripheral pulses in case of unfavorable prognosis.

3.1.5 Neurocognitive Status

An altered mental status indicates a variable impairment of consciousness that from a clinical point of view can present itself as:

- Lethargy or drowsiness: the patient has lost interest in the surrounding environment and tends to fall asleep in the absence of stimuli, but he/she can communicate.
- Delirium: the patient experiences spatial and temporal disorientation, agitation, hallucinations.
- Astonishment: the subject can be awakened only by vigorous and/or painful stimuli.

– Coma: the most severe form, in which the vigorous or painful stimuli are not able to determine the patient's awakening. Its degree of severity can be evaluated through the Glasgow Coma Scale, which, however, will not be discussed in this text.

Both respiratory and circulatory failure can have neurological effects [4].

3.1.5.1 Level of Consciousness

A rapid emergency assessment of the state of consciousness can be done by assigning the patient to one of the following categories (according to the acronym AVPU proposed by emergency pediatrics manuals):

Alert: alert patient.
Voice: it responds to verbal stimuli.
Pain: it responds to painful stimuli.
Unresponsive: the subject does not respond to any stimuli.

A child responsive only to pain or unresponsive generally has a significant degree of coma [4].

The most frequent coma etiology that we can find in cardiology is hypoxia, ischemia, infection, and metabolic and electrolyte disorders.

3.1.6 PEWS and C-CHEWS Tools

Recognizing the gravity of the situation, being timely, and appropriate in the intervention are among the factors that determine the clinical outcome of acute diseases. Some scientific evidence has shown that, compared to the evaluation of single parameters, the introduction of a multiparameter system involves a reduction in unscheduled admissions to intensive care [9]. Which is then the useful instrument to make this assessment?

Numerous publications have highlighted the need to use alarm systems, such as the early warning scores (EWS), which allow you to identify the acute stages of a disease and arrange in advance appropriate care. The National Health Service, the British national health service, has promoted the drafting of a uniform EWS for the whole nation, to be implemented in all healthcare services: a valid NEWS, for all healthcare services [10].

The NEWS basic principle is the collection of vital parameters usually and easily detected on a scale score, which allows a quick and shared assessment of the patient's clinical conditions. Benefits of early warning scores are as follows:

• Allow more opportunities for clinicians to intervene early before an arrest event
• Provide standardized tool and management algorithm for at-risk patients
• Decrease unplanned transfers between ICUs and inpatient wards
• Provide trend data for clinicians to review individual patient's scores within a given period of time [10]

3.1.6.1 Pediatric Early Warning Score (PEWS)

Following the introduction of the NEWS, special scales for the pediatric field have been introduced. Currently, the most popular one is the PEWS (Pediatric Early Warning Score). These instruments were developed within the Anglo-Saxon health system, where they have become of common practice. In Italy, only a few isolated bodies have begun to introduce them.

The early recognition of clinical deterioration should be supported by the use of indicators that are as objective, standardized, immediate as possible, and simple to read. The PEWS allows an early detection of the child's clinical worsening, and it evaluates the neurocognitive, cardiovascular, and respiratory systems (Table 3.3). To make this assessment, a pulse oximeter is sufficient. This type of detection does not represent an increased workload for nurses because the recorded data is that of usual detection.

For each item the nurse assigns a score between 0 and 3, which is augmented by 1 point in case of persistent vomiting (interpreted as index of a possible electrolyte imbalance) and use of aerosol with bronchodilators and/or adrenaline.

Table 3.3 Pediatric Early Warning Score (PEWS) [11, 12]

	0	1	2	3	Score
Behavior	• Playing • Alert • Appropriate • At baseline	• Sleep • Fussy but consolable	• Irritable/inconsolable	• Lethargic • Confused • Reduced response to pain	
Cardiovascular	• Pink • Capillary refill 1–2 s	• Pale • Capillary refill 3 s	• Gray • Capillary refill 4 s • Tachycardia of 20 above normal rate	• Gray • Mottled • Capillary refill 5 s or above • Tachycardia of 30 above normal rate or bradycardia	
Respiratory	• Within normal parameters • No retractions	• Greater than 10 above normal parameters • Use of accessory muscles • 30+% FiO_2 • 3+ L/min	• Greater than 20 above normal parameters • Retractions • 40+% FiO_2 • 6+ L/min • Trach and ventilator dependent	• Below normal parameters with retractions • Grunting • 50% FiO_2 • 8+ L/min	

Add 1 point in case of persistent vomiting (interpreted as index of a possible electrolyte imbalance) and use of aerosol with bronchodilators and/or adrenaline

On the basis of the sum of the points given, the nurse will adopt a different behavior referring to a decision algorithm that includes the intervention of health-care professionals with increasing professional skills.

Levels of Alert

0–1 (white): continue with usual nursing assessment. PEWS every 6 h.

Low 2–3 (green): consult an experienced colleague nurse who will consider whether or not to call a doctor on duty; in the absence of an experienced colleague, speak with the doctor on duty. PEWS every 3 h.

Medium 4–5 (yellow): call the doctor on duty who will decide whether or not to call a resuscitator. PEWS every hour.

High ≥ 6 (red): this should be considered an emergency, alert the entire team, resuscitation skills are required, and the patient might need to be transferred to subintensive or intensive care. Continuous monitoring.

3.1.6.2 Cardiac Children's Hospital Early Warning Score (C-CHEWS)

Most inpatient pediatric arrests are preventable by early recognition/treatment of deterioration. The majority of pediatric cardiopulmonary arrests occur on intensive care units. Hospitalized pediatric patients may have treatable symptoms present 1–16 h prior to arrest events, and early recognition and treatment of these symptoms could potentially prevent most arrests. Children with cardiac disease have the highest arrest rates. Almost two/three of arrests are considered preventable. Common causes of inpatient pediatric arrests are respiratory failure, circulatory shock (e.g., hypovolemia, sepsis, or poor cardiac function), ventricular tachycardia, or ventricular fibrillation [13].

There are many pediatric early warning score tools that are validated and in use at various institutions. C-CHEWS has excellent discrimination to identify deterioration in children with cardiac disease and performed significantly better than PEWS; C-CHEWS has a higher sensitivity than PEWS at all cut points [13].

This tool was developed to provide standardized assessment of patients at risk for cardiac arrest with goal of early intervention for preventable events. Patients are scored on a scale from 0 to 3 based on physiologic parameters and their relative deviation from baseline (Table 3.4) [13].

Patients receive an additional "1" point for staff concern and/or family concern (if family is absent, staff can add this point as appropriate) [13].

Levels of Alert

0–2 (green): continue assessment every 4 h.

3–4 (yellow): increase frequency of assessment; notify charge nurse and resident; discuss treatment plan as a team. Consider: higher level of care.

5 or > (red): clinician evaluation at bedside; notify attending physician; discuss treatment plan as a team. Consider: rapid response team. Continuous monitoring [13].

Table 3.4 C-CHEWS [13]

	0	1	2	3	Score
Behavior/neuro	• Playing/sleeping appropriately • Alert at patient's baseline	• Sleepy, somnolent when not disturbed	• Irritable, difficult to console • Increase in patient's baseline seizure activity	• Lethargic, confused, floppy • Reduced response to pain • Prolonged or frequent seizures • Pupils asymmetric or sluggish	
Cardiovascular	• Skin tone appropriate for patient • Capillary refill <2 s	• Pale • Capillary refill 3–4 s • Mild tachycardia • Intermittent ectopy or irregular heart rhythm (not new)	• Gray • Capillary refill 4–5 s • Moderate* tachycardia	• Gray and mottled • Capillary refill >5 s • Severe* tachycardia • New onset bradycardia • New onset/increase in ectopy, irregular heart rhythm, or heart block	
Respiratory	• Within normal parameters • No retractions	• Mild* tachypnea • Mild increased WOB (flaring, retracting) • Up to 40% supplemental oxygen via mask • Up to 1 L NC > patient's baseline need • Mild* desaturation (<5 below patient's baseline) • Intermittent apnea self-resolving	• Moderate* tachypnea • Moderate increased WOB (flaring, retracting, grunting, use of accessory muscles) • 40–60% oxygen via mask • 1–2 L NC > patient's baseline need • News q 1–2 h • Moderate* desaturation (<10 below patient's baseline) • Apnea requiring repositioning or stimulation	• Severe* tachypnea • RR below normal for age* • Severe increased WOB (i.e., head bobbing, paradoxical breathing) • >60% oxygen via mask • > 2L NC> patient's baseline need • News q 30 min–1 h • Severe* desaturation (<15 below patient's baseline) • Apnea requiring interventions other than repositioning or stimulation	
Staff concern		Concerned			
Family concern		Concerned or absent			
				Total	

(continued)

Table 3.4 (continued)

		Mild	Moderate	Severe
Respiratory rate and heart rate	Infant	>10% ↑ for age	>15% ↑ for age	>25% ↑ for age
	Toddler and older	>10% ↑ for age	>25% ↑ for age	>50% ↑ for age
Desaturation from patient's baseline 02 saturation	All ages	5 points	10 points	15 points

© Children's Hospital, Boston, 2011

Conclusions

In this chapter, vital signs have been considered, and their meaning has been analyzed together with their normal reference values, seeing how some of these parameters may change in childhood heart disease. The importance of vital parameter detection is emphasized: data collection is relatively simple, but this procedure should be carried out carefully because the data found can be prognostically very important in the cardiopathic child. Two multiparametric scales have been presented for parameter interpretation, PEWS and C-CHEWS, since it is now common thought that vital parameters should be analyzed under a common viewpoint compared to the single parameter analysis.

References

1. Badon P, Cesaro S. Manuale di nursing pediatrico. Milano: Casa Editrice Ambrosiana; 2006.
2. Murphy KA. Pediatric triage guidelines. St. Louis: Mosby; 1997.
3. Hockenberry MJ, et al. Wong's essentials of pediatric nursing. St Louis: Elsevier Mosby; 2005.
4. Balagna R, Benedetti M, Biban P, et al. PALS pediatric advanced life support. Elsevier – Masson; 2009.
5. Marcdante KJ, Kliegman RM, Jenson HB, Behrman RE. Nelson Manuale di Pediatria. Milano: Elsevier; 2012.
6. National High Blood Pressure Education Program Working Group on High Blood Pressure in Children and Adolescents. The fourth report on the diagnosis, evaluation, and treatment of high blood pressure in children and adolescents. Pediatrics. 2004;114:555–76.
7. Puglierin A. Misurazione della temperature corporea in sala operatoria. Società Italo Svizzera Studi Ipotermia. 2013.
8. Sessler DI. Temperature monitoring and perioperative thermoregulation. Anesthesiology. 2008;109(2):318–38.
9. McNeill G, Bryden D. Do either early warning systems or emergency response teams improve hospital patient survival? A systematic review. Resuscitation. 2013;84:1652–67.
10. National Early Warning Score (NEWS). LINEA GUIDA. Consiglio Sanitario Regionale Regione Toscana; 2014.
11. Duncan H, Hutchison J, Parshuram CS. The Pediatric Early Warning System score: a severity of illness score to predict urgent medical need in hospitalized children. J Crit Care. 2006;21:271–8.
12. Frigato V, Vagliano L, Bondone C, et al. Studio sull'applicabilità del Pediatric Early Warning Score System nella pratica infermieristica di un ospedale pediatrico italiano. Child Nurses Ital J Pediatr Nurs Sci. 2013.
13. McLellan MC, Gauvreau K, Connor JA. Validation of the cardiac Children's hospital early warning score: an early warning scoring tool to prevent cardiopulmonary arrests in children with heart disease. Congenit Heart Dis. 2014;9(3):194–202.

Acid-Base Balance in Pediatric Congenital Heart Patients

4

Marco Ranucci

Abstract

Acid-base balance in children with congenital heart disease before and after heart surgery is of paramount importance. In general, newborns have a reduced ability to cope with metabolic acidosis, especially under parenteral nutrition. Changes in arterial pCO_2 and pH determine changes in pulmonary vascular resistances, which may trigger serious hemodynamic problems in the balance between systemic and pulmonary circulation and in case of critical pulmonary blood flow (cavopulmonary connection, Fontan circulation). In patients with tetralogy of Fallot, acidosis and hypercapnia are triggers of tet-spell crisis.

In addition to these peculiar factors, after heart surgery in congenital patients, the acid-base balance is a marker of the adequacy of cardiac output to sustain the metabolic needs. Metabolic acidosis and hyperlactatemia are among the most important indirect markers of a poor cardiac output. Maintenance of a normal acid-base balance guarantees against the risk of electrolyte concentration changes (viz., potassium) which may in turn lead to arrhythmic complications. This chapter offers a brief overview of the acid-base balance in the general physiologic setting and in the particular conditions involved in the intensive care management of congenital heart children.

4.1 The Basic Determinants of Acid-Base Balance [1, 2]

The pH of a solution depends on the concentration of H^+, and the pH is the negative logarithm of the H^+ concentration:

M. Ranucci
Cardiovascular Anesthesia and Intensive Care Department, IRCCS Policlinico San Donato, Milan, Italy

© Springer International Publishing AG, part of Springer Nature 2019
S. F. Flocco et al. (eds.), *Congenital Heart Disease*,
https://doi.org/10.1007/978-3-319-78423-6_4

$$pH = -\log_{10}\left[H^+\right]$$

The lower the pH, the more acid is the solution. A neutral solution has a pH of 7.0. Values below 7.0 are defined as "acid solutions" and greater than 7.0 as "basic solutions."

The normal pH of the human body extracellular fluids is 7.35–7.45, so it is moderately basic.

The equation ruling the pH value in the human body is the Henderson-Hasselbalch equation:

$$pH = pK_\alpha + \log_{10}\left[\frac{A^-}{HA}\right]$$

or

$$pH = pK_\alpha + \log_{10}\left[\frac{HCO_3^-}{\alpha pCO_2}\right]$$

where $pK_\alpha = 6.1$, HCO_3^- is 24 mmol/L, $\alpha = 0.03$, and $pCO_2 = 40$ mmHg.
Therefore:

$$7.4 = 6.1 + \log_{10}\frac{24}{1.2} = 6.1 + \log_{10}\left[20\right] = 6.1 + 1.3$$

From the above equation, it is easy to understand that the main determinants of the pH are the HCO_3^- content (bicarbonates ions) and the arterial pCO_2, being the pK of the solution (6.1) and the α (coefficient of solubility of the CO_2, 0.03) constant values.

Changes in the bicarbonate ions concentration and pCO_2 will determine changes in the pH value. If one of the two factors remains constant, increases in bicarbonate ions or decreases in pCO_2 will determine an alkalosis and decreases in the bicarbonate ions or increases in pCO_2 an acidosis.

4.2   How to Interpret an Arterial Blood Gas Analysis (BGA) Output [3]

Arterial BGA is one of the most common point-of-care laboratory tests in the cardiac pediatric intensive care unit (CPICU). Congenital heart patients usually receive several arterial BGA tests during the first 24 h after surgery and during mechanical ventilation. BGA includes a number of parameters directly or indirectly related to the acid-base balance:

pH
HCO_3^- (mmol/L)
$PaCO_2$ (mmHg)

Base excess (BE)
Blood lactates (mmol/L)
Na⁺ and K⁺.

The BE is the concentration of H^+ ions required to lead the pH of blood to 7.4. From this perspective, it is around zero if the pH is close to 7.4, positive in case of alkalosis, and negative in case of acidosis. However, the BE may be positive or negative even if the pH is far from 7.4, whenever compensatory mechanism(s) are in action.

To correctly interpret an arterial BGA output, the following steps should be followed:

(a) Look at the pH first, and assess if it is in the normal range (7.35–7.45) or acid (<7.35) or basic (>7.45).
(b) Look at the HCO_3^-, and assess if it is normal (22–26 mmol/L), decreased (<22 mmol/L), or increased (>26 mmol/L).
(c) Look at the BE, which is usually positive if the HCO_3^- is positive and negative if the HCO_3^- is negative; the normal range is −2 to +2.
(d) Look at the pCO_2, and assess if it is in the normal range (35–45 mmHg), decreased (<35 mmHg) or increased (>45 mmHg).
(e) Look at the additional parameters of blood lactates and K⁺. The first may be useful in case of metabolic acidosis; the second may represent a warning sign when outside the normal range as a consequence of acidosis/alkalosis (see later on).

Depending on the combination of the pH, HCO_3^-, and pCO_2 values, different conditions are diagnosed (see Figs. 4.1 and 4.2). The BE value is used to establish the degree of acidosis/alkalosis and the following therapeutic interventions.

Clinical condition	pH	PaCO₂	HCO₃⁻
Respiratory acidosis	⬇⬇	⬆⬆	═
Respiratory alkalosis	⬆⬆	⬇⬇	═
Metabolic acidosis	⬇⬇	═	⬇⬇
Metabolic alkalosis	⬆⬆	═	⬆⬆

Fig. 4.1 Uncompensated respiratory and metabolic acid-base disturbances

Clinical condition	pH	PaCO$_2$	HCO$_3^-$
Partially compensated respiratory acidosis	⬇ (red)	⬆⬆ (green)	⬆ (blue)
Partially compensated respiratory alkalosis	⬆ (green)	⬇⬇ (red)	⬇ (blue)
Partially compensated metabolic acidosis	⬇ (red)	⬇ (blue)	⬇⬇ (red)
Partially compensated metabolic alkalosis	⬆ (green)	⬆ (blue)	⬆⬆ (green)

Fig. 4.2 Partially compensated respiratory and metabolic acid-base disturbances. Green or red arrows are the primary disturbance; blue arrows are compensatory mechanisms

Figure 4.1 presents uncompensated acid-base balance disturbances. However, under a number of circumstances, active compensatory mechanisms are activated by the primary disturbances, and it is more common to find partially compensated conditions, as depicted in Fig. 4.2.

Finally, there are extremely severe conditions where instead of a reciprocal compensation of the metabolic and respiratory mechanisms, there is a combined effect: A typical case is severe acidosis due to a combination of respiratory and metabolic acidosis.

4.3 Acute Disturbances of the Acid-Base Balance [3, 4]

4.3.1 Respiratory Acidosis

Respiratory acidosis results from an increased PaCO$_2$. The PaCO$_2$ depends on the CO$_2$ production (VCO$_2$) and the pulmonary ventilation (V_E), following the equation:

$$PaCO_2 = \frac{VCO_2}{V_E}$$

Normally, the V_E is spontaneously adapted to the VCO$_2$ (for increasing values of VCO$_2$) in order to maintain the PaCO$_2$ at a normal value.

Whenever the V_E is inadequate to match the VCO$_2$, a respiratory acidosis occurs. This may happen in a spontaneously ventilating patient in case of poor mechanical ventilation due to a reduced function of the respiratory muscles. However, even an apparently normal V_E may result in an inadequate CO$_2$ clearance when the alveolar component of the ventilation (V_A) is reduced. This, in turn, may derive from disturbances in the ventilation/perfusion ratio at an alveolar level (e.g., in case of respiratory distress syndrome, poor pulmonary blood flow).

Table 4.1 Main causes of respiratory acidosis in congenital heart patients in the pediatric cardiac intensive care unit

Ventilation	Cause of respiratory acidosis
Spontaneous	Respiratory distress syndrome
	Poor pulmonary blood flow
	Poor respiratory muscle function
	Pulmonary edema
	Opioid overdose
Mechanical	Excessive dead space in the respiratory circuit (connectors, filters)
	Low tidal volume/respiratory rate in volume controlled ventilation
	Low pressure support in pressure controlled ventilation

In mechanically ventilated patients, an increased $PaCO_2$ may derive from an excessive dead space (at the level of the respiratory circuit) or from an inadequate pulmonary ventilation.

The main causes of respiratory acidosis in the setting of PCICU are listed in Table 4.1.

4.3.2 Respiratory Alkalosis

Respiratory alkalosis is a rare disorder in spontaneously ventilating pediatric patients. It can however be found as a compensative reaction to hypoxemia or hypermetabolic conditions (sepsis).

It is more common as an iatrogenic disorder in case of excessive ventilation in mechanically ventilated patients.

4.3.3 Metabolic Acidosis

This important disorder is caused by an insufficient oxygen delivery (DO_2) to the peripheral organs. As so, it is an almost invariable finding in every kind of shock.

In the setting of cardiac surgery congenital heart patients, the most common condition leading to a metabolic acidosis is cardiogenic shock. During cardiogenic shock, the cardiac output is reduced, and the DO_2 is inadequate to guarantee the organs' oxygen needs (VO_2). Therefore, the energy required to maintain the cell metabolism is partially guaranteed by the anaerobic metabolism, which leads to lactic acid formation, hyperlactatemia, and an excessive H^+ formation. Blood lactates increase, and the HCO_3^- is decreased, with a resulting negative BE.

Even in the presence of a normal cardiac output, this condition may appear whenever the metabolic needs are increased, like in septic shock.

Renal and liver failure may be responsible for metabolic acidosis. In the first case, it is basically due to an inadequate ability of the kidney to retain HCO_3^- and in the second to a decreased lactate clearance.

The main causes of metabolic acidosis are listed in Table 4.2.

Table 4.2 Main causes of metabolic acidosis in congenital heart patients in the pediatric cardiac intensive care unit

Acute renal failure
Acute liver failure
Cardiogenic shock
Hypovolemic shock
Hyperlactatemia
Profound anemia (rare)
Septic shock
Fever

4.3.4 Metabolic Alkalosis

The most common mechanism leading to metabolic alkalosis in the PCICU is the overuse of loop diuretics. The inhibition of Cl^- ions reabsorption at the level of the kidney loop leads to a compensatory influx of H^+ and K^+ in the urine. This determines a pattern of hypokalemic alkalosis.

4.3.5 Interaction Between Acid-Base Balance and Electrolytes

Due to the strict intercorrelation between H^+ ions concentration and transmembrane exchange of ions regulated by electrical forces, changes in H^+ concentrations (and therefore of pH) lead to changes in other ion concentrations. This is particularly important with respect to K^+ concentration, given the paramount role of K^+ in regulating the heart rhythm. Basically, it can be said that acidosis is accompanied by hyperkalemia and alkalosis by hypokalemia, due to redistribution between the intracellular and extracellular space. Both these conditions may represent a dangerous and even life-threatening condition. Hyperkalemia may lead to asystolic cardiac arrest, whereas hypokalemia triggers arrhythmias and ventricular fibrillation.

4.4 Acid-Base Balance in the Newborn

Newborns have serum bicarbonate lower than the adults. This is due to poor bicarbonate reabsorption at the level of the proximal tubule of the kidney. Moreover, there is a poor ability of the kidney to excrete acids [5].

The newborn survive this "acidosis pattern" by assuming base equivalents contained in the mother's milk [5, 6].

An additional factor leading to acidosis in newborns is the loss of bicarbonates due to gastroenteric disturbances. In case of diarrhea, pancreatic bicarbonates are lost.

These considerations should be taken into account in newborns under total parenteral nutrition. Additionally, this developmental pattern of the acid-base balance justifies the poor infant's ability to recover from metabolic acidosis generated by cardiogenic shock and sepsis or from the administration of amino acids in the parenteral nutrition [7–9].

4.5   Special Conditions Related to Congenital Heart Disease

There are a number of cardiocirculatory conditions in the congenital heart patients which link acid-base disturbances to hemodynamics.

Hypercapnia and acidosis trigger tet-spell crisis in patients with tetralogy of Fallot. Bicarbonate administration may prevent or treat tet-spell crisis during induction of anesthesia or whenever additional factors (pain, anxiety) trigger the crisis.

In patients with a critical pulmonary circulation (e.g., cavopulmonary connection and moreover Fontan circulation), hypercapnia increases the pulmonary resistances and impairs the pulmonary blood flow. This activates a vicious circle where the poor pulmonary blood flow leads to venous blood stagnation, hypercapnia, low values of end-tidal CO_2, and veno-arterial CO_2 gradient.

In patients with single-ventricle circulation and pulmonary-systemic blood flow sustained by the same vascular axis (truncus arteriosus; stage I Norwood correction), the $PaCO_2$ is a strong regulator of the pulmonary blood flow and therefore of the systemic blood flow. Hyperventilation and hypocapnia lead to an excessive pulmonary blood flow, reduced systemic blood flow, and coronary flow steal.

To a lesser extent, a similar situation is faced in the presence of systemic-pulmonary shunts surgically positioned.

Patients with left-to-right shunt (ventricular septal defect, atrioventricular canal, and others) have an increased pulmonary blood flow. This is actually compensated by a higher V_E and V_A in the spontaneously ventilating patients. In patients under mechanical ventilation, ventilator volumes higher than normal are required to match the increased pulmonary blood flow.

These patients typically experience an increased amount of pulmonary secretions which may lead to a poor alveolar gas exchange and respiratory acidosis. A careful care of the airways with frequent suction of the secretions is often required.

Severe aortic coarctation of the newborn may manifest with dramatic signs of metabolic acidosis once the ductus arteriosus closes. This is due to a poor or absent perfusion of the visceral vessels and the lower body; the only reasonable approach is an emergent surgical correction if the pharmacological attempts to reopen the ductus arteriosus fail.

4.6   Correction of Acid-Base Disturbances

As a general rule, the maintenance of a correct acid-base balance is mandatory in the treatment of congenital heart patients before, during, and after surgery. Last, but not least, it should be always considered that the cerebral blood flow is strongly ruled by the pH and the $PaCO_2$. Hypocapnia and alkalosis may determine critical levels of cerebral blood flow.

In turn, profound acidosis (pH < 7.10) will result in an impaired myocardial contractility, vasodilation, poor response to cathecolamines, and coagulation factors impairment.

A comprehensive analysis of the therapeutic interventions to correct acid-base balance disturbances goes beyond the purposes of the present chapter. However, a reasonable first step is to identify the leading cause of the disturbance and to treat it. This may be relatively easy for respiratory acidosis. In spontaneously ventilating patients, a careful clearance of the airways may be sufficient in patterns of minor severity. Supportive measures, namely, tracheal intubation and mechanical ventilation, are required in the most severe cases. The use of noninvasive ventilator supports is more adequate to treat hypoxia than hypercapnia.

Metabolic acidosis due to cardiocirculatory failure should not be treated symptomatically by a simple bicarbonate replacement. The leading cause should be identified (hypovolemia, cardiac failure, vasoplegia, septic shock, etc.), and an appropriate cardiocirculatory support should be established. In the more severe cases, extracorporeal circulatory support may be required. The use of bicarbonates should be restricted to severe acidosis ($pH < 7.15$) always considering that lactic acidosis buffering will produce an excess of CO_2 which needs to be cleared out by ventilation.

References

1. Gilfix BM, Bique M, Magder S. A physical chemical approach to the analysis of acid-base balance in the clinical setting. J Crit Care. 1993;8:187–97.
2. Gluck SL. Acid-base. Lancet. 1998;352:474–9.
3. Haber RJ. A practical approach to acid-base disorders. West J Med. 1991;155:146–51.
4. Narins RG, Emmett M. Simple and mixed acid-base disorders: a practical approach. Medicine (Baltimore). 1980;59:161–87.
5. Rector FC. Sodium, bicarbonate, and chloride absorption by the proximal tubule. Am J Physiol Renal Physiol. 1983;244:F461–71.
6. Nagami G. Renal ammonia production and excretion. In: Seldin DW, Giebisch G, editors. The kidney: physiology and pathophysiology. New York: Lippincott, Williams and Wilkins; 2000. p. 1995–2013.
7. Baum M, Quigley R. Postnatal renal development. In: Seldin DW, Giebisch G, editors. The kidney: physiology and pathophysiology. New York: Lippincott, Williams and Wilkins; 2000. p. 703–26.
8. Baum M, Quigley R. Maturation of proximal tubular acidification. Pediatr Nephrol. 1993;7:785–91.
9. Day R, Franklin J. Renal carbonic anhydrase in premature and mature infants. Pediatrics. 1951;7:182–5.

Cardiac Medications: Dosages, Preparation and Administration

5

Grandi Nadia

Abstract

The paediatric and developing age cardiology and heart surgery are the units where I am working. Users are from neonates (most of them with prenatal diagnosis) up to adults, considering that our patients are congenital heart disease patients. As hereby we will only discuss the therapeutic approach, I would like to emphasise that for nurses it is mandatory to know the most used drugs and, in this specific case, to which category the cardiac drugs belong (antiarrhythmic, adrenergic, inotropic, anticoagulant, antiplatelet, beta-blocker, diuretics, vasodilators, ACE inhibitors, cortisone-like drugs, analgesic, antipyretic, immunosuppressant, antibiotics (Cardiologia pediatrica, McGraw-Hill, Milan, p. 333–8, 1998)), its usage, function, any precaution, side effects, administration and storage. The friendly leaflet and its consultation can help us when there is a lack or a doubt regarding a medication. Considering that for newborn patients it is not always suggested on the leaflet the recommended dosage, a hospital treatment form is usually available in the paediatric unit to allow all the staff to check safely all dosages. In this chapter I will discuss about dosages, preparation and administration of the therapy to cardiopath patients.

5.1 Introduction

First of all is to remind that, in general, children have higher sensibility to medications, as their pharmacokinetics processes are different to the adult one because of their organs immaturity. So drug effects in newborns and children could be overly

G. Nadia
Pediatric and Developing Age Cardiology and Heart Surgery Unit, Department Cardiovascular and Thoracic, University Hospital Policlinico Sant Orsola Malpighi, Bologna, Italy

© Springer International Publishing AG, part of Springer Nature 2019   105
S. F. Flocco et al. (eds.), *Congenital Heart Disease*,
https://doi.org/10.1007/978-3-319-78423-6_5

intense and prolonged, as the collateral effects could be stronger. Aged patients too have the same sensibility to medications because of organs' deterioration, often added to multiple diseases or to a worsening of these diseases. Regarding children it should be taken into account some other parameters like body weight (most of the paediatric drugs are prescribed as mg/kg/24 h), body surface area and some data regarding adsorption, hepatic metabolism, renal excretion and blood-brain barrier. Thus reactions to medications in children are not as predictable as in adult patients. In neonates and above all in suckling infants, many hepatic functions are reduced: many enzymatic systems are still absent or uncompleted, and drug renal elimination is still limited, which is the reason for the major sensibility to nephrotoxic drugs. Starting from the age of about 1 year, many pharmacokinetics parameters are similar to the adult ones, so drug responses in children over 1 year old are more similar to adult responses than to neonatal responses. Farther it is important to remind that often for the children, we need to use adult medications fractionated according to the baby's body weight. It is implied that the paediatric unit deserves a separate discussion about therapy preparation and taking of it. Some drugs (e.g. antibiotics, antiasthma and analgesics) could be also used with indication, dosage and target different from the one indicated on the leaflet. In this case scientific evidences able to motivate the choice should support the doctor's prescription [1].

5.2   Dosages

As the paediatric unit concerns patients from birth to adolescent age, nurses will face prescriptions completely different according to the age and the body weight of patients: grammes become milligrammes or gamma with several decimal numbers that can lead to errors. In this case math is applied to pharmacology, and it is strictly suggested to all nurses to update their knowledge and to revise the main principles of math based on roman numbers, fractions, decimals, percentages, rations, proportions and unit of measurement. Regarding the decimal metric system, it is necessary that nurses know the main measures of capacity (from litre to millilitre) and the main measures for weight (kilogramme, gramme, milligramme, microgram or gamma and nano).

A good knowledge of the conversion system allows us to change the unit of measurement easily, from a smaller to a bigger one (dividing or moving decimal to the left) and contrariwise from a bigger to a smaller one (multiplying or moving decimal to the right). It is important to know that measures of capacity (ml) are used both for liquid medications and to indicate the amount of cream, gel or ointment. Whilst regarding infusions, there exists a formula to quickly calculate the delivery rate, it is necessary to divide the total volume to be infused, expressed as ml, with the infusion time expressed as minutes, and the result should be multiplied by 60.

Careful calculations should be done to obtain very low-dose medications when it is not commercially available with the required concentration; thus it is necessary to dilute the drug by adding an amount of solvent, calculating the proportion and aspiring the quantity necessary to dispense.

There exists some international standard measures for the dosage of some drugs, for example, for insulin 1 mL = 100 U, whilst for heparin 1 mL = 5000 U.

Moreover to calculate the electrolytes' concentration (e.g. sodium chloride, potassium chloride, calcium chloride, calcium gluconate, sodium bicarbonate), milliequivalents are used. To remind that usually commercially available injections expressed as mEq/ml are highly concentrated, not to be used before a suitable dilution and than should be slowly administrated. This is especially for potassium chloride.

A special discussion should be done for all medications expressed as gamma, as they require a careful attention during prescription and preparation. In the paediatric cardiology unit, it is used to prescribe micrograms or gamma/kg/min. In this case it is important that nurses know the calculations done by doctors, so they may know the right dosage for any age. And anyway, to decrease the risk of error, it is important to do these complicated calculations with double check. The most used drugs are prostaglandins, dopamine, dobutamine, isoprenaline, noradrenaline, adrenaline and sodium nitroprusside. To prepare these drugs, there exists a schedule that allows nurses to quickly extrapolate the right amount to administrate to babies or how to calculate this dose based on proportions that can be easily used by skilled operators.

During the prescription doctors should legibly write the full name of the patient, date of birth, potential allergies, name of drug using the full name of the molecule without abbreviations, pharmaceutical form, route of administration (os, iv, etc.), numbers of administrations, doses and time. Then the doctor should write the date and sign. Regarding infusions it would be correct if next to the dosage, expressed as mg or gamma, the doctor writes the total volume to be administrated expressed as cc or ml and the hourly rate, if it is a continuous infusion. Before any administration nurses should question themselves if the prescribed dose is correct and not only execute the prescription; this is to avoid any therapeutic errors that can lead to worrying consequences. After the administration of the prescribed drug, nurses must also affix their signature.

Sometimes calculations and preparation of medications have to be done in an urgency-emergency situation, often characterised by chaos and unrest that can lead to confusion. Three basic aspects characterise the emergency situation: division of roles, staff coordination and space organisation; this is to allow each worker to focus on his skills and competences without hindering nobody else. In order to reach this coordination and to avoid using in a hurry vital drugs, in our unit, divided in the two sectors (hospital stay and semi-intensive care unit), there are two emergency trolleys, one each sector, with a set of emergency drugs (atropine, isoprenaline, adrenaline, calcium chloride, sodium bicarbonate) ready to be used in syringes marked with the name of the drug and a red spot. These drugs are daily prepared, usually at the same time. In paediatric unit preparation, administration of medications in emergency situation could be a bigger problem than in adult unit; this is because not all drugs used in an adult patients can be used in paediatric patients; children cannot always use the same dosages than for adults, and for children the dose of drug must be calculated according to the children's body weight that often in emergency situation is unknown. Thus workers must be fast and accurate; must know calculations, proportions and equivalences; must have precise competences and skills; and must be ready to face both expected drug reactions and any adverse effects. I would like to underline that in case of critical patients, for example, for the intubated ones, the emergency drug set is ready to be used next to the patient, and over the medication listed above, the set includes fentanyl, midazolam and vecuronium bromide, diluted according to the patient body weight.

5.3   Preparation

When nurses know what should be administrated to patient, the right dose and how to administrate it, they should prepare the therapy in a quite space, for example, in the nurses' room, where they can find a good concentration without distractions or external stimulus to avoid any error that can lead to a danger for patients. It is absolutely forbidden to prepare the therapy in advance and let it lie whether in nurses' room or next to the patient's bed.

Mistakes could generate along all the chain, including drugs storage (expiry date, storage condition), prescription (readable and without abbreviations), preparation (if necessary to do a double check with a colleague) and administration (to be sure about the right drug, right dose, right route of administration, right time and right patient). Nurses should monitor all these steps because they must have all the knowledge about the diagnosis of the patient, any potential allergy and about the prescribed drugs. Nurses' responsibility is also the close monitoring of the patient after taken the therapy (therapy efficacy or adverse effects).

According to my experience, the risk of errors is higher and remarkable during paediatric patient discharge, for many reasons: the hurry during discharging, the parents' anxiety, the huge load of information given in the last minute and the therapy explanation are not always easy and understandable because of many information about dilutions and proportions and often including mince, mix and solution to be prepared inside a syringe. Furthermore all these difficulties are still higher when the paediatric patients belong to a different ethnicity, so a cultural mediator must be present, and the therapeutic education should be longer and extended to many family members. In this case it would be better to speak with the family well in advance. For sure it is not always possible to start in advance with the family therapeutic education because therapy could change during the stay in the hospital with the risk of explaining different calculations and dilutions. In any case after it is well explained and showed to relatives how to handle medications, it would be suitable that relatives prepare the drug under the nurse's supervision to verify their comprehension. Moreover parents are taught how to face problems that can happen during the therapy administration, like vomiting or a minimal exit of drugs from the mouth, or what to do if a child presents any fever or diarrhoea and if drugs should be taken during fasting, full stomach or either. In our unit, when the patient is discharged, we give him/her the discharging letter and a paper where we write together with parents how to dilute the oral therapy in a very practical way, shifting milligrammes to millilitres and teaching them how to use a syringe for liquid preparation. This paper is signed by the operator, copied and added to the medical record as evidence of what have been done.

Conversely in case of heart transplanted paediatric patients, the therapeutic education for parents starts when health condition appears compatible with a short discharge. In this case the ratio of patient-nurse is 1:1, so the time taken for parents' education is high and includes observation, practical execution of parents under nurses' supervision and finally independent execution; all these steps are monitored and recorded on a proper paper kept in the patient's room.

5.4 Administration

Those approaching for the first time at paediatric unit, and in this particular case to the paediatric cardiology, think that calculations, dosages, preparations, dilutions, counting and proportions are the most difficult tasks, requiring a huge amount of time and high concentration. In the beginning I too was thinking the same, but very soon I realised that the most difficult thing in the paediatric unit is the administration of oral therapy to children. When I speak about "children" I include people with huge age difference, i.e newborns until first/secon childwood. It is well known that the therapy administration is one of the main, if not the principal, responsibilities of nurses. This is because over the therapy preparation, it is required to establish a relationship with paediatric patients based on collaboration, complicity and emotional bond that allows patients to be in an emotional balance and tranquillity during the administration of medications. For sure it could be useful to know the child's cognitive development, as divided by Piaget in four phases [2]. It is important to explain all the procedures in detail to patients, though children's reactions could be refusals and moods that nurses should ignore. We suppose to use an easy and direct language without confounding children with too many requests. We should use techniques of distraction, because it is clear that recreational activities may become a means of relationship with children. Allowing children to handle medical material (e.g. gauze, patches, syringes, etc.) could reduce the anxiety related to the medical procedures [3]. Not less important is the parents' role to which we should previously explain what we want to do so they can help us during the drug administration phase. Clearly the more aged and independent the patient is, the more the nurse should look for his collaboration.

5.4.1 Oral Administration

With youngest patients, mainly until the school age, without gastric problems, it is better to use oral therapy, that is, capsules emptied of their content or tablets chopped with specific mortars or pulverisers. The powder obtained could be diluted in water or any glucose solution or by using syrups, vials or any solution that allows the deglutition. It is better to avoid mixing drugs with any liquid usually taken by babies, like milk or juice; this is to reduce the risk that the child rejects these foods over time. Patients should stand or sit and be informed about everything that is happening. With time and with parents's support, it will be possible to know if our patient prefers a pharmaceutical form to another. For example, I met babies preferring the chopped tablet of ranitidine from the syrup, but this was found by attempts, above all if the patient is not able to speak yet. If the child vomits right after the drug administration, it is important to inform the doctor and repeat the administration. The administration of the oral therapy can be employed by syringes, spoons or glasses according to the patient's age. In case of patients with gastric trouble, the nasogastric tube helps nurses in drug administration, but it is important to observe some rules both for the treatment safety and to avoid the tube obstruction. Through the nasogastric tube, it is possible to administrate tablets, capsules and all the oral liquid drugs. Concerning capsules content should be used, while tables should be chopped as fine as possible. With controlled or modified release drugs, micro-encapsulated granules and gastro-resistant tablets are an exception: once chopped or out of their enclosure, these drugs modify their pharmaceutical characteristics, like resistance to gastric juices and/or rate of absorption, making the treatment less effective. All medications should be dissolved in water before administration. This decreases the hyperosmolarity of the solution and helps the administration of pulverised drugs. To avoid any interaction between medications and feeding solutions, it is better to suspend the nutrition, wash the nasogastric tube, administer drugs, wash the tube again and restart the feeding. This also avoids any tube obstruction. For the same reason, it is better to avoid mixing drugs with the food of the patient. If the child has the nasogastric tube for decompression purpose after the drug administration, the tube should be closed for at least 30 min to allow the drug to be absorbed. In case of obstruction of the tube, it could be useful to wash it with warm water, alternating gentle pressures and aspirations. In case of very young babies, where reduced doses of medications are required, it is suitable to obtain from the central pharmacy galenical products or powdered drugs previously dosed with precision or intravenous drugs already prepared in syringes ready to be administrated.

5.4.2 Headset and Ophthalmic Administration

The headset, ophthalmic or mucosal administration is very difficult to perform because often it requires strong movements against patients which usually do not agree and are somewhat frightened. For the correct administration of headset drops, it is suggested to gently push down and forward the pinna by holding the child lying. For the ophthalmic installation, the patient should lie down, and by gently pulling the lower eyelid, the nurse should instil drops or apply the prescribed ointment.

5.4.3 Rectal Administration

For rectal drugs, usually administrated when drugs cannot be adsorbed orally, often necessary are the child's contention and the collaboration of parents. Moreover, for this more cruel administration route, it is mandatory that nurses act safely and fast to avoid further traumatic reactions in patients. The child should be placed on his stomach or on his back with legs raised, keeping for a while the buttocks tightened after inserting suppository of paracetamol or a rectal tube to administer drugs such as valium or midazolam.

5.4.4 Inhaled Administration

Children feel like inhaled therapy is a friend/enemy, for instance, nebulised aerosol, above all, because of the mask that should be well attached to the face. If the inhaled therapy is properly introduced, for example, like a game, in children under 6 years old, it could be considered as an amazing moment during which they try to capture all the mist coming off the mask. Otherwise it is necessary to nebulise drugs, whilst children are sleep. In older children, the use of the mouthpiece is recommended; however it does not exclude the use of the mask if the patient prefers it.

5.4.5 Intramuscular Administration

Because of the pain, intramuscular administrations are mainly avoided. But when it is not possible to shift to some other administration routes or when it is necessary to have a fast absorption, patients should be well positioned, and nurses should inject quickly and safely drugs in the right muscles, chosen according to the age of the patient: quadriceps femoris muscle if under 3 years old and dorsogluteal muscle if over 3 years old. To be taken into account is the patient's weight as well as the age. It would be good to consider also that the intramuscular adsorption in newborns is slow and irregular, while in aged babies it becomes faster.

5.4.6 Subcutaneous Administration

The same consideration should be done for the subcutaneous injections of insulin or heparin: once the injection site is chosen, nurses should act safely, without hesitation and without massaging the injection site after. Remember that this route of administration has a slower adsorption compared to the intravenous administration and is used only for small volumes of medication. In children it is preferred to use the front of the thighs [4].

5.4.7 Intravenous Administration

Therapy administration is easier when patients already have a venous access, either peripheral or central. These accesses can be used to administrate emergency drugs, hydrating solutions or blood products. Regarding the peripheral venous access positioning, once the right insertion point on intact skin is identified, it is necessary to evaluate the patient's collaboration; otherwise get help from another colleague, and ask parents to participate and keep the baby as calm as possible. It is not necessary to persist in attempts; it is preferable to ask for some help to colleagues or to the anaesthetist. Once the catheter is well placed and the patency is checked, it should be fixed with tape or sometimes by using rigid splints. When it is possible, it is preferable to avoid placing the catheter over joints or in the dominant hand. The upper limbs are the first to be considered, above all, in aged children; instead in newborns it is preferable to use lower limb veins, like saphenous vein, without excluding scalp veins, though in our unit they are not used. In case these veins are not available, it is possible to ask doctors to cannulate the external jugular vein. Over the following days, it is necessary to check the insertion site and keep the catheter's patency by washing it with sodium chloride solution. Regarding the therapy administration, it will be the nurses' responsibility to know what solutions are compatible to be infused through a peripheral vein, according to pH and osmolarity (indicating the concentration of dissolved particles in a solution). Nurses should know which medicines might cause phlebitis and if drugs should be injected by slow bolo or by fast injection. It is important that nurses know differences among isotonic, hypotonic or hypertonic solutions and that osmolarity is one of the main factors to cause chemical phlebitis. Main liquids used as solvents are glucose 5% and sodium chloride 0.9%, belonging to isotonic solutions, but it should be known that some drugs could precipitate or be deteriorated by glucose 5% or sodium chloride 0.9%. Close attention must be given to the external solution appearance: generally it should be clear, colourless or pale and free from precipitates, with the exception of some particular drugs with specific opalescence or colourings features. Obviously the risk of phlebitis increases when pH (which must be included between 5 and 9) and osmolarity (which must be not higher than 600 mOsm/L) of the intravenous solution differ from the blood one. Regarding the infusion rate, it should consider several factors: osmolarity (hypertonic solutions should be infused slowly), characteristics of the molecules, cardiopath patient conditions to avoid overloading volumes, venous access calibre to know the correct flow rate (mL/min), infusion site condition and total volume to be infused. Often, in the paediatric unit, drugs are further diluted before the injection, in order to facilitate the fractioning of the dose. To underline that pharmacological response could change if some medications are administrated alone or as combination with some other drugs, it is mandatory for nurses to check if any drugs are incompatible or if their combination may influence processes of absorption, distribution, metabolism and excretion or threaten to cause embolism, toxicity, ineffectiveness or occlusion of the catheter. It is the nurses' task to know and consult the chart of drug interactions and incompatibility. This chart shows if two drugs are compatible within the same infusion, if they cannot be diluted in the same drip and must be administered with two different infusion sets or even if incompatibility in the same infusion is not at the tap. A careful consultation of these schedules can definitely help nurses in the usage of drugs and their preparation, decreasing the risk of errors and adverse events. Obviously these tools must be constantly supplemented and updated without ever falling into the stillness of the information. It is understood that whilst not all infusions may be administered through a peripheral vein catheter, the problem does not occur when the child has a central venous catheter, either in internal jugular vein (for older children), subclavian vein, femoral vein (in case of emergency quickly accessed) or umbilical vein (in infants). According to the patient age, the doctor will decide the most suitable type of venous access.

Conclusions

Whatever therapy must be prepared, first of all the nurse must wash his hands carefully and then, if necessary, he should use gloves, and he should strictly comply with the aseptic techniques for the preparation of intravenous infusions, as well as disinfection of the skin in case of cutaneous injections. The pharmacological therapy safety in childhood is still a big target, with the purpose of decreasing, or better to delete, the therapeutic mistakes, as it has been demonstrated that errors in paediatric patients occur three times over than in adult patients and above all in intensive care unit [5]. When we speak about therapeutic mistakes, we speak about errors which occurred during prescription, preparation, distribution, administration or monitoring of medications. In this context nurses have a very important role, because they act as the last check for any mistakes and for the monitoring of any side effects. This critical role is based on nurses' pharmacological knowledge [6]. Moreover sharing any mistakes that occurred with all team could help to avoid the repetition of the same mistake, giving a profitable teaching.

References

1. Mirabile L, Baroncini S. Rianimazione In Eta'pediatrica. Milan: Springer. p. 651–8.
2. Thompson ED, Ashwill JW. Manuale Di Pediatria Puericultura Clinica E Assistenza, Edises; 2000. p. 329–35.
3. Benini S. Pedagogia E Infermieristica In Dialogo, Clueb; 2006. p. 224–7.
4. Huband S, Trigg E. Nursing Pediatrico, Linee Guida E Procedure Per L'ospedale E Il Territorio. Milan: Mcgraw-Hill; 2001.
5. IPASVI/ECM/RIVISTA L'INFERMIERE N.4-2011/Errore Terapeutico In Neonatologia: Si Puo'limitarlo Con La Gestione Informatica Del Processo Farmacologico? p. 21–7.
6. Benner P. L'Eccellenza Nella Pratica Clinica Dell'infermiere, L'apprendimento Basato Sull'esperienza. Milan: McGraw-Hill; 2003. p. 93–8.

Fluid and Electrolyte Balance

6

Alessandra Rizza and Zaccaria Ricci

Abstract

The appropriate evaluation and maintenance of fluid and electrolyte balance in children with congenital heart disease are a fundamental aspect of everyday clinical practice. Fluids are continuously administered for the most reasons: nutrition, drug administration, and fluid resuscitation. Their amount and biochemical composition have been associated with several important outcomes in the pediatric and adult cardiac surgery populations. For example, even if human albumin and crystalloids remain the first choice for cardiopulmonary bypass priming and volume replacement, uncertainty currently concerns third-generation hydroxyethyl starches. Secondly, appropriate and timely fluid resuscitation may improve patients' survival, but an incorrect fluid therapy in pediatric intensive care setting can significantly impact several organ functions. Hence, the fluid status assessment and management during perioperative period in pediatric cardiac surgery are a clinical challenge: there is no consensus regarding the optimal definition of fluid overload, which also varies by calculations and by the time frame during which fluid balance is assessed. Furthermore, the estimation of intravascular volume to guide fluid therapy is typically based on clinical assessment and on standard hemodynamic and perfusion parameters, but these parameters could be inadequate in children affected by congenital heart disease.

Similarly, derangements of potassium, sodium, calcium, phosphate, and magnesium (both above and below the normal range) are extremely common in this population and require strict monitoring and careful intervention.

This chapter will review the current evidence concerning perioperative fluid and electrolyte management, assessment, outcomes, and treatment in critically ill children undergoing congenital heart surgery.

A. Rizza · Z. Ricci (✉)
Department of Cardiology and Cardiac Surgery, Pediatric Cardiac Intensive Care Unit,
Bambino Gesù Children's Hospital, IRCCS, Rome, Italy

© Springer International Publishing AG, part of Springer Nature 2019
S. F. Flocco et al. (eds.), *Congenital Heart Disease*,
https://doi.org/10.1007/978-3-319-78423-6_6

115

6.1   Introduction

Perioperative fluid and electrolyte management is part of everyday routine clinical practice in pediatric cardiac surgery patients. Nonetheless, the type of fluids (colloids vs. crystalloids), the ideal composition of solutions, and the amount of fluids that should be administered are currently debated. In cardiac surgery patients, the distribution of fluids and electrolytes in the intravascular or extravascular space depends on a number of intra- and postoperative factors that highly influence the pathophysiology of body fluid kinetic: cardiopulmonary bypass (CPB) (starting, conducting, and weaning), CPB priming solution (volume and composition), cardioplegic solutions (volume, composition, and temperature), CPB circuits and artificial lungs, thermal management, and vasoactive and inotropic drugs. Patients' age is another key factor determining different fluid kinetics during cardiac surgery. Furthermore, perioperative clinical events (including the need for fluid replacement) frequently cause electrolyte derangements including potassium, calcium, sodium, phosphate, and magnesium shifts above and below the normal range: monitoring such elements normal serum concentration is not standardized and needs careful bedside alertness.

This chapter will focus on fluid and electrolyte management during and after pediatric cardiac surgery in two separate sections: (1) issues related to fluid management and goal-directed fluid administration and (2) electrolyte balance and derangement correction.

6.2   Fluid Balance

6.2.1   The Choice of Fluids in Pediatric Heart Surgery

In pediatric heart surgery, intraoperative management of intravascular fluids is a priority: the relatively elevated blood loss amount and the high ratio between the CPB circuit priming volume and the circulating blood volume complicate the management of hemodilution. Human albumin (HA) is commonly used in pediatric cardiac surgery for CPB priming: it has the advantage to delay the absorption of circulating fibrinogen and to reduce the platelet activation through the pre-coating of the CPB circuit [1]. Although HA has demonstrated several beneficial effects compared to crystalloids, synthetic colloids may provide a valuable alternative for intraoperative fluid replacement during pediatric cardiac surgery [2, 3]. Van der Linden et al. [3] confirmed the equivalence between 6% HES 130/0.4 and 5% HA in children aged 2–12 years undergoing cardiac surgery with CPB: these authors examined the total volume of colloid infusion for intraoperative volume replacement including priming of the extracorporeal circuit. The two treatments resulted equivalent in terms of volume expansion, but intraoperative fluid balance (FB) was less positive in the HES group. Furthermore, no difference was found regarding hemodynamic parameters, the use of vasoactive drugs, blood losses, blood products' transfusions, renal function, increase of renal biomarkers, and adverse events up to postoperative day 28. However, the small sample size of the study precluded any firm conclusion regarding HES's safety. The group recently retrospectively reviewed a largest database (1495 cardiac surgery children operated between 2002 and 2010) [4]. During the study period, the CPB circuit was primed primarily with 4% HA—between 2002 and 2005—and with 6% HES 130/0.4 after that period. HES and HA administration was limited to 50 mL/kg/day. They confirmed that the use of HES was safe. In addition, intraoperative use of HES was associated with significantly lower intraoperative FB, perioperative blood losses, volume of blood products, and transfusion rate. No difference of incidence of postoperative renal failure, morbidity, or mortality was observed. However, part of these results may be attributable to the modification, over time, of CPB management: CPB priming volume was reduced due to miniaturization of the circuitry, and a lower exposition to blood products was likely caused by a change in institutional practice. It must be acknowledged that these results are in line with other previous small studies [5, 6].

Regardless of the perioperative phase, it should be considered that cardiac surgery patients may be admitted to the pediatric intensive care unit (PICU) soon after birth. A state of elevated metabolism and a high percentage (up to 80%) of extra- and intracellular water is a typical condition of the first days of life: these features tend to progressively decrease with age until the lowest percentage during adulthood and senescence [7]. Extra- and intracellular electrolyte composition is similar in children and adults, but liver mass (glycogen stores) and muscle mass (protein stores) are lacking in newborns, who are therefore less able to maintain, through glycogenolysis and gluconeogenesis, normoglycemia during fasting [7]. As a matter of fact, however, the administration of normal saline (NaCl 0.9%) is the most commonly used intravenous solution in the world. A great amount of concern on saline use was recently described by a big observational study on patients undergoing major surgery who received either saline or a balanced crystalloid solution: patients who received saline did worse on every evaluated outcome (mortality, complications, infections, renal failure requiring dialysis, blood transfusion, electrolyte disturbance, acidosis, and re-intervention rate) [8]. There is currently no strong evidence of potential harm by saline on pediatric patients: however, renal damage and acidosis secondary to unbalanced crystalloids' administration should be carefully taken into consideration, and balanced solution should be reasonably preferred in all children.

6.2.2 Fluid Overload in Pediatric Cardiac Surgery

Fluid overload (FO) is a common occurrence in the early postoperative period in pediatric cardiac surgery, and it may range up to 50% of patients, depending on the type of surgery and age [9–11]. Generally, patients who are sicker at PICU admission require more volume for stabilization, and in this setting an early aggressive fluid administration may be lifesaving. However—after hemodynamic stabilization—an excessively positive FB may impact organ function and negatively influence outcomes of critically ill patient [12, 13]. Children undergoing cardiac surgery are at risk of developing FO, due to surgery-associated inflammatory condition, eventual increased capillary permeability, and consequent fluid extravasation into the extracellular compartment: this cascade ultimately causes increased extravascular lung water and global tissue edema [13, 14]. In the early postoperative period, the low cardiac output syndrome (LCOS), surgical blood losses, and eventual hemodynamic instability may require a large amount of fluid administration and transfusions, which further contribute to FO [15]. Finally, it should be considered that mechanical ventilation induces increase of antidiuretic hormone (ADH) secretion [7].

Reliable monitoring of the FB in critically ill children is very important to detect a potential FO. However, it is unclear which is the most precise measure of FB in PICU. The most common and easy method used for FB estimation is to compute daily weight gain and/or loss indexing it as a percentage of PICU admission [16]. A FO between 5 and 10% is considered pathologic, and Sutherland clearly showed that for each 1% increase in severity of fluid overload, an additional 3% risk of mortality is observed [17]. Bontant et al. recently evaluated the accuracy of the mostly used methods in PICU [18]: the fluid intake minus output (FIMO) and FIMO adjusted for insensible fluid loss (AFIMO) were compared to body weight changes in 60 children at PICU admission and 24 h later. The median age of this population was 304 days (39–1565), and the median weight was 9.2 (4.4–17.8). In line with previous data in neonates [19], there was poor agreement between FIMO/AFIMO methods calculated by nurses and body weight changes. Therefore, FIMO/AFIMO calculations may be reserved for the most severely ill patients in whom body weight measurement is strictly contraindicated [18].

The importance of an accurate FB assessment relies on the awareness that FO is a widely acknowledged risk factor of poor outcome with deleterious multiorgan effects both in children and adults [12, 17, 20, 21]. FO negatively affects pulmonary function in all mechanically ventilated and spontaneously breathing patients, whether or not they have acute lung injury (ALI) [13]. According to another author [9] FO occurred early postoperatively also in pediatric cardiac surgery patients, while negative fluid balance tended to occur by PICU day 4. Hassinger et al. [11] in a prospective observational study of 98 pediatric patients (2 weeks–18 years) showed that early FO increases the rate of postoperative AKI and that the occurrence of FO more often preceded AKI than followed it. Avoiding aggressive fluid administration (less than 50 mL/kg) in the first few days after surgery in these high-risk patients could potentially mitigate poorer outcomes.

6.2.3   Goal-Directed Therapy and Fluid Responsiveness in Children

Clinical assessment of hemodynamic status, based on physical examination and routine monitoring, could be inadequate especially in children [22]. Hence, other than the correct assessment of FB and FO, also intravascular volume and predictors of the "fluid responsiveness" (increase in cardiac output/index after volume loading) would be needed for hemodynamic optimization in critically ill patients: the so-called goal-directed therapy (GDT).

Numerous hemodynamic variables have been evaluated to predict fluid responsiveness (Table 6.1): *static variables* include heart rate (*HR*), systolic arterial blood pressure (*SAP*), preload pressure such as central venous pressure (*CVP*) and pulmonary artery occlusion pressure (*PAOP*), left atrial pressure (*LAP*, frequently monitored by the placement of a surgical catheter intraoperatively), echocardiographic, and Doppler measurement such as left ventricular end-diastolic area-*LVEDA*, stroke volume index-*SVI* (defined as ejected systolic volume indexed on body surface area), and corrected flow time-c*FT* (a Doppler measurement derived from the beginning to the end of the aortic velocity waveform in the descending thoracic aorta). *Dynamic variables* instead reflect the cyclical changes in left ventricular SV induced by mechanical ventilation (Table 6.1). All these ventilation-induced variations in SV result in cyclic modifications of aortic blood flow, arterial blood pressure, and plethysmographic waveform amplitude. As a general principle, the more the variation, the more the hypovolemia, and this variation is quantified by the percentage difference (*ΔSV%*) between the maximal and minimum value measured in a single breath. The definition of "response" is based on a change in SV increase of 10–15% (according to different studies). Fluid type used for bolus (usually 10 mL/kg) could be a crystalloid or colloid or a blood product, which is usually infused in 10–15 min. Little is known in the literature of pediatric perioperative setting, as far as volume status and fluid responsiveness assessment are concerned [23–34]. The ΔVpeak is the most reliable parameter for fluid responsiveness evaluation in children, as shown in the greatest number of studies [22]. The ΔVpeak is determined from pulsed Doppler of aortic blood flow during the respiratory cycle; the maximum and minimum peak aortic blood flow velocities are measured. However, ΔVpeak measurement depends on the measurement skill of the echocardiographer, and it could be affected by arrhythmias, heart rate, and mechanical ventilation. In addition, it should be considered that children have higher chest wall and lung compliance than adults: hence, the intrathoracic pressure with normal tidal volume ventilation may not cause a significant variation of hemodynamic variables. During pediatric cardiac surgery, all dynamic variables cannot be used, by definition, when the chest is open (intraoperative and complicated postoperative periods). Furthermore, children have higher arterial compliance than adults, and the magnitude of changes in arterial pressure induced by ventilation may be smaller in a more compliant vascular system: this may explain why dynamic preload variables based on arterial blood pressure do not predict fluid responsiveness in children.

It must be finally acknowledged that, at the PICU bedside, in the absence of other recommended GDT parameters that should reliably guide clinicians in hemodynamic optimization, CVP and LAP are certainly the most routinely used preload variables guiding physicians in fluid replacement prescription.

Table 6.1 Static and dynamic hemodynamic variables

Name/acronym	Definition	Measurement method	Explanation/calculation
Static variables	Hemodynamic parameters measured at a single point in time	–	–
CVP	Central venous pressure	Catheter into the right atrium (generally via superior vena cava)	None
SAP	Systolic arterial pressure	Invasive or noninvasive systemic blood pressure	None
PAOP	Pulmonary artery occlusion pressure	Pulmonary artery catheter	None
LAP	Left atrial pressure	Catheter into the left atrium (generally surgical)	None
GEDVI	Global end-diastolic volume index	Transpulmonary thermodilution (PiCCO)	None
LVEDA	Left ventricular end-diastolic area	Echocardiography	None
SVI	Stroke volume index	Echocardiography	Aortic valve area x velocity-time integral of aortic blood flow/body surface area
FTc	Flow time corrected	Echocardiography/esophageal Doppler	Doppler measurement of duration of flow during systole corrected for heart rate in the descending thoracic aorta
PV	Peak velocity	Echocardiography esophageal Doppler	Highest blood velocity detected during systole in the descending thoracic aorta
Dynamic variables	Hemodynamic parameter reflecting the cyclical changes induced by mechanical ventilation	–	–
SVV	Stroke volume (SV) variation	PiCCO, LiDCO, MostCare	SV at the beginning and at the end of respiratory cycle $SV_{max} - SV_{min}/SV_{max} \times 100$
SPV	Systolic pressure (SP) variation	PiCCO, LiDCO, MostCare	SP at the beginning and at the end of respiratory cycle $SP_{max} - SP_{min}/SP_{max} \times 100$
PPV	Pulse pressure (PP) variation	PiCCO, LiDCO, MostCare	PP (the difference between the systolic and diastolic pressure) at the beginning and at the end of respiratory cycle $PP_{max} - PP_{min}/PP_{max} \times 100$

Table 6.1 (continued)

Name/ acronym	Definition	Measurement method	Explanation/calculation
Δup–Δdown		Invasive arterial cannula and standard monitor	Difference between maximal SAP and SAP at end-expiratory pause
ΔPOP	Pulse oximeter plethysmograph (POP) amplitude variation	Masimo pulse oximeter	$POP_{max} - POP_{min}/POP_{max} \times 100$
PVI	Plethysmograph variability index	Masimo pulse oximeter	$PVI_{max} - PVI_{min}/PVI_{max} \times 100$
ΔVPeak	Respiratory variation in aortic blood flow peak velocity	Echocardiography	Pulsed Doppler during the respiratory cycle $(Vpeak_{max} - Vpeak_{min})/$ $[(Vpeak_{max} + Vpeak_{min})/2]$: ΔVpeak is measured as the average of three consecutive breaths
SDV	Stroke distance (SD) variation	Echocardiography	Systolic velocity integral variation over respiratory cycle $SD_{max} - SD_{min}/SD_{max} \times 100$
ΔIVCD	Inferior vena cava diameter (IVCD) variation	Echocardiography	Respiratory variation of IVCD $(IVCD_{max} - IVCD_{min})/$ $[(ICVD_{max+min})/2]$

6.2.4 Fluid Removal in AKI Children

Loop diuretics (LD) are the mainstay of pharmacological fluid removal therapy in infants and children undergoing cardiac surgery particularly after complex procedures when the risk of FO is increased [35]. Furthermore LD are needed for left and right ventricular failure (in order to decrease pulmonary and systemic venous congestion, ventricular filling pressures, and hypervolemia) [36]. Few literature exists about appropriate clinical use of diuretics (e.g., regarding intermittent intravenous doses or continuous infusion) in pediatric patients undergoing cardiac surgery. The commonly used LD in PICU are furosemide, ethacrynic acid (EA), bumetanide, and acetazolamide. High-dose IV furosemide was showed effective and safe for reducing FO in unstable post-cardiac surgery infants by van der Vorst et al. [37] Clinical effects of LD continuous infusion has recently been compared in 74 infants undergoing cardiac surgery [38]. This prospective randomized double-blinded study demonstrated that EA continuous infusion induces at postoperative day (POD) 0 a urine output (UO) significantly higher than furosemide (6.9 (3.3) vs. 4.6–2.3 mL/kg/h, respectively); lower doses of EA compared to furosemide (0.22 (0.13) mg/kg/h vs. 0.33 (0.19 mg/kg/h), respectively) were needed to achieve similar UO, and EA induced a significantly more negative FB at POD 0. A recent retrospective analysis showed that bumetanide continuous infusion is also a safe, potent, and effective diuretic in pediatric critically ill patients [39].

Patients with symptomatic FO in addition to severe AKI characterized by conventional indications for RRT initiation (hyperkalemia, uremia, acidosis) or with low probability of immediate response to pharmacological therapy should be urgently referred for RRT [40]. Although there are currently no clear indications on pediatric RRT start, in a recent retrospective study, Modem showed that an early start (2 days from PICU admission) was beneficial with respect to later timing [41]. Intervening prior to development of significant FO may be more clinically effective than attempting an aggressive fluid removal after a severe FO has developed [42].

6.3   Electrolyte Balance

6.3.1   Hypernatremia

Routine intravenous fluid choices in cardiac surgery children should be always supplemented with dextrose and sodium: consensus opinion in critically ill children is shifting toward isotonic intravenous fluids in the perioperative period to avoid hyponatremia, and the more ideal intravenous fluid choice to reduce the likelihood of hyperchloremic acidosis (due to intravenous normal saline) could be a dextrose-added lactated Ringer's solution. To be certain of making an adequate fluid choice, it should be recommended to daily monitor glucose and electrolytic levels [7]. After cardiac surgery children are prone to hypo- and hypernatremia—in case of free water repletion and dehydration, respectively—and to inappropriate secretion of antidiuretic hormone.

Hypernatremia is defined as a serum or plasma sodium greater than 150 mEq/L. The plasma tonicity is mainly due to sodium salts in the extracellular space. As a result, serum or plasma sodium is used as a surrogate for assessing tonicity:

$$\text{Plasma tonicity} = 2 \times \left[\text{Na}\right] + \left[\text{glucose}\left(\text{mg}/\text{dL}\right)/18\right].$$

Plasma tonicity is tightly regulated by the release of *antidiuretic hormone (ADH)* from the posterior pituitary promoting water retention and by *thirst-prompting water ingestion*. These homeostatic mechanisms are similar in adults and children, resulting in a normal range of plasma sodium between 135 and 145 mEq/L that does not vary by age.

Etiology—hypernatremia can be separated in three mechanisms:

- Water loss or hypotonic fluid loss that is not replaced. Sources of hypotonic body fluid losses include gastrointestinal fluids, dilute urine, and skin loss. Excessive urinary free water loss may be caused by disorders with impaired urinary concentration defects (e.g., diabetes insipidus).
- Inadequate water intake that fails to replace ongoing normal fluid losses will result in increases in hypernatremia.

- Excessive salt intake relative to water ingestion. After complex congenital heart surgery (CHS), hypernatremia can also occur from urinary water losses due to renal excretion of nonelectrolyte, non-reabsorbed solutes, such as mannitol or glucose (due to hyperglycemia). Iatrogenic causes of hypernatremia after CHS include the administration of sodium bicarbonate infusions for metabolic acidosis. Compared with older children and adults, infants and young children are at increased risk for hypernatremic hypovolemia because they have a higher ratio of surface area to volume, resulting in greater insensible water losses from the skin, and while their thirst mechanism is intact, they are unable to communicate their need for fluids. Clinical findings are generally manifested by neurological symptoms as water moves out of brain cells leading to cerebral contraction [43].

Management: In any child with significant volume depletion, first management steps should be directed toward ensuring cardiovascular stability. With the restoration of effective intra-arterial volume, the focus turns to providing enough free water to correct the hypernatremia. The volume of free water to be provided can be calculated using this formula:

$$\text{Free water deficit in liters} = \text{Total body water}\left(\text{TBW}\right) \times \left(\left[\text{current plasma Na} / 140\right] - 1\right).$$

Estimating the TBW as 60% of the child's weight in kilograms (0.6 L/kg) is a reasonable starting point for the purposes of calculating fluid replacement. Thus, in a 6 kg infant with a plasma sodium of 160, the free water deficit is (0.6 L/kg) × (6 kg) × ([160/140]−1) = 0.51 L or 510 mL. The **normal saline (0.9% saline)** is isotonic in patients with normal plasma sodium; however, it is a hypotonic fluid for children with hypernatremia and can be used as initial rehydration fluid in this setting. Enteral fluids including oral rehydration therapy are also typically hypotonic fluids. The recommended rate of correction **does not exceed a fall of sodium greater than 0.5 mEq/L per hour** (e.g., 10–12 mEq/L per day), due to the risk of cerebral edema [44].

6.3.2   Hyponatremia

Hyponatremia is defined as a serum or plasma sodium less than 135 mEq/L and is among the most common electrolyte abnormalities in children. Hyponatremia is caused by an imbalance in the body's handling of water, resulting in a relative deficit of effective plasma tonicity to TBW.

Etiology: Hyponatremia can be classified based on the patient's volume status, and within each category, the release of ADH may be appropriate or inappropriate.

- Hyponatremia with hypovolemia secondary to gastrointestinal or skin or losses, or diuretic therapy, induces ADH release, which is a physiologic response to maintain circulating volume. Most pediatric cases of hyponatremia are due to hypovolemic conditions that are associated with an appropriate elevation in ADH, which leads to hyponatremia.

- Hyponatremia with normovolemia due to inappropriate excess of ADH activity.
- Hyponatremia with hypervolemia is less common and is typically seen in conditions associated with reduced effective circulating volume and renal failure (due to decreased renal perfusion and stimulation of the renin-angiotensin-aldosterone axis resulting in low urinary sodium excretion, both of which contribute to a decrease in plasma sodium).

Other causes include the syndrome of inappropriate ADH secretion (SIADH), which typically occurs in normovolemic patients and is associated with several clinical conditions (pulmonary and oncologic disorders, recent surgery, central nervous system injury or infection, endocrine disorders). The presence and severity of clinical manifestations correlate with the degree of hyponatremia and its rate of decline. The range of findings varies from no symptoms (especially in patients with chronic hyponatremia, defined as duration greater than 24 h) to severe neurologic symptoms (e.g., seizure and coma) [45].

Management: Treatment of hyponatremia consists of correcting hyponatremia with one or more interventions including fluid restriction, administration of sodium chloride, and treatment of the underlying etiology.

The recommended rate of correction **must not exceed an increase of 8 mEq/L over a 24-h** period. Overly rapid correction can cause *osmotic demyelination syndrome* resulting in diffuse demyelination in the brain and the development of profound irreversible neurologic symptoms [46].

6.3.3 Hyperkalemia

Hyperkalemia is usually defined as a serum or plasma potassium greater than 5.5 mEq/L.

Etiology—Hyperkalemia is caused by derangements of the normal hemostatic mechanisms that regulate potassium balance and is due to one or a combination of the following mechanisms:

- Large increase in potassium intake. This may occur infrequently due to the infusion of parenteral nutrition or massive transfusion.
- Transcellular movement of intracellular potassium into the extracellular space can cause hyperkalemia due to either cellular injury (e.g., rhabdomyolysis, severe hemolysis) or significant shift of potassium seen in patients with metabolic acidosis or diabetic ketoacidosis.
- Decreased renal excretion of potassium is the most common cause of persistent hyperkalemia (e.g., renal disease, decreased activity to the renin-aldosterone system).
- Pseudohyperkalemia is common because hemolyzed specimens are often observed due to difficulties in obtaining blood samples, especially in infants.

Most children with hyperkalemia are asymptomatic as they have mild (serum or plasma potassium <6 mEq/L) or moderate elevations (potassium between 6 and 7 mEq/L). Clinical manifestations in children with severe hyperkalemia (potassium level > 7 mEq/L) include muscle weakness, paralysis, and cardiac conduction abnormalities.

Hyperkalemia is associated with significant and potentially life-threatening disturbances in cardiac conduction. Electrocardiographic changes reflect the impact of increasing levels of serum and plasma potassium on the electrical activity of the heart including aberrant atrial (P wave), ventricular (QRS complex) depolarization, and abnormal repolarization (T wave) [47].

Management—for patients with severe hyperkalemia (>7 mEq/L [mmol/L]) or those with lower potassium values and electrocardiographic changes indicative of hyperkalemia (e.g., peaked T waves), it is recommended administering rapid transient therapeutic interventions. These include the following:

- Slow infusion of **calcium gluconate 10%** solution at a dose of 0.5 mL/kg (maximum dose 20 mL [2 g]).
- Therapy to shift extracellular potassium into cells including (1) intravenous administration of regular **insulin and glucose** and/or (2) inhaled beta-adrenergic agonists, such as salbutamol.
- **Sodium bicarbonate** also causes transcellular potassium movement, but its beneficial effect is uncertain. As a result, it is not recommended the use of sodium bicarbonate as the sole intervention to shift potassium intracellularly.
- **Diuretics and cation exchange resin** are used in patients with persistent, moderately elevated potassium (5.5–6.5 mEq/L [mmol/L]) and as adjuncts for those with more severe hyperkalemia.
- **Dialysis** therapy is reserved for patients with persistent hyperkalemia who are unresponsive to diuretic or cation exchange therapy. In general, hemodialysis is the preferred modality to reduce potassium levels, as it is the quickest and most controlled renal replacement treatment [48].

6.3.4 Hypokalemia

Hypokalemia is defined as a serum or plasma potassium that is less than the normal value: most reference laboratories establish the lower pediatric limit of normal serum potassium between 3 and 3.5 mEq/L. However, symptoms are unlikely to occur in most healthy children until serum potassium is below 3 mEq/L.

Etiology—hypokalemia is due to one or a combination of the following mechanisms:

- Decreased potassium intake.
- Increased intracellular movement of potassium, which is called redistributive hypokalemia and is due to the following mechanisms:

- Either respiratory or metabolic alkalosis can be associated with hypokalemia. Intracellular potassium movement is promoted to maintain electroneutrality as hydrogen ions exit the cell in response to the increase in extracellular pH. In general, serum potassium concentration falls by less than 0.4 mEq/L for every 0.1 unit rise in pH.
- Insulin promotes intracellular potassium movement by increasing the activity of the Na-K-ATPase pump and is used therapeutically to treat severe hyperkalemia.
- Elevated beta-adrenergic activity or beta-adrenergic agonists.
- Excessive loss of potassium via the gastrointestinal tract (especially diarrhea), kidney (increased urinary potassium loss), or skin.

Manifestations of hypokalemia include severe muscle weakness, cardiac arrhythmias, renal abnormalities, and glucose intolerance. The risk of arrhythmias from hypokalemia is highest in patients with organic heart disease, on digoxin or antiarrhythmic drugs [49].

Management: For symptomatic patients with hypokalemia (arrhythmias, marked muscle weakness, or paralysis), potassium supplementation must be administered. In those who are unable to take oral medications, this requires intravenous (IV) administration of potassium chloride. In this setting, an infusion with a **potassium concentration of no more than 40 mEq/L is given at a rate not to exceed 0.5–1 mEq/kg of body weight per hour**. Pain and phlebitis can occur during parenteral infusion of potassium into a peripheral vein. This primarily occurs at rates above 10 mEq/h but can be seen at lower rates.

The goal is to raise the potassium level by 0.3–0.5 mEq/L. These patients require continuous ECG monitoring to detect changes due to hypokalemia and also possibly rebound hyperkalemia during replacement therapy. In asymptomatic patients, the need for potassium supplementation is based on the underlying cause and the severity of hypokalemia.

Oral potassium preparations include potassium chloride, potassium bicarbonate or its precursors (potassium citrate, potassium acetate), and potassium phosphate. Potassium chloride can be given in crystalline form (salt substitutes), as a liquid, or in a slow-release tablet or capsule. Potassium bicarbonate or its precursors are preferred in patients with hypokalemia and metabolic acidosis. Potassium phosphate should be considered only in patients with hypokalemia and hypophosphatemia [50].

6.3.5 Hypercalcemia

Calcemia is defined as a serum calcium level greater than 12 mL/dL. Within the plasma, calcium circulates in different forms. Of the plasma calcium, roughly 40% is bound to albumin; 15% is complexed with citrate, sulfate, or phosphate;

and 45% exists as the physiologically important ionized (or free) calcium. As routinely measured in the laboratory, the plasma calcium concentration includes all of the calcium in the plasma (free and bound). In general, measuring the total plasma calcium concentration is sufficient since changes in this parameter are usually associated with parallel changes in the ionized concentration. Exceptions to this commonly occur in patients with hypoalbuminemia, acid-base disorders, and chronic kidney disease (e.g., decreased serum albumin concentration will lower the total calcium concentration without affecting the ionized calcium concentration).

Most of the body calcium, as well as much of the body phosphate, exists in bone as hydroxyapatite ($Ca_{10}[PO4]_6[OH]_2$). Bone is a calcium reservoir that is involved in maintaining a normal plasma ionized calcium concentration; this process depends upon the activity of osteoblasts and osteoclasts, which are regulated by many hormones and proteins, including parathyroid hormone (PTH) and vitamin D. Only ionized (free, non-protein-bound) calcium is filtered by the glomerulus. It is estimated that 97–99% of the filtered calcium is reabsorbed in subsequent segments of the nephron.

The serum calcium concentration is regulated by multiple hormonal pathways including PTH, vitamin D, fibroblast growth factor 23 (FGF-23), calcitonin, and estrogen. PTH is released from the parathyroid chief cells, due to calcium-sensing receptor which continuously senses the serum ionized calcium concentration; this classic negative endocrine feedback loop allows for an increase in PTH secretion as serum ionized calcium decreases. Vitamin D promotes calcium and phosphorus absorption from the gastrointestinal tract. Calcitonin plays a less critical role in calcium homeostasis and acts by decreasing bone resorption by osteoclasts.

Etiology—The most common causes are:

- Increased bone resorption (e.g., hyperparathyroidism due to parathyroid hormone (PTH)-mediated activation of osteoclasts, malignancy, and thyrotoxicosis).
- Increased calcium absorption (e.g., increased calcium intake in preterm infants receiving total parenteral nutrition, hypervitaminosis A or D, milk alkali syndrome, chronic kidney diseases.
- Miscellaneous causes (rhabdomyolysis, lithium, thiazide diuretics, theophylline toxicity, adrenal insufficiency) [51].

Management: Therapy for mild and moderate hypercalcemia (Ca < 12 mg/dL and Ca 12–14 mg/dL, respectively) does not require immediate treatment. However, it is recommended to avoid volume depletion and thiazide diuretics. Severe hypercalcemia (Ca > 14 mg/dL) includes a three-pronged approach: (1) **volume expansion** with normal saline that is adjusted to maintain an adequate urine output, in association with furosemide in case of renal failure or heart failure, (2) **salmon-calcitonin**, and (3) **zoledronic acid or pamidronate** [52].

6.3.6 Hypocalcemia

Physiologic hypocalcemia refers to a reduction in the concentration of serum ionized calcium, which is closely related to the total calcium concentration. However, the relationship may vary in setting of abnormal albumin concentrations, pathologic pH, or blood transfusions (see above).

The normal ranges after 12 months of age are established as the following ranges: ionized calcium 4.6–5.2 mg/dL (or 1.2–1.3 mmol/L) and total calcium 8.5–10.5 mg/dL (or 2.1–2.6 mmol/L).

Etiology—Causes of hypocalcemia include:

- Neonatal hypocalcemia as occurs within 72 h of life, related to maternal factors (maternal diabetes), prematurity or fetal growth restriction, concurrent illness (e.g., sepsis, hyperbilirubinemia), or iatrogenic factors (e.g., bicarbonate, inadequate calcium intake).
- Cases of persistent hypocalcemia should be investigated (e.g., PTH levels) and usually are due to (i) vitamin D insufficiency or high phosphate intake.
- Low PTH (genetic mechanisms, e.g., DiGeorge syndrome, CATCH-22 syndrome, or autoimmune mechanisms).
- High PTH (e.g., hypovitaminosis D, hepatic or renal dysfunction, end-organ resistance to PTH).
- Miscellaneous (sepsis, hyperphosphatemia, hypomagnesemia, pancreatitis) [53]. Management: In asymptomatic infants, providing adequate Ca intake is suggested by initiating early feedings, if possible, or parenteral nutrition. In addition, any underlying disorder resulting in a low Ca value should be corrected. In symptomatic patients, it is recommended to provide initial parenteral Ca therapy as a **10% Ca gluconate solution at a dose of 100 mg/kg** or 1 mL/kg [54].

6.3.7 Hypermagnesemia and Hypomagnesemia

The kidney is crucial in maintaining the normal plasma magnesium concentration. In contrast to most other filtered solutes, only 10% of filtered magnesium is absorbed in the proximal tubule; most (50–70%) of the filtered magnesium is passively reabsorbed in the cortical aspect of the thick ascending limb of Henle. Loop resorption is appropriately diminished with magnesium loading, thereby allowing the excess magnesium to be excreted in the urine. Hypermagnesemia is primarily seen in the following settings:

- Renal insufficiency (plasma magnesium levels rise as renal function declines since there is no magnesium regulatory system other than urinary excretion).
- Magnesium infusion: hypermagnesemia commonly occurs when parenteral magnesium is used.
- Magnesium enemas: substantial quantities of magnesium can be absorbed from the large bowel following a magnesium enema.

- Miscellaneous causes: primary hyperparathyroidism, diabetic ketoacidosis, and tumor lysis syndrome.
- Management:

Most cases of symptomatic hypermagnesemia can be prevented by anticipation. Patients in renal failure should **not** receive magnesium-containing medications, and patients receiving parenteral magnesium for any reason should be monitored at least daily. If renal function is normal, **cessation of magnesium therapy** will allow prompt restoration of normal magnesium levels. In addition, loop (or even thiazide) diuretics can be used to increase renal excretion of magnesium.

In patients with chronic kidney disease (CKD) and also in patients with mild acute kidney injury (AKI), initial treatment consists of therapy with intravenous **isotonic fluids** (e.g., normal saline) plus a loop diuretic, in addition to cessation of magnesium-containing medications.

Dialysis may be required in patients with severe or symptomatic hypermagnesemia who have advanced CKD or who have moderate to severe AKI. Since preparation for hemodialysis often takes a long time, patients with symptomatic hypermagnesemia should be given intravenous calcium as a magnesium antagonist to reverse the neuromuscular and cardiac effects of hypermagnesemia. The usual dose is 100–200 mg of elemental calcium over 5–10 min [55].

The most common etiology of **hypomagnesemia** in newborns is transient, although rare disorders of intestinal and/or renal tubular magnesium transport can occur. In these cases, serum magnesium concentration typically is 0.8–1.4 mg/dL (0.33–0.58 mmol/L) (normal values are 1.6–2.8 mg/dL [0.66–1.16 mmol/L]).

Hypomagnesemia causes resistance to PTH and impairs PTH secretion, both of which can result in hypocalcemia. For the correction of the hypomagnesemia, magnesium sulfate solution is suggested: the dose ranges from 25 to 50 mg/kg IV over at least 2 h [56].

6.3.8 Hyperphosphatemia and Hypophosphatemia

The maintenance of calcium and phosphate homeostasis involves intestinal, bone, and renal handling of these ions.

In comparison to calcium, plasma phosphorus exists in both organic and inorganic forms, including phospholipids, ester phosphates, and inorganic phosphates. Inorganic phosphates are completely ionized, circulating primarily as HPO_4^{2-} or $H_2PO_4^-$ in a ratio of 4:1 at a plasma pH of 7.40.

Only a small fraction of the total body calcium and phosphate is located in the plasma. However, it is the plasma concentrations of ionized calcium and inorganic phosphate that are under hormonal control. Phosphorous balance, as calcium, is also primarily regulated by PTH but may also respond to fibroblast growth factor 23 (FGF-23) which promotes renal excretion of phosphorous and other phosphatonins and active vitamin D (calcitriol). The physiologic roles of other hormones (such as calcitonin and estrogens) in the regulation of calcium and phosphate balance are incompletely understood.

In contrast to the complete absorption of dietary sodium, potassium, and chloride in the gastrointestinal tract, the absorption of calcium and phosphate is incomplete due to two factors: activated vitamin D is required for intestinal calcium absorption, and calcium combines with certain anions in the intestinal lumen to form insoluble salts that are not absorbed.

Regulation of Plasma Phosphate Concentrations: although bone release and gut absorption are important in establishing the filtered load of phosphate, it is the *renal threshold for phosphate reabsorption in the proximal tubule* that is most important in determining the steady state serum phosphate concentration. In addition, although acute cellular uptake of phosphate may transiently reduce serum levels (such as might occur following acute episodes of respiratory alkalosis), steady state concentrations are most dependent upon rates of renal reabsorption:

- Low dietary phosphate intake or low serum phosphate levels increase both synthesis and insertion of transporters, leading to the almost complete reabsorption of phosphate.
- Conversely, PTH and FGF-23, the two dominant phosphaturic hormones, act by increasing phosphate excretion and lowering the plasma phosphate concentration. Thus hypocalcemia stimulates PTH release, causing secondary phosphaturia. The mechanisms by which high phosphate intake and high serum phosphate levels lead to changes in phosphatonins, active vitamin D, and FGF-23 remain uncertain [57].

Hyperphosphatemia is typically related to acute or chronic renal failure. Phosphate excretion can be increased by saline infusion if renal function is intact. Hemodialysis is often indicated in patients with hypocalcemia, particularly if renal function is impaired.

True hypophosphatemia can be induced by decreased net intestinal absorption, increased urinary excretion, renal replacement therapy, or acute movement of extracellular phosphate into the cells (the measurement of urinary phosphate excretion is useful for the differential diagnosis).

Phosphate repletion is recommended when a serum phosphate is less than 2 mg/dL (0.64 mmol/L). If the serum phosphate is 1.0–1.9 mg/dL, oral phosphate is suggested (the dose is 1 mmol/kg in three to four doses over a 24-h period). If the serum phosphate is less than 1.0 mg/dL, intravenous phosphate is suggested (the dose varies depending upon the severity of the hypophosphatemia ranges from 0.08 to 0.50 mmol/kg) [58].

Conclusions

Much work is yet to be performed in pediatric critical care setting and, specifically, in pediatric cardiac surgery as far as fluid management is concerned. As a matter of fact, current literature is mostly retrospective and likely biased in patients' selection. However, some final recommendations can be made. The choice of administered fluids is likely important, even if HA is commonly administered in clinical practice; regarding crystalloids, balanced crystalloids should be preferred. The overall amount of postsurgical fluids should be limited, especially when FB cannot be managed adequately. A fluid excess over 5% of the body weight is considered harmful for pulmonary, cardiac, and renal function, and early pharmacological and dialytic strategies in order to keep it under this level should not be delayed. Electrolytes can be deeply affected through multiple pathways in critically ill children undergoing CHS, and their serum concentrations have to be strictly monitored, and careful treatment has to be implemented.

References

1. Hanart C, Khalife M, De Ville A, et al. Perioperative volume replacement in children undergoing cardiac surgery: albumin versus hydroxyethyl starch 130/0.4. Crit Care Med. 2009;37:696–701.
2. Aubron C, Bellomo R. Infusion of hydroxyethyl starch-containing fluids. Minerva Anestesiol. 2013;79(9):1088–92.
3. Van der Linden P, De Ville A, Hofer A, et al. Six percent hydroxyethyl starch 130/0.4 (Voluven®) versus 5% human serum albumin for volume replacement therapy during elective open-heart surgery in pediatric patients. Anesthesiologica. 2013;119:1296–309.
4. Van der Linden P, Dumolin M, Van Lerberghe C, et al. Efficacy and safety of 6% hydroxyethyl starch 130/0.4 (Voluven) for perioperative volume replacement in children undergoing cardiac surgery: a propensity-matched analysis. Crit Care Med. 2015;19(1):87–97.
5. Sümpelmann R, Kretz FJ, Gäbler R, et al. Hydroxyethyl starch 130/0.42/6:1 for perioperative plasma volume replacement in children: preliminary results of a European Prospective Multicenter Observational Postauthorization Safety Study (PASS). Paediatr Anaesth. 2008;18(10):929–33.
6. Akkucuk FG, Kanbak M, Ayhan B, et al. The effect of HES (130/0.4) usage as the priming solution on renal function in children undergoing cardiac surgery. Ren Fail. 2013;35(2):210–5.
7. Carcillo JA. Intravenous fluid choices in critically ill children. Curr Opin Crit Care. 2014;20(4):396–401.
8. Shaw AD, Bagshaw SM, Goldstein SL, et al. Major complications, mortality, and resource utilization after open abdominal surgery: 0.9% saline compared to plasma-lyte. Ann Surg. 2012;255:821–9.
9. Seguin J, Albright B, Vertullo L, et al. Extent, risk factors and outcome of fluid overload after pediatric heart surgery. Crit Care Med. 2014;42(12):2591–9.
10. Hazle MA, Gajarski RJ, Sunkyung Y, et al. Fluid overload in infants following congenital heart surgery. Pediatr Crit Care Med. 2013;14:44–9.
11. Hassinger AB, Wald EL, Goodman DM. Early postoperative fluid overload precedes acute kidney injury and is associated with higher morbidity in pediatric cardiac surgery patients. Pediatr Crit Care Med. 2014;15:131–8.
12. Sinitsky L, Walls D, Nadel S, et al. Fluid overload at 48 hours is associated with respiratory morbidity but not mortality in a general PICU: retrospective cohort study. Pediatr Crit Care Med. 2015;16:205–9.
13. Arikan AA, Zappitelli M, Goldstein SL, et al. Fluid overload is associated with impaired oxygenation and morbidity in critically ill children. Pediatr Crit Care Med. 2012;13:253–8.
14. Upadya A, Tilluckdharry L, Muhalidharan V, et al. Fluid balance and weaning outcomes. Intensive Care Med. 2005;31(12):1643–7.
15. Cooper DS, Costello JM, Bronicki RA, et al. Current challenges in cardiac intensive care: optimal strategies for mechanical ventilation and timing of extubation. Cardiol Young. 2008;18(Suppl 3):72–83.
16. Goldstein SL, Somers MJ, Baum MA, et al. Pediatric patients with multi-organ dysfunction syndrome receiving continuous renal replacement therapy. Kidney Int. 2005;67:653–8.

17. Sutherland SM, Zappitelli M, Alexander SR, et al. Fluid overload and mortality in children receiving continuous renal replacement therapy: the prospective pediatric continuous renal replacement therapy registry. Am J Kidney Dis. 2010;55(2):316–25.
18. Bontant T, Matrot B, Abdoul H, et al. Assessing fluid balance in critically ill pediatric patients. Eur J Pediatr. 2015;174(1):133–7.
19. van Aspereen Y, Brand PL, Bekhof J. Reliability of the fluid balance in neonates. Acta Paediatr. 2012;101(5):479–83.
20. Brierley J, Carcillo JA, Choong K, et al. Clinical practice parameters for hemodynamic support of pediatric and neonatal septic shock: 2007 update from the American College of Critical Care Medicine. Crit Care Med. 2009;37:666–88.
21. Foland JA, Fortenberry JD, Warshaw BL, et al. Fluid overload before continuous hemofiltration and survival in critically ill children. A retrospective analysis. Crit Care Med. 2004;32:1771–6.
22. Gan H, Cannesson M, Chandler JR, et al. Predicting fluid responsiveness in children: a systematic review. Anesth Analg. 2013;117:1380–92.
23. Byon HJ, Lim CW, Lee JH, et al. Prediction of fluid responsiveness in mechanically ventilated childen undergoing neurosurgery. Br J Anaesth. 2013;110(4):586–91.
24. Raux O, Spencer A, Fesseau R, et al. Intraoperative use of transesophageal Doppler to predict response to volume expansion in infants and neonates. Br J Anaesth. 2012;108(1):100–7.
25. Singer M, Bennett ED. Non invasive optimization of left ventricular filling using esophageal doppler. Crit Care Med. 1991;19(9):1132–7.
26. Tibby SM, Hatherill M, Durward A, et al. Are transesophageal Doppler parameters a reliable guide to paediatric haemodynamic status and fluid management? Intensive Care Med. 2001;27:201–5.
27. Renner J, Broch O, Duetschke P, et al. Prediction of fluid responsiveness in infants and neonates undergoing congenital heart surgery. Br J Anaesth. 2012;108:108–15.
28. Chandler JR, Cooke E, Hosking M, et al. Volume responsiveness in children, a comparison of static and dynamic variables. In: Proceedings of the IARS 2011, Annual meeting: S-200; 2011.
29. Pereira de Souza Neto E, Grousson S, Duflo F, et al. Predicting fluid responsiveness in mechanically ventilated children under general anesthesia using dynamic parameters and transthoracic echocardiography. Br J Anaesth. 2011;106:856–64.
30. Renner J, Broch O, Gruenewald M, et al. Non-invasive prediction of fluid responsiveness in infants using pleth variability index. Anaesthesia. 2011;66:582–9.
31. Durand P, Chevret L, Essouri S, et al. Respiratory variations in aortic blood flow predict responsiveness in ventilated children. Intensive Care Med. 2008;34:888–94.
32. Choi DY, Kwak HJ, Park HY, et al. Respiratory variation in aortic blood flow velocity as a predictor of fluid responsiveness in children after repair of ventricular septal defect. Pediatr Cardiol. 2010;31:1166–70.
33. Lee JH, No HJ, Kim HS, et al. Prediction of fluid responsiveness using a non-invasive cardiac output monitor in children undergoing cardiac surgery. Br J Anaesth. 2015;29:1–7.
34. Weber T, Wagner T, Neumann K, et al. Low predictability of three different noninvasive methods to determine fluid responsiveness in critically ill children. Pediatr Crit Care Med. 2015;16:e89–94.
35. Ricci Z, Iacoella C, Cogo P. Fluid management in critically ill pediatric patients with congenital heart disease. Minerva Pediatr. 2011;63:399–410.
36. Felker GM, Kerry LL, Bull DA, et al. Diuretic strategies in patients with acute decompensated heart failure. N Engl J Med. 2011;364:797–805.
37. van der Vorst MM, van Heel Ruys-Dudok I, Kist-van Holthe JE, et al. Continuous intravenous furosemide in haemodynamically unstable children after cardiac surgery. Intensive Care Med. 2001;27:711–5.
38. Ricci Z, Haiberger R, Pezzella C, et al. Furosemide versus ethacrynic acid in pediatric patients undergoing cardiac surgery: a randomized controlled trial. Crit Care. 2015;19:2.
39. McCallister KM, Chhim RF, Briceno-Medina M, et al. Bumetanide continuous infusions in critically ill pediatric patients. Pediatr Crit Care Med. 2015;16:e19–22.

40. Goldstein S, Bagshaw S, Cecconi M, et al. Pharmacological management of fluid overload. Br J Anaesth. 2014;113:756–63.
41. Modem V, Thompson M, Gollhofer D, et al. Timing of continuous renal replacement therapy and mortality in critically ill children. Crit Care Med. 2014;42:943–53.
42. Selewski D, Cornell TT, Blatt NB, et al. Fluid overload and fluid removal in pediatric patients on extracorporeal membrane oxygenation requiring continuous renal replacement therapy. Crit Care Med. 2012;40:2694–9.
43. Forman S, Crofton P, Huang H, et al. The epidemiology of hypernatraemia in hospitalised children in Lothian: a 10-year study showing differences between dehydration, osmoregulatory dysfunction and salt poisoning. Arch Dis Child. 2012;97(6):502–7.
44. Fang C, Mao J, Dai Y, et al. Fluid management of hypernatraemic dehydration to prevent cerebral oedema: a retrospective case control study of 97 children in China. J Paediatr Child Health. 2010;46(6):301–3.
45. Choong K, Arora S, Cheng J, et al. Hypotonic versus isotonic maintenance fluids after surgery for children: a randomized controlled trial. Pediatrics. 2011;128(5):857–66.
46. Sterns RH, Hix JK, Silver S. Treatment of hyponatremia. Curr Opin Nephrol Hypertens. 2010;19(5):493–8.
47. Masilamani K, van der Voort J. The management of acute hyperkalaemia in neonates and children. Arch Dis Child. 2012;97(4):376–80.
48. Kim M, Somers MJG. Fluid and electrolyte physiology and therapy. In: McMillan JA, DeAngelis CD, Feigin RD, editors. Oski's pediatrics. 4th ed. Baltimore: Lippincott Williams and Wilkins; 2006. p. 54.
49. Mount DB, Zandi-Nejad K. Disorders of potassium balance. In: Brenner BM, editor. Brenner and rector's the kidney. Philadelphia: WB Saunders Co; 2008. p. 547.
50. Rose BD, Post TW. Hypokalemia. In: Rose BD, Post TW, editors. Clinical physiology of acid-base and electrolyte disorders. 5th ed. New York: McGraw-Hill; 2001. p. 836.
51. Maier JD, Levine SN. Hypercalcemia in the intensive care unit: a review of pathophysiology, diagnosis, and modern therapy. J Intensive Care Med. 2015;30(5):235–52.
52. Bilezikian JP. Management of acute hypercalcemia. N Engl J Med. 1992;326(18):1196–203.
53. Marx SJ, Bourdeau JE. Calcium metabolism. In: Maxwell MH, Kleeman CR, Narins RG, editors. Clinical disorders of fluid and electrolyte metabolism. 4th ed. New York: McGraw-Hill; 1987.
54. Thomas TC, Smith JM, White PC, Adhikari S. Transient neonatal hypocalcemia: presentation and outcomes. Pediatrics. 2012;129(6):e1461–7.
55. Greenberg MB, Penn AA, Whitaker KR, et al. Effect of magnesium sulfate exposure on term neonates. J Perinatol. 2013;33(3):188–93.
56. Mordes JP, Wacker WE. Excess magnesium. Pharmacol Rev. 1977;29(4):273.
57. Blaine J, Chonchol M, Levi M. Renal control of calcium, phosphate, and magnesium homeostasis. Clin J Am Soc Nephrol. 2015;10(7):1257–72.
58. Bergwitz C, Jüppner H. Phosphate sensing. Adv Chronic Kidney Dis. 2011;18(2):132–44.

Nutrition Management: Parenteral and Enteral Nutrition and Oral Intake

7

Piyagarnt Vichayavilas and Laura Kashtan

Abstract

Infants and children with congenital heart disease are contended with growth challenges. The causes are multifactorial and contributed by hypermetabolism, poor feeding, limited tolerance to feeding, and iatrogenic caloric deficits from procedural interruptions and fluid volume restriction that are inherent in the intensive care unit. Providing enteral and parenteral nutrition support, with attentive surveillance to nutrition delivery, can mitigate growth faltering in this population.

7.1 Introduction

Malnutrition is a well-known consequence of congenital heart disease [1–7]. Inadequate energy intake and delivery are present in both the preoperative [8] and postoperative phase [4, 9–14]. Intake often remains insufficient with resulting 20–74% of patients requiring assisted feeding device, for either partial or full gavage feeds upon hospital discharge [11, 15–21]. For families, this is a stressful component of care [22, 23]. Even when intake appears adequate for age, growth faltering may still persist [24]. In the hospital setting, malnutrition increases the risk of infection [20, 25] and length of hospital stay [4, 20, 26]. After discharge, the effects of malnutrition can persist into the social environment, with links to impaired

P. Vichayavilas (✉) · L. Kashtan
Department of Clinical Nutrition, Children's Hospital Colorado,
Aurora, CO, USA
e-mail: Piyagarnt.Vichayavilas@childrenscolorado.org;
laura.kashtan@childrenscolorado.org

© Springer International Publishing AG, part of Springer Nature 2019
S. F. Flocco et al. (eds.), *Congenital Heart Disease*,
https://doi.org/10.1007/978-3-319-78423-6_7

cognitive ability [27, 28] and arithmetic performance [29], reduced motor skills [19], and increased behavioral problems [28].

With advancements in technology, expertise, and postoperative care, children with complex heart disease are now expected to survive. Decreasing morbidity and improving quality of life are emerging indicators of an institution's success [30, 31]. Passive acceptance of growth failure is being replaced by appraising how to manage these complex nutritional needs to improve outcome. Growth and feeding are often impeded by a unique set of nutrition challenges: hemodynamic instability, concern for mesenteric compromise, fluid overload, tachypnea, hypermetabolism, vocal cord injury, neurological dysfunction, chylous effusion, protein-losing enteropathy, and other genetic syndromes that may hamper nutrition provision. Arbitrating these heterogeneous nutrition demands with appropriate enteral and parenteral nutrition support, combined with careful surveillance of nutrition delivery and weight gain, is a modifiable intervention that can positively affect outcome.

7.2 Energy

Reports on energy requirements in infants and children with congenital heart disease have varied. Both normal and hypermetabolism have been discussed [9, 32–37]. Some reports have been on total energy expenditure (TEE), while others have been on resting energy expenditure (REE). The difference is important to note (Fig. 7.1) because the interpretation exerts an important role when assessing energy requirement for nutrition support of a critically ill child.

In adults, energy requirement (ER) is the predicted average energy intake needed for the maintenance of energy balance and health defined by age, gender, weight and height, and physical activity [38]. Total energy expenditure (TEE) is the amount of energy spent in a typical day. Thus in energy balance, in non-pregnant and non-lactating adults, ER = TEE.

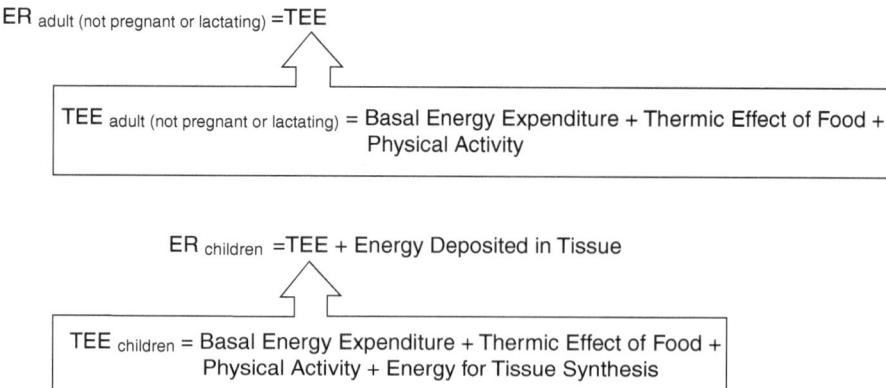

$ER_{\text{adult (not pregnant or lactating)}} = TEE$

$TEE_{\text{adult (not pregnant or lactating)}}$ = Basal Energy Expenditure + Thermic Effect of Food + Physical Activity

$ER_{\text{children}} = TEE$ + Energy Deposited in Tissue

TEE_{children} = Basal Energy Expenditure + Thermic Effect of Food + Physical Activity + Energy for Tissue Synthesis

Fig. 7.1 Components of energy requirement in adults and children

However, in children, additional calories are needed to support growth—energy required for tissue synthesis (a component of TEE) and also the energy that is deposited in those tissues: ER = TEE + energy deposited in tissue [39]. Therefore, energy intake minus TEE is the "spare energy" available for weight gain. Some studies have shown that this "spare energy" is lower in children with congenital heart disease either due to insufficient intake to make up for increased energy demand [40], higher cost of physical activity [41], or caloric loss from vomiting [42].

Growth is an energy-consuming process. Neonates and young children are at exceptional risk for malnutrition due to low reserves and greater energy demand per kilogram body weight. Caloric requirements for growth are high during the first 3 months of life, 35% of TEE (40% during the first month) and drop to 3% at 12 months of age [38, 39]. The early months of life thus present a sensitive time during which energy deficits can have significant growth consequences.

7.3 Nutrition Support

Energy requirements vary throughout the course of critical illness. Energy needs do not correlate well with diagnosis or severity of illness, and clinicians often fail to correctly predict the degree of altered metabolism [43, 44]. As over- and underfeeding are both deleterious, and predictive equations often failing to accurately calculate resting energy expenditure [9, 43, 45–49], the gold standard is to use indirect calorimetry to prevent unbalanced caloric delivery [50]. In the absence of the device or the child not meeting criteria for this testing, calculated REE is the alternative (examples of some equations are in Table 7.1). REE, whether derived from predictive equations or obtained via indirect calorimetry measurement, is insufficient to promote growth (compare REE to TEE in Tables 7.1 and 7.2 below). Care must be taken to not extrapolate REE to TEE or to daily energy requirement as this underestimates total energy required for growth [51].

Evaluating the advancement of nutrition support and growth of a critically ill child requires knowledge of the different phases of critical illness: acute, stable, and recovery phase. The acute phase is characterized by the requirement for, or

Table 7.1 Common predictive equations for calculating resting energy expenditure

Formula	Age (years)	Equation Male	Female
WHO [52]	0–3	$(60.9 \cdot W_{kg}) - 54$	$(61.0 \cdot W_{kg}) - 51$
	3–10	$(22.7 \cdot W_{kg}) + 495$	$(22.5 \cdot W_{kg}) + 499$
	10–18	$(17.5 \cdot W_{kg}) + 651$	$(12.2 \cdot W_{kg}) + 746$
Schofield [53]	0–3	$(0.167 \cdot W_{kg}) + (15.174 \cdot H_{cm}) - 617.6$	$(16.252 \cdot W_{kg}) + (10.232 \cdot H_{cm}) - 413.5$
	3–10	$(19.59 \cdot W_{kg}) + (1.303 \cdot H_{cm}) + 414.9$	$(16.969 \cdot W_{kg}) + (1.618 \cdot H_{cm}) + 371.2$
	10–18	$(16.25 \cdot W_{kg}) + (1.372 \cdot H_{cm}) + 515.5$	$(8.365 \cdot W_{kg}) + (4.655 \cdot H_{cm}) + 200.0$

Table 7.2 Energy requirement for healthy children, FAO/WHO/UUN Joint Commission[a]

Age		Male, kcal/kg			Female, kcal/kg		
		Total energy expenditure[b,c]	Energy deposited in tissue	Daily energy requirement	Total energy expenditure[d,e]	Energy deposited in tissue	Daily energy requirement
Infant	0–1 month	66.8	46.1	113	65.7	40.9	107
	1–2 months	70.5	33.3	104	69.3	31.3	101
	2–3 months	72.8	22.1	95	71.5	23.0	95
	3–4 months	74.2	7.6	82	73.2	10.6	84
	4–5 months	75.3	6.0	81	74.3	8.2	83
	5–6 months	76.0	4.5	81	75.1	6.4	81
	6–7 months	76.6	2.0	79	75.7	2.6	78
	7–8 months	77.0	1.9	79	76.2	2.1	78
	8–9 months	77.4	1.6	79	76.7	1.8	78
	9–10 months	77.8	2.3	80	77.0	2.1	79
	10–11 months	78.0	2.2	80	77.3	1.7	79
	11–12 months	78.3	2.3	81	77.6	1.6	79
Toddler and adolescent	1–2 years	81.2	1.2	82	78.8	1.3	80
	2–3 years	82.7	0.8	84	79.6	0.9	81
	3–4 years	79.0	0.8	80	75.8	0.7	77
	4–5 years	76.2	0.6	77	73.3	0.6	74
	5–6 years	73.9	0.6	74	71.0	0.5	72
	6–7 years	71.9	0.6	72	68.7	0.6	69
	7–8 years	70.0	0.6	71	66.0	0.7	67
	8–9 years	67.9	0.6	69	63.1	0.8	64
	9–10 years	66.0	0.6	67	60.0	0.8	61
	10–11 years	63.9	0.7	65	57.1	0.7	58
	11–12 years	61.8	0.7	62	54.2	0.6	55
	12–13 years	59.5	0.7	60	51.4	0.6	52
	13–14 years	57.3	0.7	58	48.8	0.5	49
	14–15 years	55.0	0.6	56	46.6	0.4	47
	15–16 years	52.9	0.5	53	45.1	0.2	45
	16–17 years	51.2	0.4	52	44.3	0.1	44
	17–18 years	50.1	0.2	50	44.1	0	44

[a]Adapted from Joint FAO/WHO/UUN Expert Consultation, human energy requirements, Tables 3.2, 4.2, and 4.3 [39]

[b]TEE, male, 0–12 months, $-99.4 + (88.6 \cdot W_{kg})$

[c]TEE, male, 1–18 years, $310.2 + (63.3 \cdot W_{kg}) - (0.263 \cdot W_{kg^2})$

[d]TEE, female, 0–12 months, $-99.4 + (88.6 \cdot W_{kg})$

[e]TEE, female, 1–18 years $263.4 + (65.3 \cdot W_{kg}) - (0.454 \cdot W_{kg^2})$

escalation of, vital organ support [32]. Growth is suspended as energy is used to fuel the stress response [34]. Overfeeding may worsen clinical outcome and not attenuate any weight loss. The practice of applying a stress factor to REE is discouraged during the acute phase of critical illness. However, adequate protein should be provided: 3–4 g/kg for low birth weight infants, 2–3 g/kg for term neonates, and 1.5 g/kg for older children [54]. Jaksic and colleagues reported that stressed neonates on extracorporeal life support (ECLS)—an extremely catabolic intervention—did not demonstrate elevated REE compared to hemodynamically stable, TPN-fed, non-ventilated surgical neonates [34]. Providing caloric excess in patients on ECLS has been reported to increase protein turnover, resulting in a more net negative nitrogen balance [55]. Teixeira-Cintra et al. reported that in ventilated young children (63% were on neuromuscular blockade) who underwent cardiac surgery, delivery of at least 55 kcal/kg and 1 g/kg protein is associated with anabolism [56]. It is so far inconclusive whether hypermetabolism is present post cardiopulmonary bypass (CPB). One study reported that bypass increases REE (CPB, 74 kcal/kg; no CPB, 68 kcal/kg), while another reported no difference between children undergoing bypass compared to those not needing bypass surgery. This could be related to the time of measurement as REE is elevated immediately after bypass surgery and decreases with time from bypass [9, 57]. When the acute phase subsides, with commencement of the stable and recovery phase, this marks the time when aggressive nutrition support is indicated [32]. Additional calories should be added to support recovery and promote growth. Depending on requirement, at this time REE × 1.3–2 is recommended [32]. Estimated energy requirement per age (Table 7.2) can also be used. Again, this is a starting point as these energy requirements were derived from healthy children and may not be appropriate for children with complex nutritional needs.

Children with congenital heart disease often need more calories than their age-matched counterpart. In children with hypoplastic left heart syndrome (HLHS), it is recommended to advance feeds to a goal of 100–120 kcal/kg, utilizing feeding concentrations between 24 and 27 kcal/oz, with subsequent adjustments if weight gain is under 20–30 g/day [58, 59]. The presence of hypermetabolism appears to depend on whether there is concomitant congestive heart failure or pulmonary hypertension [24, 37]. Caloric requirements up to 150 kcal/kg have been reported in some children. This elevated energy need normalizes after surgery, with reported REE comparable to healthy children at 1 week, 3 months, and 6 months after surgery [60–62]. Subsequent catch-up growth is seen in some children [62, 63]. For those with significant growth deficits, continued high caloric delivery should be continued to provide energy for accelerated growth until target weight is achieved.

7.4 Enteral and Parenteral Nutrition

In the cardiac intensive care unit, various factors compete with the delivery of adequate nutrition. Hemodynamic instability, concern for intestinal hypoperfusion, electrolyte abnormalities, fluid volume limitations, and interruptions for procedures are common instances that may preclude or minimize advancement to full and sustained nutrition delivery. In the preoperative phase, it is common for caregivers to hold enteral therapy while a child is receiving prostaglandin due to the concern for intestinal hypoperfusion, despite little evidence to support this practice. Howley and colleagues reported that 56% of respondents in the United States and 9% of those internationally surveyed withheld enteral therapy in prostaglandin-dependent neonates [64]. A small number of studies have demonstrated the safety of enteral feeding on prostaglandin. Toms and colleague reported no case of necrotizing enterocolitis in a group of patients with HLHS receiving low volume feeds [20]. Natarajan et al. reported that out of 52 patients on PGE, 100 mL/kg was achieved in 75% of patients, and 29% reached full feeds before surgery, with one case of NEC that occurred in a patient with HLHS [18], a known risk factor for NEC [65, 66]. Feeding prostaglandin-dependent infants remain controversial and not fully elucidated. However, it appears that enteral feeding prostaglandin-dependent infants is safe in some cases and can be initiated in those who are hemodynamically stable [67].

In cases where enteral feeding is hazardous, especially in infants with single ventricle heart defects, parenteral nutrition should be started early [67, 68]. Children in the intensive care unit are known to not meet their nutrition requirements [4, 9, 11–14] and accumulate substantial feeding interruptions for tests, procedures, deterioration in medical status, and gastrointestinal intolerances [14]. These cumulative deficits are associated with declines in weight-for-age (WAZ) and arm circumference z-scores [69]. Starting parenteral nutrition early is a reasonable intervention to lessen the consequence of short-term and long-term malnutrition. In the short term, malnutrition and poor weight gain have been shown to increase the risk of postoperative infection [20], increase need for prolonged respiratory support [70], and increase length of hospital stay [20, 26]. Low WAZ has also been shown to increase mortality at 1 year of age [70], increase length of hospital stay after bidirectional Glenn [71, 72], and increase risk of infection after Fontan procedure [73]. Providing adequate calories via parenteral nutrition is thus a modifiable intervention that may diminish the effect of malnutrition in this fragile population.

However, parenteral nutrition is not without liability, and care must be taken to balance the risks and benefits of this nutrition therapy. A recent multinational study showed that withholding parenteral nutrition for 7 days reduced the amount of time spent on the ventilator, risk for central line infection, and the need for renal replacement therapy [74]. It is not evident whether the delay in provision of parenteral nutrition poses growth consequences in neonates that rely on intravenous nutrition. Reducing morbidity and improving growth in the intensive care unit are not competing interests but rather interventions that should coincide. Institution-based feeding protocols have been shown to improve nutrition delivery [75] and decrease the incidence of NEC [75, 76]. Guidelines that detail criteria for parenteral nutrition support and advancement of enteral nutrition may help focus parenteral nutrition to only those who depend on it while minimizing exposure to those who may not benefit from IV nutrition support.

7.5 Necrotizing Enterocolitis, Chylous Effusion, and Feeding Device

The high incidence of feeding and gastrointestinal complication in children with HLHS, and their disproportionate utilization of nutrition-related resources, warrants a separate discussion regarding common nutrition considerations post stage 1 palliation. The incidence of NEC in children with congenital heart disease is between 0.3 and 7% [65, 77–80]. For children with single ventricle heart defects, the risk increases to 7.6–18%. NEC is a rare but serious complication with reported mortality rate between 19 and 38% [65, 81–83]. Children who have lower weight or gestational age [65, 82, 83] exhibit cardiac failure [78, 79], are diagnosed with HLHS, truncus arteriosus or aortopulmonary window, or have other single ventricle heart defects are at increased risk for NEC [65, 77]. The mechanism is not thoroughly understood but is thought to be related to impaired mesenteric perfusion [76, 84, 85], opposed to the feeding of an immature gut in preterm and very low birth weight neonates.

In the neonatal literature, human milk feeding rather than infant formula is associated with the prevention of NEC [86, 87]. However, this has not been verified in children with congenital heart disease. In this population, it does not appear that type of feed (breastmilk, standard or hydrolyzed formula) is protective against NEC [76, 81]. When diagnosed, medical NEC is treated with 7–14 days bowel rest, gastric decompression, broad-spectrum antibiotics, and parenteral nutrition support. Surgical NEC involves laparotomy and resection of perforated or necrotic tissue. Parenteral nutrition is the modality of nutrition support while enteral feeds are held. Feeding protocols have been described to decrease the incidence of NEC [75, 76]; however, there are no published guidelines for enteral nutrition support post-medical or surgical treatment of NEC in children with congenital heart disease. It seems reasonable to resume feeding per institution-based guidelines with close monitoring of feeding tolerance.

Chylothorax is another well-recognized complication after cardiothoracic surgery. Conservative management with dietary modification, with or without concurrent non-surgical medical management, is often sufficient [88–91] (Table 7.3). In the case of protracted chylous drainage, surgical therapy is the next course of treatment.

Table 7.3 Chylous effusion, nutrition intervention

| Type | Enteral nutrition | | Parenteral nutrition |
	Formula	Breastmilk	
Infant to toddler	• ↑MCT ↓LCT infant formula • Nonfat formula if needed[a]	• Fortified defatted human milk with additional formula as needed • Not recommend defatted human milk without fortification	• Standard parenteral nutrition per age • Continue to provide IV lipids (no restrictions)
Toddler to adolescent	• ↑MCT ↓LCT pediatric or adult formula • Nonfat formula if needed[a] • Low fat diet	Not applicable	• Standard parenteral nutrition per age • Continue to provide IV lipids (no restrictions)
Vitamin and supplement	• Consider additional vitamin D per age • If on nonfat formula or nonfat diet, provide water-soluble fat-soluble vitamin	• Consider additional vitamin D per age • Consider water-soluble fat-soluble vitamin if low volume delivery	Standard IV dosing per age

[a]Monitor biochemical markers or signs of essential fatty acid deficiency

Nutrition management begins with a high medium-chain/low long-chain triglyc-eride (↑MCT/↓LCT) diet. Since MCTs are absorbed and transported through the portal vein rather than the lacteals, this dietary modification should minimize the contribution of flow through the thoracic duct. For infants receiving breastmilk or formula, therapy includes (1) fortified-defatted human milk mixture [92, 93], (2) ↑MCT/↓LCT formula [88–91], or (3) both. Due to the large contribution of fat in human milk, volume yield and caloric concentration are significantly reduced after the fatty layer is skimmed off—10–13 kcal/oz [92, 94]. Thus a combination of fortified-defatted human milk, with supplemental ↑MCT/↓LCT formula, is often necessary to return adequate volume for daily intake. For children and adolescents who are not receiving formula, a low fat diet is recommended. Added MCTs can provide supplementary calories, but it will not serve as an essential fatty acid (EFA) source.

There is no consensus to what constitutes a low fat diet. There is also no agree-ment on the duration of modified diet therapy. Reports of a successful therapy course between 10 days and 6 weeks have been documented [88–91, 95, 96]. When considering this dietary intervention, caution is advised to ensure that adequate long-chain fat be delivered. It would be reasonable to prescribe a diet that meets at least the minimum requirements for these long-chain fats to prevent EFA deficiency.

Linoleic Acid (LA) and α-Linolenic (ALA) are long-chain fats; they are considered essential because they cannot be synthesized by humans and must be sourced through the diet. The American Society for Parenteral and Enteral Nutrition (ASPEN) recommends 2–4% of total calories from LA and 0.25–0.5% from ALA [97]. The Institute of Medicine (IOM) recom-mends 4.4–4.6 g/day LA and 0.5 g/day ALA for infants, and 10–16 g/day LA and 1–1.6 g/kg ALA for children and adolescents [38].

In the case where a very reduced fat or a nonfat diet is trialed, it is prudent that the duration of therapy be minded. Since some dietary fat is required for the absorp-tion of fat-soluble vitamins, consider supplementation with a water-soluble formu-lation of fat-soluble vitamins when intake of fat is minimal. Without any fat, infants can show biochemical signs of EFA deficiency within 1 week [98] and 2–4 weeks in children and adults [99, 100]. Intravenous lipids should be considered during a prolonged course of fat absent diet to prevent the development of EFA deficiency. Enteral therapy should be trialed first. When dietary therapy fails, full parenteral nutrition is recommended.

These complications can contribute to the delay in progression of oral feeds. Twenty to 74% of patients require an assisted feeding device for either partial or full gavage feeds upon hospital discharge. The incidence is higher in children with single ventricle physiology, up to one-half to three-fourths of cases requiring tube feeding support [11, 15–21]. Some studies have shown that increased risk adjust-ment for congenital heart surgery (RACHS-1) score and longer ventilator time is associated with feeding failure [11, 19]. Children with congenital heart disease are often discharged at a WAZ lower than their admit score (Δ, −1.0 to −1.5) [13, 17, 25, 101]. Poor postoperative growth, delayed postoperative nutrition, hemodynamically significant AV valve regurgitation, long postoperative ventilation time, and requirement of additional central venous line have been associated with decreased WAZ [17, 25]. This may reflect a sicker group of patients susceptible to growth failure despite efforts paid to improve nutrition delivery, and the placement of a feeding tube itself may not sufficiently mitigate weight loss [17]. Involvement of an interdisciplinary care that includes feeding therapists and dietitians may help with the early identification of patients with feeding failure and with consequent interventions that may improve weight gain and decrease the length of hospital stay.

Conclusion

Children with congenital malformed hearts have a tradition of expected growth delay. Present-day, poor growth is no longer regarded as unavoidable. While some remain malnourished and do continue to have gastrointestinal and feeding complications, many are able to grow normally. At a time when increasing interest is paid to decreasing morbidity and improving quality of life, vigilance to nutrition and growth is an integral part of care that can have a positive impact on the child's recovery from the intensive care unit and provides continued support for his/her development.

References

1. Cameron JW, Rosenthal A, Olson AD. Malnutrition in hospitalized children with congenital heart disease. Arch Pediatr Adolesc Med. 1995;149(10):1098–102.
2. Mitchell IM, et al. Nutritional status of children with congenital heart disease. Br Heart J. 1995;73(3):277–83.
3. Okoromah CA, et al. Prevalence, profile and predictors of malnutrition in children with congenital heart defects: a case-control observational study. Arch Dis Child. 2011;96(4):354–60.
4. Toole BJ, et al. Perioperative nutritional support and malnutrition in infants and children with congenital heart disease. Congenit Heart Dis. 2014;9(1):15–25.
5. Vaidyanathan B, et al. Malnutrition in children with congenital heart disease (CHD) determinants and short term impact of corrective intervention. Indian Pediatr. 2008;45(7):541–6.
6. Vaidyanathan B, et al. What determines nutritional recovery in malnourished children after correction of congenital heart defects? Pediatrics. 2009;124(2):e294–9.
7. Varan B, Tokel K, Yilmaz G. Malnutrition and growth failure in cyanotic and acyanotic congenital heart disease with and without pulmonary hypertension. Arch Dis Child. 1999;81(1):49–52.
8. Hansen SR, Dorup I. Energy and nutrient intakes in congenital heart disease. Acta Paediatr. 1993;82(2):166–72.
9. De Wit B, et al. Challenge of predicting resting energy expenditure in children undergoing surgery for congenital heart disease. Pediatr Crit Care Med. 2010;11(4):496–501.
10. Gebara BM, Gelmini M, Sarnaik A. Oxygen consumption, energy expenditure, and substrate utilization after cardiac surgery in children. Crit Care Med. 1992;20(11):1550–4.
11. Kogon BE, et al. Feeding difficulty in newborns following congenital heart surgery. Congenit Heart Dis. 2007;2(5):332–7.
12. Li J, et al. Energy expenditure and caloric and protein intake in infants following the Norwood procedure. Pediatr Crit Care Med. 2008;9(1):55–61.
13. Nicholson GT, et al. Caloric intake during the perioperative period and growth failure in infants with congenital heart disease. Pediatr Cardiol. 2013;34(2):316–21.

14. Schwalbe-Terilli CR, et al. Enteral feeding and caloric intake in neonates after cardiac surgery. Am J Crit Care. 2009;18(1):52–7.
15. Anderson JB, et al. Variation in growth of infants with a single ventricle. J Pediatr. 2012;161(1):16–21.e1; quiz 21.e2–3.
16. Davis D, et al. Feeding difficulties and growth delay in children with hypoplastic left heart syndrome versus d-transposition of the great arteries. Pediatr Cardiol. 2008;29(2): 328–33.
17. Medoff-Cooper B, et al. Weight change in infants with a functionally univentricular heart: from surgical intervention to hospital discharge. Cardiol Young. 2011;21(2):136–44.
18. Natarajan G, Reddy Anne S, Aggarwal S. Enteral feeding of neonates with congenital heart disease. Neonatology. 2010;98(4):330–6.
19. Sables-Baus S, et al. Oral feeding outcomes in neonates with congenital cardiac disease undergoing cardiac surgery. Cardiol Young. 2012;22(1):42–8.
20. Toms R, et al. Preoperative trophic feeds in neonates with hypoplastic left heart syndrome. Congenit Heart Dis. 2015;10(1):36–42.
21. Williams RV, et al. Factors affecting growth in infants with single ventricle physiology: a report from the pediatric heart network infant single ventricle trial. J Pediatr. 2011;159(6):1017–22. e2.
22. Stewart J, et al. Caregiver anxiety due to interstage feeding concerns. Congenit Heart Dis. 2015;10(2):E98–106.
23. Medoff-Cooper B, et al. Feeding, growth, and nutrition in children with congenitally malformed hearts. Cardiol Young. 2010;20(Suppl 3):149–53.
24. Menon G, Poskitt EM. Why does congenital heart disease cause failure to thrive? Arch Dis Child. 1985;60(12):1134–9.
25. Anderson JB, et al. Poor post-operative growth in infants with two-ventricle physiology. Cardiol Young. 2011;21(4):421–9.
26. Costello CL, et al. Growth restriction in infants and young children with congenital heart disease. Congenit Heart Dis. 2015;10(5):447–56.
27. Grantham-McGregor SM, Walker SP, Chang S. Nutritional deficiencies and later behavioural development. Proc Nutr Soc. 2000;59(1):47–54.
28. Dykman RA, et al. Behavioral and cognitive status in school-aged children with a history of failure to thrive during early childhood. Clin Pediatr (Phila). 2001;40(2):63–70.
29. Black MM, et al. Early intervention and recovery among children with failure to thrive: follow-up at age 8. Pediatrics. 2007;120(1):59–69.
30. Jacobs JP, Wernovsky G, Elliott MJ. Analysis of outcomes for congenital cardiac disease: can we do better? Cardiol Young. 2007;17(Suppl 2):145–58.
31. Tchervenkov CI, et al. The improvement of care for paediatric and congenital cardiac disease across the World: a challenge for the World Society for Pediatric and Congenital Heart Surgery. Cardiol Young. 2008;18(Suppl 2):63–9.
32. Joosten KF, Kerklaan D, Verbruggen SC. Nutritional support and the role of the stress response in critically ill children. Curr Opin Clin Nutr Metab Care. 2016;19(3):226–33.
33. Preiser JC, et al. Metabolic response to the stress of critical illness. Br J Anaesth. 2014;113(6):945–54.
34. Jaksic T, et al. Do critically ill surgical neonates have increased energy expenditure? J Pediatr Surg. 2001;36(1):63–7.
35. Coss-Bu JA, et al. Resting energy expenditure and nitrogen balance in critically ill pediatric patients on mechanical ventilation. Nutrition. 1998;14(9):649–52.
36. Jones MO, et al. The metabolic response to operative stress in infants. J Pediatr Surg. 1993;28(10):1258–62; discussion 1262–3.
37. Farrell AG, et al. Large left-to-right shunts and congestive heart failure increase total energy expenditure in infants with ventricular septal defect. Am J Cardiol. 2001;87(9):1128–31, A10.
38. Dietary reference intakes: the essential guide to nutrient requirements. Washington, D.C.: The National Academies Press; 2006.

39. Food and Agriculture Organization of the United Nations. Joint FAO/WHO/UUN Expert Consultation, Human energy requirements. 2004. http://www.fao.org/docrep/007/y5686e/y5686e00.htm#Contents. Reproduced with permission.
40. Leitch CA. Growth, nutrition and energy expenditure in pediatric heart failure. Prog Pediatr Cardiol. 2000;11(3):195–202.
41. Ackerman IL, et al. Total but not resting energy expenditure is increased in infants with ventricular septal defects. Pediatrics. 1998;102(5):1172–7.
42. van der Kuip M, et al. Energy expenditure in infants with congenital heart disease, including a meta-analysis. Acta Paediatr. 2003;92(8):921–7.
43. Mehta NM, et al. Cumulative energy imbalance in the pediatric intensive care unit: role of targeted indirect calorimetry. JPEN J Parenter Enteral Nutr. 2009;33(3):336–44.
44. Mehta NM, et al. Energy imbalance and the risk of overfeeding in critically ill children. Pediatr Crit Care Med. 2011;12(4):398–405.
45. Kaplan AS, et al. Resting energy expenditure in clinical pediatrics: measured versus prediction equations. J Pediatr. 1995;127(2):200–5.
46. Sentongo TA, et al. Resting energy expenditure and prediction equations in young children with failure to thrive. J Pediatr. 2000;136(3):345–50.
47. Vazquez Martinez JL, et al. Predicted versus measured energy expenditure by continuous, online indirect calorimetry in ventilated, critically ill children during the early postinjury period. Pediatr Crit Care Med. 2004;5(1):19–27.
48. Taylor RM, et al. Can energy expenditure be predicted in critically ill children? Pediatr Crit Care Med. 2003;4(2):176–80.
49. Coss-Bu JA, et al. Resting energy expenditure in children in a pediatric intensive care unit: comparison of Harris-Benedict and Talbot predictions with indirect calorimetry values. Am J Clin Nutr. 1998;67(1):74–80.
50. Mehta NM, Compher C, A.S.P.E.N. Board of Directors. A.S.P.E.N. Clinical Guidelines: nutrition support of the critically ill child. JPEN J Parenter Enteral Nutr. 2009;33(3):260–76.
51. Leitch CA, et al. Increased energy expenditure in infants with cyanotic congenital heart disease. J Pediatr. 1998;133(6):755–60.
52. Consultation, F.W.U.E. Energy and protein requirements. Estimates of energy and protein requirements of adults and children. 1985. http://www.fao.org/docrep/003/aa040e/AA040E06.htm#ch6.
53. Schofield WN. Predicting basal metabolic rate, new standards and review of previous work. Hum Nutr Clin Nutr. 1985;39(Suppl 1):5–41.
54. Agus MS, Jaksic T. Nutritional support of the critically ill child. Curr Opin Pediatr. 2002;14(4):470–81.
55. Shew SB, et al. The determinants of protein catabolism in neonates on extracorporeal membrane oxygenation. J Pediatr Surg. 1999;34(7):1086–90.
56. Teixeira-Cintra MA, et al. Monitoring of protein catabolism in neonates and young infants post-cardiac surgery. Acta Paediatr. 2011;100(7):977–82.
57. Floh AA, et al. Systemic inflammation increases energy expenditure following pediatric cardiopulmonary bypass. Pediatr Crit Care Med. 2015;16(4):343–51.
58. Hehir DA, et al. Feeding, growth, nutrition, and optimal interstage surveillance for infants with hypoplastic left heart syndrome. Cardiol Young. 2011;21(Suppl 2):59–64.
59. Schwarz SM, et al. Enteral nutrition in infants with congenital heart disease and growth failure. Pediatrics. 1990;86(3):368–73.
60. Irving SY, et al. Resting energy expenditure at 3 months of age following neonatal surgery for congenital heart disease. Congenit Heart Dis. 2013;8(4):343–51.
61. Trabulsi JC, et al. Total energy expenditure of infants with congenital heart disease who have undergone surgical intervention. Pediatr Cardiol. 2015;36(8):1670–9.
62. Nydegger A, et al. Changes in resting energy expenditure in children with congenital heart disease. Eur J Clin Nutr. 2009;63(3):392–7.
63. Hulst J, et al. Malnutrition in critically ill children: from admission to 6 months after discharge. Clin Nutr. 2004;23(2):223–32.

64. Howley LW, et al. Enteral feeding in neonates with prostaglandin-dependent congenital cardiac disease: international survey on current trends and variations in practice. Cardiol Young. 2012;22(2):121–7.
65. McElhinney DB, et al. Necrotizing enterocolitis in neonates with congenital heart disease: risk factors and outcomes. Pediatrics. 2000;106(5):1080–7.
66. Carlo WF, et al. Persistent diastolic flow reversal in abdominal aortic Doppler-flow profiles is associated with an increased risk of necrotizing enterocolitis in term infants with congenital heart disease. Pediatrics. 2007;119(2):330–5.
67. Medoff-Cooper B, Ravishankar C. Nutrition and growth in congenital heart disease: a challenge in children. Curr Opin Cardiol. 2013;28(2):122–9.
68. Slicker J, et al. Nutrition algorithms for infants with hypoplastic left heart syndrome; birth through the first interstage period. Congenit Heart Dis. 2013;8(2):89–102.
69. Hulst JM, et al. The effect of cumulative energy and protein deficiency on anthropometric parameters in a pediatric ICU population. Clin Nutr. 2004;23(6):1381–9.
70. Mitting R, et al. Nutritional status and clinical outcome in postterm neonates undergoing surgery for congenital heart disease. Pediatr Crit Care Med. 2015;16(5):448–52.
71. Anderson JB, et al. Lower weight-for-age z score adversely affects hospital length of stay after the bidirectional Glenn procedure in 100 infants with a single ventricle. J Thorac Cardiovasc Surg. 2009;138(2):397–404.e1.
72. Menon SC, et al. Clinical outcomes and resource use for infants with hypoplastic left heart syndrome during bidirectional Glenn: summary from the Joint Council for Congenital Heart Disease National Pediatric Cardiology Quality Improvement Collaborative registry. Pediatr Cardiol. 2013;34(1):143–8.
73. Anderson JB, et al. Low weight-for-age z-score and infection risk after the Fontan procedure. Ann Thorac Surg. 2011;91(5):1460–6.
74. Fivez T, et al. Impact of withholding early parenteral nutrition completing enteral nutrition in pediatric critically ill patients (PEPaNIC trial): study protocol for a randomized controlled trial. Trials. 2015;16:202.
75. Braudis NJ, et al. Enteral feeding algorithm for infants with hypoplastic left heart syndrome poststage I palliation. Pediatr Crit Care Med. 2009;10(4):460–6.
76. del Castillo SL, et al. Reducing the incidence of necrotizing enterocolitis in neonates with hypoplastic left heart syndrome with the introduction of an enteral feed protocol. Pediatr Crit Care Med. 2010;11(3):373–7.
77. Becker KC, et al. Necrotizing enterocolitis in infants with ductal-dependent congenital heart disease. Am J Perinatol. 2015;32(7):633–8.
78. Mukherjee D, et al. Outcomes analysis of necrotizing enterocolitis within 11 958 neonates undergoing cardiac surgical procedures. Arch Surg. 2010;145(4):389–92.
79. Cheng W, Leung MP, Tam PK. Surgical intervention in necrotizing enterocolitis in neonates with symptomatic congenital heart disease. Pediatr Surg Int. 1999;15(7):492–5.
80. Leung MP, et al. Necrotizing enterocolitis in neonates with symptomatic congenital heart disease. J Pediatr. 1988;113(6):1044–6.
81. Luce WA, et al. Necrotizing enterocolitis in neonates undergoing the hybrid approach to complex congenital heart disease. Pediatr Crit Care Med. 2011;12(1):46–51.
82. Weiss SL, et al. Comparison of gastrointestinal morbidity after Norwood and hybrid palliation for complex heart defects. Pediatr Cardiol. 2011;32(4):391–8.
83. Jeffries HE, et al. Gastrointestinal morbidity after Norwood palliation for hypoplastic left heart syndrome. Ann Thorac Surg. 2006;81(3):982–7.
84. Pickard SS, et al. Short- and long-term outcomes of necrotizing enterocolitis in infants with congenital heart disease. Pediatrics. 2009;123(5):e901–6.
85. Iannucci GJ, Oster ME, Mahle WT. Necrotising enterocolitis in infants with congenital heart disease: the role of enteral feeds. Cardiol Young. 2013;23(4):553–9.
86. Lucas A, Cole TJ. Breast milk and neonatal necrotising enterocolitis. Lancet. 1990;336(8730):1519–23.

87. Cristofalo EA, et al. Randomized trial of exclusive human milk versus preterm formula diets in extremely premature infants. J Pediatr. 2013;163(6):1592–1595 e1.
88. Biewer ES, et al. Chylothorax after surgery on congenital heart disease in newborns and infants—risk factors and efficacy of MCT-diet. J Cardiothorac Surg. 2010;5:127.
89. Milonakis M, et al. Etiology and management of chylothorax following pediatric heart surgery. J Card Surg. 2009;24(4):369–73.
90. Densupsoontorn NS, et al. Management of chylothorax and chylopericardium in pediatric patients: experiences at Siriraj Hospital, Bangkok. Asia Pac J Clin Nutr. 2005;14(2):182–7.
91. Cormack BE, et al. Use of Monogen for pediatric postoperative chylothorax. Ann Thorac Surg. 2004;77(1):301–5.
92. Fogg KL, et al. Feasibility and efficacy of defatted human milk in the treatment for Chylothorax after cardiac surgery in infants. Pediatr Cardiol. 2016;37(6):1072–7.
93. Lessen R. Use of skim breast milk for an infant with Chylothorax. ICAN Infant Child Adolesc Nutr. 2009;1(6):303–10.
94. Wang CD, et al. Creamatocrit and the nutrient composition of human milk. J Perinatol. 1999;19(5):343–6.
95. Katanyuwong P, Dearani J, Driscoll D. The role of pleurodesis in the management of chylous pleural effusion after surgery for congenital heart disease. Pediatr Cardiol. 2009;30(8):1112–6.
96. Panthongviriyakul C, Bines JE. Post-operative chylothorax in children: an evidence-based management algorithm. J Paediatr Child Health. 2008;44(12):716–21.
97. The A.S.P.E.N. pediatric nutrition support core curriculum. In: Corkins MR, editor. American Society for Parenteral and Enteral Nutrition: United States of America; 2010.
98. Tashiro T, et al. The effect of fat emulsion (Intralipid) on essential fatty acid deficiency in infants receiving intravenous alimentation. J Pediatr Surg. 1976;11(4):505–15.
99. Barr LH, Dunn GD, Brennan MF. Essential fatty acid deficiency during total parenteral nutrition. Ann Surg. 1981;193(3):304–11.
100. Goodgame JT, Lowry SF, Brennan MF. Essential fatty acid deficiency in total parenteral nutrition: time course of development and suggestions for therapy. Surgery. 1978;84(2):271–7.
101. Kaufman J, et al. Improved nutrition delivery and nutrition status in critically ill children with heart disease. Pediatrics. 2015;135(3):e717–25.

Respiratory Physiotherapy After Paediatric Cardiac Surgery: The Interaction between Physiotherapist, Nurse and Parent

8

Davide Girelli

Abstract

Technically, paediatric rehabilitation is not different from adult rehabilitation. The main difference consists in the possibility of establishing a verbal communication. This is difficult, if not impossible, in the paediatric patient since the abilities of verbal expression and comprehension are not completely developed, especially during the neonatal period.

The main purpose in the context of paediatric cardiac surgery is to guarantee the patient a better future quality of life. Recognizing the clinical conditions of rehabilitative interest and the management of anxiety and fears of the relatives of the young patients represents additional difficulties. The fundamental difference with the adult patient is that this one can communicate his or her own perceptions, fears, difficulties and hopes but even his or her own symptoms. So the keywords in the rehabilitative treatment of the newborn are *imagination and simplicity*. The treatment includes the aid in enforcing motoric planning and execution. In paediatric rehabilitation, *careful observation* is one of the central competences of the physiotherapist [1].

8.1 Respiratory Physiotherapy After Paediatric Cardiac Surgery

Right from the arrival in the cardiac paediatric surgery ward, the newborn-infant-child can be "mobilized" even in the presence of drainages, catheters and other devices [2].

D. Girelli
Pediatric and Adult Congenital Heart Centre, IRCCS Policlinico San Donato,
Milan, Italy

© Springer International Publishing AG, part of Springer Nature 2019   149
S. F. Flocco et al. (eds.), *Congenital Heart Disease*,
https://doi.org/10.1007/978-3-319-78423-6_8

In our operating unit, the term "mobilization" means:

- Lateral decubitus: a support is positioned behind the back, one between the legs and one under the head (if newborn, ties are fine).
- Prone posture: the head facing one side and the arms positioned in "reflex of the fencer", positioning a wedge under the abdomen if a slope position is needed.
- Leaning on parent's arms: the child can be held by the parents in the absence of chest drainages or if trained in executing this manoeuvre.
- Seated: obviously, it depends on the age; newborns must not be seated, not even at home.

The *early mobilization* in the child (even more than in the adult) is of main importance to prevent and, in some cases it's the only non-invasive method at disposition, to solve some of the most common complications after the cardiac surgery operation [3, 4].

At the beginning it is carried out from the technical staff (physiotherapists and nurses) and then it is explained to the parents so that they can realize these manoeuvres many times during the course of the day, defeating the typical post-operative fears like: "What if I break something in my child wound?" and "It is better for the child to stay still and motionless rather than hurting him/her". So they are actively involved in the post-operative caregiving.

Another advantage in the parent-child interaction is the greater ease for the child in trusting his or her parents instead of a stranger, often doing more willingly some exercises if it is the parent himself or herself to accompany and guide him or her in the execution [5].

Independently of the haemodynamic, the precautions are very few:

- Ensure the real length of the ways of infusion and drainages, so it is possible to understand how much the child can be safely moved.
- Do not stretch the child by the arms.
- Always hold with one hand the cervical region and the head of a newborn-infant during every move.
- Check the appearance of cyanosis and breath difficulties.

Parents are also thought and pushed to use on their own child some simple techniques of bronchial unblock (often useful even at home, after the dismissal):

- *Clapping and/or PEP bottle.* Clapping is a technique used to detach the secretions in the first bronchial branches. In order to accurately learn the technique, parents are made tapping their own hand or thigh. All this to understand how to dose the intensity and the frequency of the percussions.
- *Nebuliser administration.* Parents are explained how to administrate the nebuliser (and carry out the cleaning of the devices used) to their children in specific moments of the day, keeping the supply vial precisely sloping, following the movements and the vivacity of their children, or while they are sleeping.

- *Oxygen therapy and/or active humidifier administration.* The children submitted to oxygen therapy (generally administrated with nose pipes and/or active humidifier), administrated in cycles or continuously, during the ADL can be disconnected from it for periods concordated with the stuff so they can go on improving their recovery and tolerance to the effort represented by the ADL. Parents are taught the opening, setting and closing of the medical gas source.
- *Nasal washings.* The use of salt solution for the nasal washing constitutes one of the optimal strategies (simple practice and minimally invasive, simple to teach to parents) to fight phlogosis in the high breath ways (tolerability, safety, cheap) [6, 7].

8.2 Transcultural Assistance

It is a relatively new concept in Italy. Degree courses sporadically dedicate space to this topic. Therefore the majority of Italian operators are in the situation of assisting foreign patients without having the background and support of a theoretical conceptual knowledge. Such situation can often bring to unsuitableness and inadequacy of the assistance and a sense of impotence and frustration for the difficult communication with the patient and his or her relatives [8]. In our paediatric unit, an increasing number of foreign children and relatives find care: to face this situation, we had to provide ourselves new competences in the interpersonal relationships, with the aim of assisting people coming from a rich cultural variety [9].

For non-Italian speakers/parents, a specific paper multitranslation (Arabic, English, French, Chinese) was created. In this paper it is briefly explained who we are, what is our work and how they can actively contribute to the psychophysical recover of their child [10]. Parents are only indicated the sentence they have to read.

The choice of the topics inserted in the translations contemplated:

- The presentation and explanation of the physiotherapist and/or nurse's role
- The parents' involvement in the treatment of the child, even in the presence of chest drainages and venous infusions (with particular attention on the *mobilizzazione* in the several positions-decubitus, on strollers, chair, high chair, in arms, until the exit from the room to recover through the playful aspect a better psycho-motor posture), the nebuliser therapy in the newborn and in the child, the bronchial unblocking and the nasal washing and the cleaning, care and disinfection of the used devices

Satisfaction about this initiative was practically total. The comprehension of the text has always been optimal. Obtaining a good adherence to the treatment improves the quality of the treatment itself, but this depends on multiple psycho- and socio-cultural factors. Defeating, at least, the linguistic problem in the case of paediatric patients permitted us in having the needed collaboration with parents [11].

8.3   Nasal Washings

The use of salt solution for nasal washing constitutes one of the optimal strategies (simple practice and minimally invasive, simple to teach to parents) to fight phlogosis in the high breath ways (tolerability, safety, cheap) [12]. Generally a syringe is filled with physiological saline (usually 5 mL for nostril if newborn or infant) which has to be instilled in each nostril. Attention must be payed not to apply excessive pressure (not with the syringe nor with the hand) in order to avoid direct mechanic irritation and painful reactions. The solution must be injected if not at body temperature (in the rear part of the nose, temperature reaches 27–30 °C), at least lukewarm.

The necessary equipment and sequence of execution are syringe, physiological sterile saline, bandages and towel to wrap the baby and contain his or her movements [13], and the procedure is:

- Prepare the necessary equipment.
- Create a favourable context for the tranquillity of the baby in order to reduce inconvenience.
- It might be appropriate to wrap the baby in a little towel to limit his or her movements.
- Position the baby laterally (on one side), possibly with the head slightly lower than the shoulders and slightly rotated downwards. The position is fundamental to guarantee the passage of the solution from one nostril to the other and so the removal of mucus.
- If the baby is in left lateral position, introduce the syringe in the right nostril at 90° compared with the face of the baby and push the physiological saline.
- Lift slightly the head of the baby to calm him or her down and/or get him/her prone and/or hold him or her.
- Clean the nose with bandages-handkerchief or draw.
- Once the baby is calm, repeat the operation in the other nostril positioning the baby on the opposite side.

8.4   Physical Therapy Techniques: Airway Clearance Therapies in the Acute Setting

Airway clearance methods are dependent on the disease process. The question arises as to what is appropriate in airway clearance in an acute disease process. The use of the appropriate airway clearance therapy in the acute setting appears to depend on the patient condition and physiotherapist preference. The common thought process with most paediatric clinicians is that "it cannot hurt, maybe it can help", but is this actually true? Studies have shown that airway clearance therapy is associated with decreased oxygen saturation, gastroesophageal reflux, fractured ribs, raised intracranial pressure and even brain injury. Selection of a best technique is currently more of an art than a science and depends greatly on the patient's underlying condition, level of functioning and understanding and ability and willingness to perform the technique and integrate it into normal daily routines [14].

There still can be uncertainty in the identification of the most suitable drain technique for the single patient because there are not studies scientifically highlighting the superior efficiency of a technique than another one in newborns or preschool children. In the little child (with insufficient ability to search for cough and expectorate), we use postural drainage with percussions and compressions since the pulmonary physiology of the child is different from that of an adult, and the chest wall is very elastic. Consequently, there is a higher effect of the percussions in children than in adults [15].

With advancing age, respiratory physiotherapy changes; the child, growing, can collaborate, and he or she can be taught techniques that direct him or her towards self-sufficiency. Training to the use of the *PEP Bottle* can begin and also training to other techniques which uses the positive expiratory pressure (on the level of the mouth) during exhale and, for that reason, very useful in case of important instability of the airway (instable bronchial walls are very simple to compress during exhaling) and the ACBT [16].

8.5 Conventional Chest Physiotherapy (C-CPT)

Traditional CPT has four components: postural drainage, percussions, chest wall vibrations and coughing [14].

8.5.1 Postural Drainage (Old Concept)

Postural drainage uses gravity to facilitate movement of secretions from peripheral airways to the larger bronchi where they are more easily expectorated [3, 6, 7]. The clinician places the patient in various positions designed to drain specific segments of the lung. If necessary, the patient may be supported by rolled towels, blankets or pillows. There are studies of the multiple variations of this technique [17]. Postural drainage can be performed with or without percussion or vibration. When accompanied by percussion or vibration, each position is maintained for 1–5 min, depending on the severity of the patient's condition. When percussion or vibration is omitted, longer periods of simple postural drainage can be performed [18].

8.5.2 Turning and Positioning

Alterations in position serve to redistribute ventilation, aid in gravitational movement of secretions towards the large airways and can foster gas-liquid pumping [19]. The benefits of frequent turning are often masked by patient decompensation during and after positioning. Increased perfusion and decreased ventilation to the dependent lung are more pronounced in small patients. Their high chest wall compliance can increase the difficulty of expanding the dependent lung. The chest wall is also more difficult to stabilize under gravitational pressure [14]. This same mechanism, however, allows for enhanced ventilation to the lung positioned up. Secretion removal in the nondependent lung is supported by increased lung recruitment, allowing for larger expiratory volume and faster flow. Small airway calibre in the lung positioned uppermost is also increased. Gravity can then assist in moving secretions through larger airways conducting higher flows [19].

8.5.3   Percussions or Tapping

Percussion is thought to loosen secretions from the bronchial walls. While the patient is in the various postural drainage positions, the therapist percusses the chest wall with a cupped hand or fingers (infants). Clinicians should not percuss over bony prominences, the spine, sternum, abdomen, last few ribs, sutured areas, drainage tubes, kidneys, liver or below the rib cage. The ideal frequency of percussion is unknown; however, some reports recommend a frequency of 5–6 Hz, whereas others recommend slower, rhythmic clapping [18, 20]. Several devices can be used for percussion, including a soft facemask or a commercially designed "palm cup" or pneumatic or electromechanical percussor. Clinicians can perform percussion with the patient positioned in various places, including their lap with infants and small children. Appropriate care must be taken to perform the therapy, allowing for the most comfort for the patient and the least amount of risk [7, 21].

8.5.4   Chest Wall Vibrations

Vibrations are an additional method of transmitting energy through the chest wall to loosen or move bronchial secretions. Unlike percussion, the therapist's hand or device does not lose contact with the chest wall during the procedure [7]. Vibrations can be performed by placing both hands (one over the other) over the area to be vibrated and tensing and contracting the shoulder and arm muscles while the patient exhales. To prolong exhalation, the patient may be asked to breathe through pursed lips. Like percussion, the ideal frequency is unknown, although some recommend 10–15 Hz [22], which can be difficult to achieve manually. It is unclear how well clinicians are able to perform vibrations effectively [21].

8.6   Active Cycle of Breath Techniques (ACBT)

Active cycle is the most used technique in Great Britain, proposed by two English therapists, J. Pryor and B. Webber, and can be considered the evolution of the forced expiration technique (TEF) [23].

It consists in a set of respiratory exercises focussed on the bronchial unblocking. The active cycle requires the use of several breathing modalities. In the practice the cycle includes:

- *Breath control.* Breath control (BC) is considered a fundamental part of the cycle, used to permit relaxation and avoid the outbreak of bronchospasm. It consists of a calm breathing executed with the high part of the chest; its duration is variable for each patient. Inhalation through the nose and expiration through pursed lips (pursed lips breathing) are taught.
- *Expansion of the chest exercises.* The exercises for the expansion of the chest (TEE) consist of deep and long inhalations followed by a teleinspiratory pause of 2–3 s and then by calm expirations. An increase of the volume of the air in the lungs is obtained, and it simplifies the activation of collateral ventilation, bringing, in this way, air behind the secretions and simplifying their removal.
- *Forced expiration technique.* The forced expiration technique (FET or *Huffing*) consists of one or two manoeuvres of forced expiration starting from a deep inhalation to facilitate the mobilization of the secretions from the most proximal airway. When the secretions reach the trachea, they can be expelled by coughing. These manoeuvres are always followed by the breath control to avoid the outbreak of bronchospasm.

The small-long huff: this will move sputum from low down in the chest. Take a small to medium breath in and then huff (squeeze) the air out until the lungs feel quite empty, as detailed above.

The big-short huff: this moves sputum from higher up in the chest, so use this huff when it feels ready to come out, but not before. Taking a deep breath in and then huff the air out quickly. This should clear the sputum without coughing.

How long should I do ACBT? Continuous exercises for about 10 min ideally until the chest feels clear of sputum.

What position should I do ACBT? The best position to do the ACBT will depend on medical condition and how well it works for the patient. It can be done in sitting or in a postural drainage position.

8.7   PEP Bottle or Blowing Bottle

The mode of action is based on an obstacle to the emission of air from the mouth that is on a respiratory load [24–26].

8.7.1   Mode of Action

Back pressure in expiratory phase opposes the physiological tendency to the reduction of the airway calibre and permits a more protracted expiration. At the same time, collateral ventilation is activated so the air can pass through the alternative ways bypassing the obstruction. In this way, it moves the secretions from the periphery to the central areas, where secretions are expelled with the FET or cough. This takes place with the same volume as the current one and makes this method accessible even to non-cooperating patients.

Aims of the treatment:

- Treat pulmonary periphery inaccessible in other ways.
- Recruit-re-expand the obstructed pulmonary periphery.
- Push the secretions from the periphery to the central airway.

PEP bottle or positive expiratory pressure through the bottle is a device consisting of a stream expiratory modulator, represented with a rubber tube 80 cm long (es. suction hose) and with a diameter of 1 cm inserted in a bottle (es. physiological of 500 mL) containing 6–8 cm of water that catches from the bottom of the bottle.

This device is based on the application of a resistance to the expiration directly proportional to the quantity of water and to the length and diameter of the tube, generating a positive pressure inside the airway during the whole expiratory phase.

8.7.2   Anatomo-physiological Principles of Functioning

- The possibility of removing the bronchial secretions of the distal airway taking advantage of the collateral ventilation, that is, ventilating and expanding the breathing units taken after the obstruction, allowing the secretions movement towards the proximal airway, where they can be eliminated through coughing and consequently enabling the expansion of the pulmonary atelectasis periphery and the recovery of its gaseous exchanges.
- The possibility of avoiding the interruption of expiratory streams in the airway with instable walls, avoiding or delaying the bronchial collapse, thanks to a more proximal movement of the moment of appearance of the point of equal pressure (EPP).
- The bubbles created by the expiration have a vibrating effect on the airway facilitating the detachment of secretions and an immediate feedback to the patient of the correct use of the device.

8.7.3   Indications

Bronchial unblocking and pulmonary re-expansion.

8.7.4   Mode of Administration

- Conscious and cooperating patient.
- The patient must inhale through the nose, maintain a 3-s inspiratory apnoea and execute an active non-forced expiration through the tube, with his or her lips well tightened, with the formation of little bubbles, concentrating on its duration more than on its entity.

- Five to ten consecutive breaths are repeated for 10–20 min three or four times a day, or if a single session lasts 5 min, it must be repeated six/eight times a day.
- The exercise can be done seated or in lateral decubitus; the training is usually done seated with the elbows laying on a flat surface.
- Depending on the effort felt by the patient during the execution, resistance can be increased or diminished, lifting or bringing towards the bottom the tube of the bottle.
- The ease and immediacy of the use represent particular features of the system.

8.7.5 Maintenance

It is important to daily replace the water and clean the tube. Do not place it near windows or under direct sunlight.

8.8 EZ-PAP

"Ez-PAP" (read "Easy-PAP") is a therapeutic device for the application of a positive pressure to the airways (PAP) during the entire breath cycle. It is a device for single patient use, realized in plastic material that, taking advantage of some physical principles, can multiply up to four times the oxygen flow or compressed air in entrance. The entrance flow can vary from 5 to 15 L/min, with pressure levels generated from the device that reach 20 cm H_2O. It is necessary to control the PAP with the help of a pressure gauge, to make sure that pressure does not become negative during the inhalation [27, 28].

8.8.1 Indications

- Pulmonary re-expansion (non-ventilated or atelectasis areas)
- Bronchial unblocking to patients with hypersecretion, combined with other techniques such as breath exercises, huffing and coughing (preventing atelectasis outbreak)

The Ez-PAP device could be used in association with a nose clip, if the person can bear it. In case of a non-cooperating patient, it is possible to replace the mouthpiece with a ventilation mask applied in the oronasal region of the subject, making sure that there are no aerial losses on the sides of the mask.

8.8.2 Mode of Administration

- *Mouthpiece* associated with a *nose clip* if the patient cooperates and can execute the entire breath cycle only oral uptake. Make sure that he or she keeps his or her lips tight to the mouthpiece.

- *Oronasal mask* in case of non-cooperating patient or with difficulties in breathing through the mouthpiece.
  Regulate the gas flow in entrance on 5 L/min and examine the generated PAP.
  Increase the flow depending on the pressures that the clinician wants to obtain and/or on the tolerance of the patient.
- *Mainly unblocking aim*: each session is composed of four/five cycles each of 2 min, followed by a half minute pause in which the patient must execute dosed exhalations and/or huffing and cough to remove secretions. The number of cycles for each session depends on the tolerance of the patient. The sessions can be repeated up to five/six times a day.
- *Mainly re-expansive aim*: each session includes several cycles, depending on the tolerance of the patient; each one lasts about 10 min, followed by a half minute pause in which the patient must execute the techniques of *mobilizzazione* of the secretions mentioned in the previous point. The sessions should be repeated every 2 h.

In both cases the patient should preferably be in seated position, but the position must be adapted to the clinical conditions and to the possibilities of the subject, assuring in any case the best possible thoracic expansion. It is suggested to use a PAP between 5 and 15 cm H2O. Execute the sessions far from meals (in case of newborns and children, it is suitable to execute these sessions before meals) [29].

8.9   Manual Hyperinflations

It is a technique used when the alteration affects the inhalation phase. It increases the efficiency of the cough helping the inhalation (increasing the inhalation ability, the amount of expelled air grows) through the application of a positive pressure to the airway, through non-invasive prosthesis (generally facial masks) or invasive (endotracheal tube or tracheostomy pipe), manually (Ambu ball or Mapleson circuit) [30].

- Facilitate inhalation by gradually insufflating greater quantities of air, detach the mask from the face and execute the manoeuvres of cough assistance (e.g. chest wall vibrations or squeezings).
- The thoracic squeeze determines a dynamic compression of the airway with further increase of the linear speed of air (consequent increase of cough efficiency). The insufflated volume can vary depending on the features of the techniques of the used ball, the manual skills of the operator and the applied technique (e.g. insufflation with one hand = variation of volumes between 400 and 800 mL, with two hands = variation of volumes between 500 and 1000 mL). Inhalation times (usually periods of 3 s for five consecutive breaths) and the pressure must be chosen depending on the features of the several patients [31].

8.10 Tracheobronchial Aspiration

It's the process of mechanical removal of the secretions, saliva, blood, vomit or other foreign matter from the tracheobronchial tree (nose, mouth, pharynx, trachea up to the carina) using an aspirating source and a tube inserted in the airway, in patients with ineffective cough and when other procedures less invasive failed or cannot be applied [32].

The aims of this manoeuvre are:

- Set free and keep airway patent removing secretions and/or foreign material (food, etc.).
- Promote and improve breath exchanges.
- Prevent from the side effects of the retention of secretions.
- Stimulate cough.
- Obtain a laboratory sample for culture tests (diagnosis).

The indications of this manoeuvre are:

- All the patients who cannot expectorate in a sufficient and independent manner.
- Patients who after the operation have inhibited reflex of the cough.
- Patients with neurological and/or muscular pathologies in which the reflex of the cough is altered because of difficulties or inability of muscular contractions involved in the mechanism of the cough.
- Patients into coma or in an altered state of consciousness (non-cooperatives).
- The bronchial aspiration *must be executed only if strictly necessary*, when the objective test indicates it.
- *It is the last manoeuvre to apply* when all the other nursing and physiotherapy procedures revealed ineffective.

The necessary equipment are:

- Sterile gloves, mask and goggles
- Physiological saline
- Aspiration source, connection tubes, Y connector and collection vase
- Sterile aspiration tube of the right calibre, double hole and blunt tip
- Sterile water to wash the aspiration system
- Hydrosoluble lubricant to reduce the traumatism of the tube against mucosa
- Oxygen source and device for oxygen therapy (e.g. Ambu ball or Mapleson circuit, with facial mask)
- Container for special waste

The hands must be accurately washed before and after the manoeuvre. During the procedure always check the ECG (if present), the pulse, the percutaneous saturation, the skin colour and the general conditions.

The sequences of execution are:

- Prepare the necessary equipment.
- Create a favourable context in order to calm the baby and reduce discomfort, oxygen him or her and where appropriate monitor him or her.
- Wear the goggles, the mask and the sterile gloves. If you use only one glove, wear it on the dominant hand. The dominant hand must stay sterile; for the other hand, a clean single-use glove can be used to protect from the contact with mucosa and secretions of the patient.
- Take the aspiration catheter extracting it with the dominant hand from the sterile package. Take the connecting tube with the other hand. Connect the catheter to the control valve of the aspiration without contaminating it.

The tube must be inserted until the tracheal carina (about three to four transverse fingers under the jugular dimple). The valuation of the depth is executed measuring with the tube distance between the tip of the nose and the earlobe and between the earlobe and a point situated three to four fingers under the jugular dimple. At this point, memorize the part of the tube that has to be out of the nostril:

- Wear the gloves, lubricate the tube and connect it to the Y connector.
- Insert it in the nostril in the direction perpendicular to the tip of the nose, and let it move forward until the glottis, where an obstruction to the descent is felt.
- At this point, stimulate the reflex of the cough, and in that moment with a *firm but delicate* manoeuvre, insert the tube in the airway until the estimated length making it stray through the vocal cords.
- *Only now* the aspiration must be activated plugging the free extremity of the Y connector.
- Bronco-aspirate rapidly for no more than 15 s.
- Withdraw the tube with active aspiration rotating it delicately. Avoid an intermittent movement of the removal of the thumb from the control of the aspiration completely because it can increase the risk of traumas and make the aspiration less efficient.
- Check the saturation, the skin tone and pulse rate and heart rhythm during the aspiration. In case of arterial hypertension provoked by the vagal stimulation, interrupt the aspiration and administrate oxygen. At the end of the aspiration, hyperoxygen the patient with 100% oxygen for a minute.
- Take off the glove from the dominant hand folding it back in order to leave the catheter in aspiration rolled in it, take off the other glove and eliminate everything in the container for special waste; clean the lumen of the connector tube draining the physiological saline or sterile water.
- Turn off the aspirator and put the patient in a comfortable position.
- Examine the characteristics of the aspired secretions: quantity, colour, consistency and, if possible, smell. Examine the efficiency of the aspiration, like the improvement of the arterial blood gases, improvement of the saturation and

reduction of the respiratory and cardiac rate and personal improvement reported from the patient.
- Wash your hands and record the executed operation.

If during the manoeuvre the child desaturates and/or becomes cyanotic, aspiration must be suspended without taking off the tube, O2 is administrated until he or she recovers an appropriate colour and saturation and only at this point the aspiration manoeuvre can begin again [33].

References

1. Giornale italiano di cardiologia. Vol. 15. aprile 2014.
2. Schaaf RC, Sherwen LN, Youngblood N. An interdisciplinary, environmentally-based model of care for children with HIV infection and their caregivers. Phys Occup Ther Pediatr. 1997;17(3):63–85.
3. Zuffo S. La fisioterapia respiratoria disostruente con PEP mask nel lattante e nel bambino non collaborante (cerebropatie di varia natura). Quaderni AITR. 1995;9(1–8):15–22.
4. Jenkins SC. Chapter 8: Pre-operative and post-operative physiotherapy—are they necessary? In: Respiratory care. Churchill Livingstone; 1991. p. 147–68.
5. Terry PB, Traytsman RJ, Newball HH, et al. Collateral ventilation in man. N Engl J Med. 1978;298:10–5.
6. Zuffo S. Fisioterapia respiratoria in terapia intensiva neonatale (TIN). Boll ARIR. 1996; anno 5, n. 1:11–20 e 27–8.
7. Review Article "Pediatric cardiac surgery: what to expect from physiotherapeutic intervention?" Braz J Cardiovasc Surg (Rev Bras Cir Cardiovasc). 2011;26(2). São José do Rio Preto Apr./June 2011.
8. Leininger M, Mcfarland MR. Transcultural nursing: concepts, theories, research and practice. 3rd ed. New York: McGraw-Hill; 2002.
9. World Health Organization. http://www.who.int.
10. The Ottawa charter for health promotion. 1986. 10-3-2012.
11. Isaacs S, Valaitis R, Newbold KB, Black M, Sargeant J. Competence trust among providers as fundamental to a culturally competent primary healthcare system for immigrant families. Prim Health Care Res Dev. 2012;13:1–10.
12. Ferrari B. Il lavaggio nasale: aspetti pratici. Riv Ital Fisioter Riabil Respir. 2007;3:18–22.
13. Marchisio P, Fusi M, Dusi E, Bianchini S, Nazari E, Principi N. Il lavaggio nasale con soluzioni saline come terapia delle infezioni delle alte vie respiratorie in etá pediatrica: dai presupposti ai metodi. Riv Ital Fisioter Riabil Respir. 2007;3:11–22.
14. Walsh BK, Hood K, Merritt G. Pediatric airway maintenance and clearance in the acute care setting: how to stay out of trouble. Respir Care. 2011;56(9):1424–40. ; discussion 1440–4. https://doi.org/10.4187/respcare.01323.
15. Hess DR. Secretion clearance techniques: absence of proof or proof of absence? (editorial). Respir Care. 2002;47(7):757–8.
16. Fink JB. Positive pressure techniques for airway clearance. Respir Care. 2002;47(7):786–96.
17. Gaskell D, Webber BA. The Brompton Hospital guide to chest physiotherapy. Oxford: Blackwell Scientific; 1973.
18. Hough A. Physiotherapy in respiratory care: a problem solving approach. London: Chapman & Hall; 1991.
19. Oberwaldner B. Physiotherapy for airway clearance in paediatrics. Eur Respir J. 2000;15(1):196–204.

20. Mellins R. Pulmonary physiotherapy in the pediatric age group. Am Rev Respir Dis. 1974;110(2):137–42.
21. Review Article. "Importance of pre- and postoperative physiotherapy in pediatric cardiac surgery". Rev Bras Cir Cardiovasc. 2009;24(3). São José do Rio Preto July/Sept. 2009.
22. Faling L. Chest physical therapy. Philadelphia: Lippincott; 1991. p. 625–54.
23. ACPRC 2011: Leaflet No. GL-05. "The active cycle of breathing techniques" recommendations from guidelines for physiotherapy management of adult, medical, spontaneously breathing patient.
24. Bellone A. Riabilitazione respiratoria – Nuovi Orientamenti, Ed. Midia, Monza (MI), Bottiglia d'acqua con il tubo; 1996.
25. Brivio A, Lazzeri M, Oliva G, Zampogna E. La disostruzione bronchiale - dalla teoria alla pratica, Ed. Masson, Milano; 2001.
26. Great Ormond Street Hospital (G.O.S.H.) for Children NHS Foundation Trust, "Bubble Pep, Information for Families" compiled by the respiratory physiotherapists, January 2014.
27. AARC clinical practice guideline: use of PAP adjuncts to bronchial hygiene therapy. Respir Care. 1993:38:516–20.
28. EzPAP package insert on Suggested Instructions for Use, DHD Healthcare Corporation.
29. Brivio A, Privitera E, Lazzeri M, Sommariva M, Repossini E, Zuffo S. Protocollo clinico pratico per l'utilizzo del presidio EzPAPTM, Rivista Italiana di Fisioterapia e Riabilitazione Respiratoria Maggio-Agosto 2013 • Numero 2.
30. Manual hyperinflation (MHI) guideline for practice. 2015.
31. de Godoy VC, Zanetti NM, Johnston C. Manual hyperinflation in airway clearance in pediatric patients: a systematic review. Rev Bras Ter Intensiva. 2013;25(3):258–62. https://doi.org/10.5935/0103-507X.20130043.
32. Craven RF, Himle CJ. Principi fondamentali dell'assistenza infermieristica. Vol. I e II. Milano: Casa editrice Ambrosiana; 2007.
33. American Association for Respiratory Care. Nasotracheal suctioning. Respir Care. 2004; 49:1080–4.

Respiratory System and Mechanical Ventilation in Patients with CHD

9

Giuseppe Isgrò and Simona Silvetti

Abstract

To manage pediatric ventilation in children with congenital heart disease, the knowing of the many differences from adult respiratory system is not enough.

In fact, into the wide contest of pediatric cardiac defect, lung and cardiac systems work affecting continuously their function. Any interventions designed to improve the function of one system may lead to unwanted effects on another. For these reasons, to have an optimal manage on this interaction, a thorough understanding of respiratory mechanics, patient-ventilator interactions, intrapulmonary gas exchange mechanisms, hemodynamics under physiologic and pathophysiologic conditions, and a complete knowledge of the procedures are therefore required and mandatory.

In this chapter are summarized the bases of the respiratory system in pediatric patients, the physiology of cardiopulmonary interaction, the principal respiratory support methods, and finally the specific considerations for each pathological cardiopulmonary interaction.

9.1 Pediatric Respiratory System

The respiratory system consists of the organs involved in the interchanges of gases. Respiratory system evolves with growing, and many changes concern anatomy airway from neonate (0–30 days) to infant (30 days–1 year), child, adolescent, and adult. Below are listed as following the principal anatomic differences among age:

G. Isgrò (✉) · S. Silvetti
Department of CardioVascular Anesthesia and Intensive Care,
IRCCS Policlinico San Donato, Milan, Italy
e-mail: giuisg@libero.it

© Springer International Publishing AG, part of Springer Nature 2019

163

S. F. Flocco et al. (eds.), *Congenital Heart Disease*,
https://doi.org/10.1007/978-3-319-78423-6_9

- The size of the neonate's head is large in relation to the body, and it can result in a natural neck flexion that could favor airway closure.
- Neonates are obligate nose breathers due to weak oropharyngeal muscle. The nose consists particularly of cartilage; the meatuses are narrow, and secretions can cause complete obstruction.
- In infants the tongue takes up more space; adenoids and tonsils are hypertrophic. These conditions can easily obstruct the airways.
- Neonate's epiglottis is floppy with omega shape; infant's epiglottis is located at C3-C4 vertebral level; the larynx has a funnel shape.
- Neonate's trachea has an ellipsoid shape and in infant has shape ring link. The diameter of the trachea evolves with growing from 4–6 mm to 10 mm in adult.
- The narrowest portion of the airway in infants and young children is at the cricoid ring.
- Bronchi are relatively wide, the muscle and elastic fibers are undeveloped, and the lobules and segmental bronchus are narrow.
- Lung volume is 250 cc at birth. Size of alveoli is small, and quantity of alveoli is relatively less than adult; maturation occurs by 8–10 years of age. Lung has high closing volume resulting in easily collapse.
- Skeletal chest is convex and short and largely cartilaginous and is too compliant.
- Chest muscles are not well developed. Neonates and infants are dependent on functional diaphragms and abdominal muscles for adequate ventilation because the accessory muscles contribute less to the overall work of breathing.

Anatomic modification can lead to important differences in physiology of the respiratory system; some of these lead children susceptible to obstruction, apnea, and quickly desaturation.

- Since birth neonates have high respiratory rate that lower with growing (neonate 35–30, infant 30–25, children 25–20, adolescents 15 breath/minute) that affects an elevated basal oxygen consumption.
- The narrow airway leads to high resistance in the respiratory system; small changes in the airway sizes due to edema, obstruction, or secretion will therefore increase seriously the resistance.
- Compliant trachea, larynx, and bronchi due to poor cartilaginous integrity allow for dynamic airway compression.
- Compliant chest wall determines low tendency of the lung to collapse.
- The relaxation volume of the infant thorax is small, resulting in a low functional residual capacity → increased tendency to collapse.

Respiratory failure is often determined by a vicious cycle: a greater negative inspiratory force "sucks in" the floppy airway and decreases airway diameter ⇒ airway collapse (due to poor cartilaginous integrity) ⇒ ⇑ resistance ⇒ ⇑ negative inspiratory force ⇒ ⇑ work of breathing ⇒ respiratory failure.

9.2   Cardiopulmonary Interaction

The heart and lung strictly interact.

Cardiac and pulmonary systems work together for the same ultimate goal, oxygen delivery (DO_2) but at the same time, the lungs impact in cardiovascular system, and the circulation can have profound effects on respiratory function.

9.2.1   Left Ventricle Preload

- The effect of pulmonary pressure on pulmonary venous flow depends on the relative filling state of the pulmonary circulation. During hypovolemic condition an increase in lung volume reduces venous return to the left ventricle, while in a fluid overloaded state, an increase in lung volume would shift blood, thus increasing pulmonary venous flow to the left ventricle [1].
- Change in lung volume can alter the diastolic compliance of the left ventricle because of direct compression of the chamber and also due to elevated right ventricular pressure that results in a conformational change of the interventricular septum [2].

9.2.2   Left Ventricle Afterload

LV afterload depends on transmural pressure. As shown in the following formula, the application of positive intrathoracic pressure during mechanical ventilation decreases the left ventricular transmural pressure and reduces the left ventricular afterload.

LV transmural pressure = systolic LV pressure − intrathoracic pressure

9.2.3   Right Ventricle Preload

Venous return is dependent on the pressure gradient between the extrathoracic veins and the right atrium. Spontaneous inspiration increases this gradient; on the opposite mechanical ventilation induces positive pressure during inspiration and applies a positive pressure on right atrium; this decreases the pressure gradient for systemic venous return and consequently also the right atrial and right ventricular filling and right ventricular stroke volume and potentially reduces cardiac output [3]. This event is less evident when patient has an elevated intravascular volume because intrathoracic pressure increases also intra-abdominal pressure with the positive effect on venous return.

9.2.4   Right Ventricle Afterload

The right ventricular afterload can be defined as the systolic wall stress on the right ventricle. The pulmonary vascular resistance (PVR) is the main determinant of right ventricular afterload. Regulation on pulmonary vascular resistance depends on many factors; positive pressure ventilation and positive end-expiratory pressure are the principal factors. In patients with low lung, positive pressure can reduce PVR and right ventricular afterload volumes by re-expanding collapsed pulmonary units, improving oxygenation and alveolar gas exchange, and finally improving right ventricular stroke volume. However, positive pressure ventilation and PEEP more often result in increased right ventricular afterload due to excessive alveolar expansion and capillary compression (zone 1 West) and also decrease venous return and cardiac output [1, 4].

- West zones. Based on the West categorization [5], the lung is divided into three vertical zones (in the erect position) based upon the relationship between the pressure in the alveoli (PA), in the arteries (PA), and in the veins (Pv): Zone 1, PA > PA > Pv; zone 2, pa > PA > Pv; and zone 3, PA > Pv > PA (Fig. 2).
  - In zone 1, the blood vessels can become completely collapsed by PA for alveolar overdistension (PEEP, low expiratory time), and blood does not flow through these regions inducing vessel occlusion → increase in PVR and ventilated but not perfused area = alveolar dead space.
  - In zone 3, the alveolus is collapsed by different conditions (pulmonary edema, pneumonia, disventilation due to secretion, sloping area), and aria does not arrive through these regions → perfused but not ventilated area = alveolar shunt → hypoxia.
- Hypoxic pulmonary vasoconstriction [6]. This phenomenon consists in a physiological response to alveolar hypoxia, thus optimizing the matching of perfusion and ventilation and maximizing arterial oxygenation. The pulmonary vasculature reacts to hypoxia with vasoconstriction. The exact mechanism is unknown but occurs when the alveolar PO_2 falls below approximately 50–60 mmHg. Hypercapnia and pulmonary arterial PH (acidosis) independently lead to vasoconstriction in pulmonary vessels. If vasoconstriction persists for a long period, a vascular remodeling leads to pulmonary hypertension that strains the right ventricle. Otherwise the impairment of this mechanism may result in hypoxemia due to a mismatch between ventilation and perfusion = shunt (perfused but not ventilated). This event occurs in all lung pathologies (e.g., pneumonia, edema, atelectasis).
- Hypoxemia, hypercapnia, and arterial PH (acidosis) independently lead to vasoconstriction in pulmonary vessels that strain the right ventricle.

9.3   Cardiopulmonary Interaction in Congenital Heart Diseases Before Surgery

Congenital heart diseases (CHD) consist of defects on the cardiac architecture which interfere with the venous drainage and pulmonary or systemic perfusion. There are several ways to classify CHD, but in terms of respiratory management, the most suitable is based on the clinical consequences of structural defects [7]:

- CHD with increased pulmonary blood flow. Communication between the left and right side accounts for a left-to-right shunt because of the gradient of resis-

tance between the great circulation and the pulmonary circulation (atrial septal defect, ventricular septal defect, atrioventricular septal defect, patent ductus arteriosus, truncus, partial anomalous pulmonary venous drainage).
- Obstruction to blood progression in systemic circulation (e.g., mitral or aortic stenosis, aortic arch obstructions, severe coarctation) with consequently overload of left atrium and the lungs.

Both could lead to pulmonary hyperflow → pulmonary hypertension → *impairment of alveolar-capillary interface diffusion, infection susceptibility, and progressive right ventricular dysfunction.*

- CHD with decreased pulmonary flow. Septal defects with an obstruction to pulmonary blood flow (tetralogy of Fallot, pulmonary stenosis with atrial septal defect, or atrioventricular septal defect) → right-to-left shunt → *part of the deoxygenated blood is forwarded to the systemic circulation → desaturation.*
- Obstruction in pulmonary circulation and no septal defect (e.g., pulmonary stenosis or pulmonary atresia).

In both conditions, there is a *decrease in pulmonary blood flow → ventilation/ perfusion mismatch.*

- "Ductus-dependent CHD": Complete obstruction in pulmonary or systemic circulation without any mixing. For example, transposition of the great arteries with septal defects. Parallel circulations with deoxygenated systemic venous blood being forwarded to the aorta and with oxygenated pulmonary venous blood being forwarded again to the lungs via the pulmonary artery, some blood mixing is guaranteed by septal defect of patent ductus.

All of these conditions need management with prostaglandin (PGE) to maintain patent arterial ductus. Dosage of PGE depends on ductus diameter and pulmonary vascular resistance.

9.4   Respiratory Support in Congenital Heart Disease

In most cases the decision to perform a respiratory support is usually based on inadequate oxygenation and ventilation (PaO_2 and PCO_2 value). Congenital heart patient should be carefully evaluated before starting a respiratory support which should be carefully considered. Taking into account that there are many conditions with an expected low PO_2 value, a hasty management (like mechanical ventilation) could lead to complex cardiovascular changes without the desired result.

1. First step is the identification of the patients that need respiratory support: complex CHD occurs immediately after birth, but neonates have physiological low PO_2 value, and oxygen saturation does not exceed 95%. In postnatal age, due to negative effects of oxygen, PO_2 shouldn't be more than 80 mmHg, and a respira-

tory support should be well considered; many patients with cyanotic CHD before surgery could have a very low PO_2 and oxygen saturation could be ductus dependent. In these patients, respiratory support could be only a short-term palliation; similarly, after surgical palliation persistent low PO_2 could be paraphysiologic; we should never attend a normal partial pressure gas value in these patients.

2. Second step is the identification of the cause of hypoxia. There are many causes of hypoxemia in CHD: Low FiO_2, hypoventilation (e.g., sedation), ventilation-perfusion mismatch (see above), impaired alveolar-capillary interface diffusion (e.g., pulmonary hypertension, fibrosis, pulmonary edema, interstitial pneumonia, etc.), and pulmonary hypoperfusion.

3. Third step is to perform the correct respiratory support at the adequate time:
   - To assure an adequate inspiratory oxygen pressure → oxygen supplementation.
   - To move gas between the atmosphere and the alveoli → improve ventilation.
   - To improve the oxygen diffusion into blood → reduces PVR with nitric oxide (NO_2) or other drugs such as milrinone, bosentan, and sildenafil; optimizing medical therapy with antibiotics or diuretics as final step to consider pulmonary support with ECMO.
   - To improve ventilation/perfusion mismatch → improve ventilation avoiding alveolar atelectasis; improve perfusion avoiding too high pulmonary pressure ventilation (PPV); or when it is possible and useful, support pulmonary perfusion by arterial ductus flow with prostaglandin (PGE).
   - Consider **cardiac surgery** when cardiac and respiratory support fails.

9.5 Oxygen Supplementation

There are many tools to provide oxygen supplementation. The principal methods adopted in pediatric population are:

- Nasal cannula: most patients tolerate this device well, and it is simpler to use than a mask. Oxygen can be supplied from at a rate of 1–6 liters/minute (L/min); this provides an approximate FiO_2 of 0.24–0.50, but the exact concentration depends on the flow rate and on the patient's rate.
- Simple face mask: Fits over the nose and mouth and provides a FiO_2 of 0.35–0.60. It's not possible to check the effective oxygen concentration.

To minimize drying of nasal and upper airway secretions, the flow rate should be lower than 2 L/min, or a humidification system is needed.

- Face mask Venturi delivers an accurate oxygen concentration from 24 to 60% with predetermined flow rates.
- High-flow nasal cannula is a heated, humidified, and blended air/oxygen delivered via nasal cannula at different flow rates ≥ 2 L/min, delivering both high concentrations of oxygen and potentially continuous distending pressure [8]. It has several advantages over conventional "low-flow" oxygen therapy in terms of humidification, oxygenation, gas exchange, and breathing pattern and is an alternative of

nasal continuous positive pressure (NCPAP), less tolerant, and more invasive. In infants, flow rates are greater than 2 L/min; in children, flow rates are greater than 6 L/min [9] and may be adjusted to body weight, thus closer to 1 L/kg/min. The gas temperature is set around 37 °C in order to reach optimal humidification.

- Oxyhood: a plastic device that fits over the head and shoulders of infant. It is usually used for pediatric patients who have airway inflammation, croup, or other respiratory infections. It provides oxygen, humidification, and a cool environment to help control body temperature. When using a hood, it is important to ensure that there is enough space between the curve of the hood and the child's neck to allow carbon dioxide to escape.

9.6 Mechanical Ventilation

The goals of mechanical ventilation are to decrease the work of breathing, to support gas exchange, and to allow the patient to recover from respiratory failure.

A careful attention should be given to avoid damaging the lungs by potentially injurious mechanical ventilation especially in neonates and infants. Furthermore, in the postoperative cardiac surgery period, setup ventilation support requires a solid basic understanding of the respiratory system and cardiopulmonary physiology (see above). The predominant effect of these interactions depends on several factors including the function of venous capacitance arterial vascular resistance, pulmonary vascular function, and right and left ventricular diastolic and systolic function.

9.6.1 Invasive Mechanical Ventilation

Mechanical ventilation can be broadly classified into two major categories based upon the size of the delivered inflation: one is conventional mechanical ventilation that delivers tidal volumes, which are within the normal physiological range, and the other is the high-frequency ventilation that delivers much smaller tidal volumes.

The principal classification of conventional ventilation is pressumetric and volumetric modality. With the first one, we can't decide the final total volume, and the pressure is a constant; with the second one, the volume is a constant, but the pressure can change. Changes in volume or pressure depend on several factors (tube diameter, airway resistance, opened or closed chest wall, interference with patient when lacking adequate sedation, etc.).

Pressure- or volume-limited time-cycled modes can be employed with similar results, provided tidal volumes are maintained at approximately 8 mL/kg, and driving pressures (plateau pressures—PEEP) are kept in the 15–25 cm H_2O range. PEEP is applied to prevent de-recruitment during exhalation and is generally started between 4 and 6 cm H_2O [10]. Age-appropriate inspiratory times (only in controlled ventilation)[1] and appropriate FiO_2 are also used.

---

[1] Inspiration time (IT) sec: neonates, 0.4; infants, 0.6; child, 0.7; adolescent and adult, 0.9.

However, ventilation support has different hemodynamic impacts in different kinds of CHD and should be tailored to the specific patient condition (see "specific consideration").

9.6.2 NCPAP

In neonates and infants, the use of nasal prongs to provide nasal continuous positive airway pressure (NCPAP) was described by Kattwinkel et al. in 1973 [11] but has become extremely popular over the past few years. The use in general pediatric population is growing in order to minimize lung damage, its benefits in patients with CHD is even more because of minimize also the potential hemodynamic side effects. The indications of NCPAP in CHD are the same than in general populations, after extubation and for apnea events (induced also by PGE infusion) are the two more frequents.

Various types of NCPAP are available, and their differences must be understood to use each of them correctly and optimally. Types of CPAP used in neonates include:

- Continuous flow CPAP: use a preset flow of gas to maintain CPAP through nasal prongs. CPAP delivered is dependent upon the flow rate and the resistance created by the exhalation valve. It is easy to use and has a pressure stability. Because of the presence of an exhalation valve, patients must exhale against a fixed resistance, thus resulting in a higher induced work of breathing.
- Variable flow CPAP: incorporates a flow driver that delivers fresh gas through a breathing circuit to a dual injector generator with a specially designed nasal prongs (Fig. 9.1a). Gas enters at the point of the interface on inspiration, and shunts flow away through an expiratory gas channel as the patient desires on exhalation. CPAP levels are stabilized and maintained by a change in the flow rate at the generator with little variability, unless there is a leak at the patient's interface. Require a specific equipment (Fig. 9.1b) such as flow drivers, generators, and circuits.

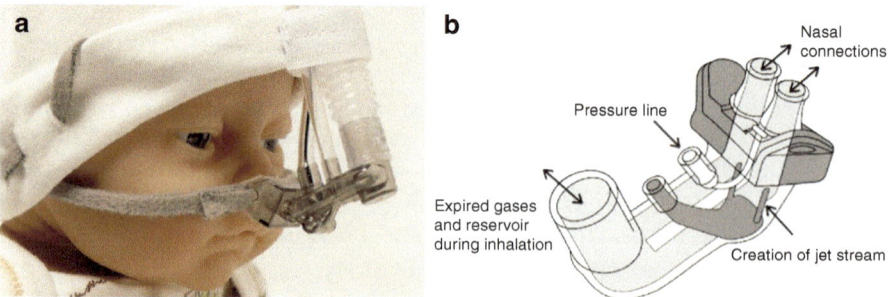

Fig. 9.1 (**a**) NCPAP variable flow, equipment. (**b**) Infant flow valve

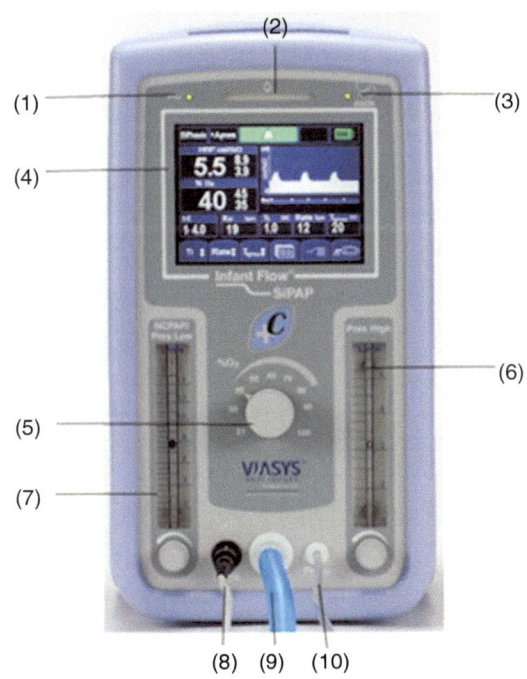

1) Power LED

2) Alarm Warning Bar

3) Transducer Interface LED

4) LCD Touch Screen

5) % O2 Control

6) Pres High Flow Meter

7) nCPAP Pres Low Flow Meter

8) Transducer Interface Connection

9) Circuit Connection Inspiratory Limb

10) Connection Proximal Pressure Line

Fig. 9.2 SiPAP machine (VIASYS)

- Bi-level CPAP (Fig. 9.2) allows spontaneous breathing at two levels of pressure; rate and time at the higher level are operator dependent. The goal of this bi-level CPAP is to achieve some higher level of alveolar recruitment and prevent alveolar collapse with continuous lower level of pressure.
- Synchronized noninvasive positive pressure ventilation: Baseline CPAP pressures are typically set at +5 cmH$_2$O, while inspiratory pressures may range from 10 to 20 cmH$_2$O. A ventilator requires a minimum driving gas flow of 8 L/min to accomplish the desired pressure.
- High-flow nasal cannula; see above.

9.7   Specific Considerations

By summarizing this chapter, we can conclude with some specific considerations.

Mechanical ventilation of the uncomplicated patient following surgical procedures is not much different than that employed in surgical patients with normal lungs.

In all conditions (presurgery or postsurgery) where the cardiac output of patients is partitioned into pulmonary (Qp) and systemic (Qs) components, the proportion of each is dependent on the amount of anatomical restriction to flow and the vascular resistances of the respective components. The respiratory support should manage following the effects showing in Fig. 9.3.

Intervention	PVR	SVR	Qp:Qs
Increase MAP	Increase	No effect	Decrease
Increase PEEP	Increase	No effect	Decrease
Hyperventilation	Decrease	Increase	Increase
Increase $PaCO_2$	Increase	Decrease	Decrease
Increase FiO_2	Decrease	Increase	Increase
Sub-atmospheric FiO_2	Increase	Decrease	Decrease

PVR, pulmonary vascular resistance; SVR, systemic vascular resistance; Qp:Qs, ratio of pulmonary to systemic blood flow; MAP, mean airway pressure; PEEP, positive end-expiratory pressure; $PaCO_2$, partial pressure of arterial carbon dioxide; FiO_2, fraction of inspired oxygen.

Fig. 9.3 Effects of different interventions on pulmonary and systemic circulation

9.7.1 Open Chest

Some patients might require delayed sternal closure after cardiac surgery; in these patients great attention should be given to the proper choice of ventilator settings because the lack of opposing forces from the intact chest wall can lead to significant hyperinflation and volutrauma without increase in pressure value. Tidal volume should set between 8 and 10 mL/kg of dry body weight; further reduction can lead to de-recruitment and atelectasis. The PEEP should be set slightly higher to prevent de-recruitment during exhalation due to lower lung recoil force [10].

9.7.2 Pulmonary Hyperflow

When an uncorrected pulmonary hyperflow (left to right shunt, IVD, PDA) is present, low pCO_2, high FiO_2, and all conditions that reduce pulmonary vascular resistances should be avoided. These conditions should be managed as follows:

- Increase in PVR (pCO_2 target 50 mmHg, FiO_2 21%).
- Reduce systemic pressure to minimize the shunt.

The same management should be used when an uncorrected pulmonary hyperflow is the cause of pulmonary hypertension. Furthermore, in this condition should be avoided all of the drugs that reduce pulmonary resistance. Drugs as iNO or milrinone should be used when the defects are corrected.

9.7.3 Diastolic Dysfunction

In hypertrophic cardiomyopathy or in tetralogy of Fallot, there is invariably some degree of diastolic dysfunction. Ventricular diastolic dysfunction is usually managed as follows:

- Improving ventricular preload with fluid challenge and concomitant low PPV to avoid reduction of venous return.
- Improving contractility and decreasing afterload usually using milrinone or iNO_2.

9.7.4 Blalock-Taussig Shunt

The cardiac output of patients following shunt palliation is partitioned into pulmonary (Qp) and systemic (Qs) components. The Qp/Qs is influenced by the size (diameter) and length of the shunt, systemic vascular resistance, and pulmonary vascular resistance. Hyperventilation increases pulmonary flow and reduces systemic and coronary perfusion. To avoid that, the ventilator should be adjusted to achieve a pH of 7.4, $PaCO_2$ of 40 torr, and PaO_2 of 40 torr. This translates to an arterial oxygen saturation of approximately 75% and a Qp:Qs near 1 [10].

9.7.5 Glenn

Following the Glenn procedure, the flow coming from the superior vena cava goes directly to the pulmonary artery, so the lung vascularization depends on cerebral (preload) and pulmonary resistance (afterload).

Hyperventilation and alkalosis not only cause a decrease in pulmonary vascular resistance but also a reduction in cerebral blood flow and venous return; it decreased systemic oxygen saturation.

On the other hand, a mild degree of hypercapnia can increase cerebral blood flow and increase venous return from the superior vena cava and pulmonary blood flow, thus increasing systemic oxygenation. If an increase in pulmonary vascular resistance has a negative effect on afterload, the use of inhaled nitric oxide has been used to selectively relax the pulmonary vascular bed [12–14].

High pulmonary airway pressure should be avoided.

9.7.6 Fontan

Following Fontan procedure, common causes for persistent hypoxemia in the patient include elevated pulmonary vascular resistance and obstruction at the site of the cavo-pulmonary anastomosis.

After Fontan, the management should be:

- Volume optimization: pulmonary circulation is high dependent on the central venous pressure because all systemic venous return must overcome the resistance of the pulmonary circulation without the assistance of a subpulmonic pumping chamber.
- Extubation as soon as possible: in the absence of contraindications, the patients should be extubated in the operating room or shortly after arrival in the pediatric cardiac intensive care unit.
- Avoid increase in PVR:
  - Avoid hypoxia: those who require continued ventilation should have adequate PEEP to minimize atelectasis.
  - Avoid elevate mean airway pressure to avoid hyperinflation.

→ PEEP is generally set at 3–5 cmH$_2$O, and effective tidal volumes of approximately 8 mL/kg are employed [10].

References

1. Michard F, Teboul JL. Using heart-lung interactions to assess fluid responsiveness during mechanical ventilation. Crit Care. 2000;4:282–9.
2. Shekerdemian L, Bohn D. Cardiovascular effects of mechanical ventilation. Arch Dis Child. 1999;80:475–80.
3. Pinsky MR. Determinant of pulmonary flow variation during respiration. J Appl Physiol. 1984;56:1237–45.
4. Venus B, Cohen LE, Smith RA. Hemodynamics and intrathoracic pressure transmission during controlled mechanical ventilation and positive end-expiratory pressure in normal and low compliant lungs. Crit Care Med. 1988;16:686–90.
5. West J, Dollery C, Naimark A. Distribution of blood flow in isolated lung; relation to vascular and alveolar pressures. J Appl Physiol. 1964;19:713–24.
6. Sommer N, Dietrich A, Schermuly RT, Ghofrani HA, Gudermann T, Schulz R, Seeger W, Grimminger F, Weissmann N. Regulation of hypoxic pulmonary vasoconstriction: basic mechanisms. Eur Respir J. 2008;32:1639–51.
7. Thiene G, Frescura C. Anatomical and pathophysiological classification of congenital heart disease. Cardiovasc Pathol. 2010;19:259–74.
8. Mayfield S, Jauncey-Cooke J, Hough JL, Schibler A, Gibbons K, Bogossian F. High-flow nasal cannula therapy for respiratory support in children. Cochrane Database Syst Rev. 2014;(3):CD009850.
9. Lee JH, Rehder KJ, Williford L, Cheifetz IM, Turner DA. Use of high flow nasal cannula in critically ill infants, children, and adults: a critical review of the literature. Intensive Care Med. 2013;39:247–57.
10. Caliumi-Pellegrini G, Agostino R, Orzalesi M, Nodari S, Marzetti G, Savignoni PG, Bucci G. Twin nasal cannula for administration of continuous positive airway pressure to newborn infants. Arch Dis Child. 1974;49:228.
11. Rotta AT, de Carvalho WB. Mechanical ventilation following cardiac surgery in children. Curr Respir Med Rev. 2012;8(1):44–52.

12. Bradley SM, Simsic JM, Mulvihill DM. Hyperventilation impairs oxygenation after bidirectional superior cavopulmonary connection. Circulation. 1998;98:II372–6; discussion II6–7
13. Bradley SM, Simsic JM, Mulvihill DM. Hypoventilation improves oxygenation after bidirectional superior cavopulmonary connection. J Thorac Cardiovasc Surg. 2003;126:1033–9.
14. Gamillscheg A, Zobel G, Urlesberger B, et al. Inhaled nitric oxide in patients with critical pulmonary perfusion after Fontan-type procedures and bidirectional Glenn anastomosis. J Thorac Cardiovasc Surg. 1997;113:435–42.

Cardiac Arrhythmias and Their Non-Pharmacological Treatment: An Overview

Vincenzo Pazzano, Fabio Anselmo Saputo, Letizia Verticelli, Ilaria Tamburri, and Antonio Longoni

Abstract

Arrhythmias represent a significant cause of morbidity and mortality in CHD. They can occur in each phase of the natural history of the disease, from the prenatal period to the late follow-up. Their relevance is increasing especially as a consequence of the good results achieved by corrective surgery, with more and more patients reaching adulthood with the possibility of developing long-term complications, often represented by arrhythmias. Their substrate can depend on the congenital abnormality itself or on surgical scars consequent to its correction, or both. To understand mechanisms underlying arrhythmias, knowledge of the physiology of the normal cardiac conduction system is necessary. This chapter gives an overview of different arrhythmias and their incidence according to the subtype of CHD, also providing basic concepts about their non-pharmacological treatment, in particular cardiac pacing for the treatment of bradyarrhythmias and ablation and ICD implantation for the treatment of tachyarrhythmias. Special emphasis is given to the particular features that arrhythmias have when they occur in congenitally abnormal hearts and in particular to the peculiar aspects of device implantation and arrhythmia ablation in the field of CHD compared to normally structured hearts.

V. Pazzano · F. A. Saputo (✉) · L. Verticelli · I. Tamburri · A. Longoni
Arrythmia Unit, Medical-Surgical Department of Paediatric Cardiology, Bambino Gesù Children's Hospital and Research Institute, Rome, Italy
e-mail: vincenzo.pazzano@opbg.net; fabioanselmo.saputo@opbg.net; ilaria.tamburri@opbg.net; antonio.longoni@opbg.net

© Springer International Publishing AG, part of Springer Nature 2019
S. F. Flocco et al. (eds.), *Congenital Heart Disease*,
https://doi.org/10.1007/978-3-319-78423-6_10

10.1   Introduction

The great progress made in the last decades in the field of cardiology and cardiac surgery for the treatment of congenital heart disease (CHD) has dramatically improved the survival rate of children born with such abnormalities (with a prevalence of approximately 0.5–1/1000 live birth) [1]. On the other hand, the increase in life expectancy is associated with a higher incidence of late complications, particularly represented by arrhythmias. Rhythm disturbances can occur at the very beginning of the natural history of CHD or complicate the postoperative course after surgery. Furthermore, they also represent the main cause of late morbidity several years after surgical correction.

10.2   Pathophysiology

Congenital heart disease (CHD) can cause arrhythmias through different mechanisms. Both structural abnormalities themselves and their associated anomalies, such as chamber hypertrophy/dilatation consequent to impaired hemodynamics or myocardial scar resulting from surgery performed for disease correction, can lead to alteration of the normal electrical impulse formation and/or conduction.

Although more frequent in anatomically complex CHD (such as TGA or CHD with single-ventricle physiology), arrhythmias can also occur in moderate (such as ToF, Ebstein's anomaly) or simple (ASD, VSD) lesions and represent an important cause of morbidity throughout all the natural history of CHD. Particularly, an acute arrhythmic event can complicate the course of a repaired congenital heart defect potentially causing a sudden death in patients otherwise in a relatively good hemodynamic status and no or only little symptoms. Thus, it is clear why a focus on arrhythmias, with identification of patients at high risk, prevention, and proper diagnosis and treatment, is fundamental for the management of CHD [2–5].

To better understand the mechanisms underlying arrhythmias, it is necessary to remind some basic concepts about the physiology of the cardiac electrical conduction system.

Normally, the cardiac electrical impulse is generated by the sinoatrial (SA or Keith-Flack) node [6], a group of cells characterized by the intrinsic ability to spontaneously generate an action potential (see further) wich propagates to the surrounding myocardium travelling through "preferential pathways" of specialized conducting tissue, reaching the atrioventricular (AV or Aschoff-Tawara) node [7] which in the normal heart is the only electrical connection between atria and ventricles (otherwise isolated by fibrous tissue). On the surface ECG, the impulse propagation to the atria is represented by the P wave, and the propagation through the AV node corresponds to the PR interval. The AV node "filters" electrical stimuli (i.e., can prevent some impulses from reaching the ventricles if they have an excessively high rate—thus protecting the ventricular myocardium from arrhythmic triggers) and continues with the His-Purkinje system, composed by the His bundle [8], the right and left bundle branches (the latter further divided in anterior and posterior fascicles), and the Purkinje fibers [9]. This system allows the electrical impulse to reach all the ventricular myocardium almost simultaneously (normally, in less than 100 ms), corresponding to a "narrow" QRS on the surface ECG.

When the electrical impulse reaches a cardiac cell, it starts the action potential, leading to a flow of positive ions through the cell membrane from outside to inside. This process leads to the muscular cell contraction (excitation-contraction coupling) and is followed by repolarization: an opposite flow of positive ions from inside to outside the membrane restoring the initial condition. Atrial repolarization is not visible on the surface ECG, while ventricular repolarization is represented by the T wave.

Normal values of heart rate and ECG intervals according to age are summarized in Tables 10.1 and 10.2.

Arrhythmia is defined as a condition in which the cardiac impulse formation and propagation does not follow the pathways just described, and/or intervals have abnormal values. The present chapter gives an overview of different arrhythmia types and pathophysiology, their incidence according to the subtype of CHD, and basic concepts about their non-pharmacological treatment.

Table 10.1 Heart rate, PR, and QRS intervals

Age	Heart rate	PR interval (ms)	QRS interval (ms)
<7 days	90–160	80–150	30–80
1–3 weeks	100–180	80–150	30–80
1–2 months	120–180	80–150	30–80
3–5 months	105–185	80–150	30–80
6–11 months	110–170	70–160	30–80
1–2 years	90–165	80–160	30–80
3–4 years	70–140	90–170	40–80
5–7 years	65–140	90–170	40–80
8–11 years	60–130	90–170	40–90
12–15 years	65–130	90–180	40–90
>16 years	50–120	120–200	50–100

Derived from Sharieff GQ, Rao SO. The pediatric ECG. Emerg Med Clin North Am 2006; 24; 196

Table 10.2 QTc interval

Age	QTc (boys ± SD)	QTc (girls ± SD)
6 months to 1 year	390 ± 20	400 ± 40
1–3 years	390 ± 20	400 ± 10
3–5 years	390 ± 20	380 ± 10
5–8 years	390 ± 20	390 ± 20
8–12 years	390 ± 20	390 ± 20
12–16 years	400 ± 20	400 ± 20
16–18 years	390 ± 30	410 ± 10

Derived from Krasemann T. et al. "Changes of the corrected QT interval in healthy boys and girls over day and night" European Heart Journal; doi: https://doi.org/10.1093/eurheartj/ehn452

10.3   Classification of Arrhythmias

Arrhythmias are divided into brady- (or hypokinetic) and tachyarrhythmias (or hyperkinetic).

Bradyarrhythmias can be caused by reduced impulse generation, delay/block of its propagation, or both. Examples are AV block, with defective conduction across the AV node, or sinus node dysfunction. They can be the consequence of a congenital abnormality of the conduction system, but they are more frequently caused by iatrogenic damage after surgery.

Tachyarrhythmias can be the consequence of increased automatic activity (i.e., abnormal generation of the impulse), altered conduction, or triggered activity.

Abnormal impulse generation can be the consequence of a tissue mechanical damage, often due to surgical lesion, and leads to tachycardia arising from myocardial areas other than the sinoatrial node (e.g., atrial ectopic or junctional) with a rate exceeding sinus rate. Postoperative junctional ectopic tachycardia (JET) is usually a consequence of irritation of the nodal myocardium, occurs immediately after heart surgery, and is typically transient. However, if particularly fast, it can lead to cardiac decompensation. On the other hand, it can represent the first sign of a postoperative heart block.

The typical example of altered conduction leading to a tachyarrhythmia is reentry, consisting in impulse propagation as a continuous loop through a closed circuit, which can be constituted by two different electrical pathways connected at the two ends (e.g., the AV node and an abnormal atrioventricular accessory pathway), around the tricuspid annulus in atrial flutter or around a myocardial scar (usually consequent to surgical lesion—"incisional" tachycardia) which can be localized both in the atrium (leading to intraatrial reentrant tachycardia, IART) and in the ventricle (leading to ventricular tachycardia—VT—potentially degenerating to ventricular fibrillation, VF).

Triggered activity is the consequence of a cell depolarization (afterdepolarization) in a critical phase of the action potential in which the cell has not yet completed its repolarization, causing electrical instability. A condition in which the repolarization time is prolonged, typically predisposing to such arrhythmias, is the long QT syndrome.

Arrhythmia classification according to the ANMCO-AIAC (Italian National Association of Hospital Cardiologists and Italian Association of Arrhythmology and Cardiac Pacing) task force is reported in Table 10.3.

10.4   Arrhythmias in Different Settings of Congenital Heart Disease

Type of arrhythmia and incidence vary according to the underlying CHD [10].

Table 10.3   Classification of arrhythmias according to ANMCO-AIAC task force

Bradycardias
- Sinus bradycardia
- Sinoatrial dysfunction
- Sinoatrial block
- I degree AV block
- II degree (Mobitz 1, also called Wenckebach; Mobitz 2: 2:1, advanced) AV block
- III degree (complete) AV block

Premature ectopic beats
- Supraventricular
- Atrial
- Junctional
- Ventricular (PVCs)

Tachycardias
- Non-sustained (<30 s)
- Sustained (>30 s)
- Permanent
- Iterative (consisting of frequent short episodes interposed with sinus rhythm)
- Paroxysmal (sudden beginning and interruption)

Supraventricular tachycardia (SVT)
- Sinus tachycardia
- Atrial tachycardia (AT)
- Atrial flutter
- Typical (common and uncommon)
- Atypical
- Atrial fibrillation (AF)
- Atrioventricular nodal reentrant tachycardia (AVNRT)
- Typical (slow-fast)
- Atypical (fast-slow or slow-slow)
- Atrioventricular reentrant tachycardia (AVRT)
- AVRT through concealed accessory pathway
- Orthodromic AVRT in WPW syndrome
- Antidromic AVRT in WPW syndrome
- Permanent junctional reciprocating tachycardia (PJRT) or Coumel type, with reentry through a decremental accessory pathway
- Junctional ectopic tachycardia (JET)

Ventricular tachycardia (VT)
- Sustained monomorphic ventricular tachycardia
- Bundle branch reentrant ventricular tachycardia
- Ventricular outflow tachycardia
- Fascicular VT
- Polymorphic VT
- Torsade de pointes VT
- Accelerated idioventricular rhythm
- Ventricular fibrillation (VF)

10.4.1 Atrial Septal Defect

The most frequent rhythm disorder associated to this condition is sinus node dysfunction. Alteration of the sinus physiology is due to mechanical damage consequent to SVC incannulation or suture of the patch, with highest incidence (about 5% of corrected subjects) in sinus venous ASD or with associated partial abnormal pulmonary venous return. Other possible arrhythmias are supraventricular tachycardias. AF is more frequent in case of history of arrhythmias prior to correction, atrial dilatation, late correction, or LV dysfunction. Atrial flutter can be typical, with macroreentry around cavo-tricuspidal isthmus, or atypical around patch or atriotomy scar: in this case atrial heart rate is lower, with the risk of 1:1 AV conduction and higher ventricular rate [11, 12]. Ectopic atrial tachycardias often originate from caval veins incannulation sites. In patients with non-repaired ASD, incidence of SVT reaches 10% before the age of 40 [13, 14].

10.4.2 Complete AV Canal Defect

The most common arrhythmia in this setting is AV block caused by surgical suture performed for patch apposition, favored by an atypical position of the AV node and His bundle, often dislocated toward the CS os. Transient postoperative AV block can occur in up to 30% of cases. Permanent AV block can occur immediately after surgery (7–10% of cases) but also later during follow-up (2–5%) [15]. There are also possible supraventricular arrhythmias, similarly to what described for ASD, and ventricular arrhythmias (up to 1/3 of cases, mainly PVCs) especially in case of ventricular dysfunction.

10.4.3 Ventricular Septal Defect

Various conduction defects can occur, from simple bundle branch block to complete AV block, especially in membranous subaortic defects corrected with a transventricular approach. Incidence of transient postoperative AV block ranges from 5 to 30%, while permanent complete AV block occurs in 1–3% of cases [16]. Ventricular arrhythmias occur in 3–6% of uncorrected VSDs while in repaired VSD are more frequent in patients treated with a transventricular approach compared with the combined transatrial-transpulmonary approach [17].

10.4.4 Tetralogy of Fallot

In this condition, characterized by malalignment of the ventricular septum, the His bundle is displaced posteriorly and inferiorly, with consequent high incidence of congenital conduction defects, mainly RBBB but also possible bifascicular (i.e., RBBB + left anterior or posterior fascicular block) or AV block. In the postoperative setting, the incidence of transient AV block is around 25%, with 50% of bifascicular block and approximately 2% of patients with permanent complete AV block [18–20]. Supraventricular arrhythmias (atrial flutter, IART, and AF) are facilitated by atrial enlargement consequent to tricuspidal regurgitation, with an incidence ranging from 10 to 50% according to duration of postoperative follow-up [21]. On the other hand, ToF is one of the CHD with the highest incidence of sudden death consequent to malignant ventricular arrhythmias, mainly originating with a mechanism of reentry around surgical scars in the RV. Sudden cardiac death (SCD) can occur late after correction, with a rate of 1.2% at 10 years and total incidence ranging from 0.6 to 6% [21, 22]. Many efforts have been made to detect predictors, with different factors identified: surgical (older age at repair, type of surgical approach, previous shunt, reinterventions, duration of postsurgical follow-up); electrophysiological (QRS duration, QT and QRS dispersion, history of non-sustained VT), and hemodynamic (RV dilatation, pulmonary regurgitation, high LV end diastolic pressure, right/left ventricular dysfunction). Additional electrophysiological tests such as programmed ventricular stimulation (PVS) or electroanatomical mapping of the RV can help to identify with further accuracy patients at high-risk, candidates for ICD implantation [23].

10.4.5 Transposition of the Great Arteries

In congenitally corrected TGA, abnormalities of the electrical conduction system are frequent, with a 15–25% incidence of AV block [24, 25]. In surgically corrected TGA (especially if corrected with atrial switch), the sinoatrial node can suffer from ischemia due to damage to the sinoatrial node artery, with sinus node dysfunction. Atrial fibrosis consequent to surgical scar and chamber dilatation can lead to focal atrial tachycardia, IART/atrial flutter or AF. Incidence of such arrhythmias is significantly lower in patients corrected with arterial switch. Ventricular arrhythmias can occur as a consequence of systemic right ventricle dysfunction/dilatation after atrial switch or myocardial ischemia consequent to coronary compression after arterial switch [26].

10.4.6 Physiologically Univentricular Heart Post-fontan Operation

The typical arrhythmia in this case is sinus node dysfunction, with an incidence of up to 50% in the long-term postoperative follow-up, caused by direct lesion to the sinoatrial node artery in the site of connection of the conduit to the right atrium. AV block can occur immediately after surgery with an incidence of approximately 10% [27, 28]. Moreover, surgical lesion can lead to fibrous tissue formation, constituting the substrate for atrial tachyarrhythmias, especially reentrant tachycardias (IART, atrial flutter), which represent an important cause of morbidity during follow-up [29–31].

10.4.7 Ebstein's Anomaly

The displacement of the tricuspid valve is often associated with the presence of right atrioventricular accessory pathways causing ventricular pre-excitation (detectable at the ECG during sinus rhythm) and predisposing to atrioventricular reentrant tachycardia (Wolff–Parkinson–White syndrome) in up to 20% of cases [32]. Compared to the WPW syndrome in structurally normal hearts, Ebstein's anomaly carries higher risk of multiple accessory AV pathways and Mahaim fibers (sharing with the AV node decremental properties and characterized by only antegrade conduction) [33].

10.5 Non-pharmacological Treatment of Arrhythmias

10.5.1 Bradyarrhythmias

The treatment of bradyarrhythmias is essentially based on antibradycardia pacing, with implantation of a pacemaker, a device capable of detecting spontaneous cardiac electrical activity and giving impulses if intrinsic activity is defective. Such systems are provided with leads reaching one or more cardiac chambers (single chamber—atrial or ventricular, dual chamber, or biventricular pacemaker) in different ways (intracavitary, with a transvenous course, or epicardial).

Cardiac pacing in children and in CHD patients in general can be particularly difficult. Cardiac pacing in children and CHD patients in general can be particularly challenging, non only for the small dimensions of the heart in the young, but also for the peculiar characteristics of the pediatric patients, more vulnerable to trauma and infections. Body growth can cause displacement or damage to the system, with consequent dysfunction. Moreover, considering young age at implantation, the life expectancy of the patient can exceed the predicted lifespan of the leads, physiologically subject to consumption. Finally, while in the normal heart pacemakers are typically implanted transvenously, in CHD the complexity of cardiac anatomy can make very hard if not impossible to get an access to the heart chambers cavities.

Bradyarrhythmias requiring electrical pacing are basically sinus node dysfunction and AV block. SA node dysfunction is treated with atrial pacing (single-chamber atrial pacemaker is the system of choice in case of preserved AV conduction), while in presence of complete AV block, especially in the absence of adequate junctional escape rhythm, ventricular pacing is needed. In this case, a single chamber ventricular system warrants an adequate ventricular rate, while a dual chamber (atrial-ventricular) system gives in addition atrial-ventricular synchrony, optimizing diastolic ventricular filling. Moreover, atrial pacing can be part of tachyarrhythmia therapy, helping to prevent (or in some cases interrupting, with high rate pacing) ectopic atrial rhythms or atrial reentrant arrhythmias/AF.

Endocardial leads are implanted reaching the right cardiac chambers (or the left ventricle through the coronary sinus draining in the right atrium) transvenously, mostly through a subclavian/axillary puncture. The pulse generator is placed in a subcutaneous (alternatively, submuscular) pocket in the prepectoral subclavian area, usually on the left side. Endocardial leads are preferred as data available in literature show a better performance and longevity compared to the epicardial leads. However, these studies have a follow-up that rarely exceeds 15 years, a period that can be considered still too short compared to the young age and long life expectancy at the time of implantation [34–40].

The implantation of epicardial pacing leads (requiring thoracotomy, with the pacemaker generator placed in an abdominal pocket) is often a forced choice, driven by the impossibility of placing a transvenous system due to anatomical reasons. Examples are represented by abnormal venous return preventing access from the superior vena cava (status post-Fontan or post-Glenn operation) or presence of intracardiac shunt predisposing to paradoxical embolism originating from the right-sided leads (especially, but not only, in the presence of a right-to-left shunts) [41]. Moreover, a contraindication to transvenous pacing can be represented by young age: this technique is usually avoided in patients below 15–20 kg of weight, for potential long-term complications such as tricuspid valve damage leading to regurgitation [42], occlusion of relatively small venous axis [43], and high risk of lead damage or fracture consequent to body growth. In this category of patients, it is important to consider the higher adverse impact of leaving an abandoned lead in a small heart (especially if the implantation of a new one is needed) or the high risk of an extraction procedure. Thus, epicardial pacing is often the preferred approach in young children with CHD, postponing the implantation of a transvenous system at an older age (usually, waiting as long as possible until the inevitable occurrence of dysfunction of the epicardial lead, damaged in consequence of body growth). Moreover, a factor driving the choice (and also the time) of an epicardial approach can be represented by the need for cardiac surgery for other reasons (i.e., for repair or residual defect correction), allowing the performance of the two procedures at the same time.

Finally, it is necessary to remind potential complications related to cardiac pacing. Besides intra-/periprocedural surgical complications, long-term complication associated to cardiac pacing in general is represented by system damage, displacement, or infection. Another possible complication is chamber dilatation and contractile dysfunction, particularly in case of chronic ventricular pacing, as a consequence of impulse formation and propagation through pathways different from the physiologic cardiac conduction system. In CHD in particular, compared to pacing in structurally normal hearts, the existence of an optimal ventricular pacing site has not been demonstrated, and a narrow paced QRS does not necessarily correspond to a better outcome in terms of contractility preservation [44]. However, contractile dysfunction consequent to long-term right ventricular pacing, occurring approximately in 6% of cases, is significantly correlated to catheter placement in RV free wall compared to RV apex or left ventricle (via the coronary sinus) [45].

10.5.2 Tachyarrhythmias

Pharmacological therapy of tachyarrhythmias is usually associated with the need for a long-term (potentially life-long) drug therapy, with the risk of incomplete efficacy or side effects also including pro-arrhythmic effects. Thus, a definitive treatment abolishing the arrhythmic substrate is the alternative of choice, especially considering the good efficacy and safety reached with the current techniques. Surgical ablation is an option, but percutaneous catheter ablation represents the gold standard at the moment, both for supraventricular and ventricular arrhythmias.

Transcatheter ablation consists in the destruction of a small portion of cardiac tissue responsible of an arrhythmia, i.e., the origin of a focal arrhythmia (consequent to increased automatism) or part of the circuit responsible for a reentrant arrhythmia, such as an accessory atrioventricular conduction pathway in AVRT.

According to the energy used, there are two different techniques of ablation: radiofrequency (RF) ablation and cryoablation. In both cases, the tip of a catheter is placed on a site recognized critical for initiation or propagation and persistence of an arrhythmia, and the energy delivered causes tissue necrosis with subsequent replacement with fibrous tissue, unable to generate or propagate electrical impulses. In RF ablation, the energy used is based on alternate electrical current causing coagulative necrosis. On the other hand, cryoablation creates a lesion by reducing the tip of the catheter to temperatures that reach -80 °C, with subsequent intracellular crystallization. The lesion created with this process is more homogeneous compared to RF but less deep. The main advantage provided by cryoablation is the possibility of creating a reversible lesion (with temperatures of $-30/-50$ °C and short ablation time). Thus, when the ablation site is particularly close to vulnerable sites as the AV node (i.e., in AVNRT slow pathway ablation), cryoablation allows to test the effect of an ablation on a specific site (so-called cryomapping), with the possibility of stopping it in case of evidence of side effects (e.g., AV block), with subsequent regression of the damage. On the other hand, if the cryomapping shows no occurrence of side effects, it is possible to further reduce the temperature of the catheter tip creating an irreversible damage (cryoablation). Another quality of cryoablation is that once the catheter tip has reached low temperatures, it adheres to the endocardial surface, so there is no risk of catheter instability or displacement during ablation. The negative aspects of cryoablation are longer procedure times, as each ablation needs from 4 to 8 minutes to be effective, higher stiffness of the catheter, and the impossibility to create deep lesions.

As previously described, to perform a successful ablation, it is necessary to localize an area which is crucial for arrhythmia initiation or propagation. This is done analyzing the local electrograms registered at the tip of the catheters, traditionally moved in the heart under fluoroscopy guide. However, a very important contribution has come from tridimensional electroanatomic mapping systems, which allow the creation of a 3D map which reconstructs chamber geometry. Then, according to different color codes, it is possible to depict areas of different local voltages (e.g., normal vs reduced, corresponding to electrical scars), put tags on specific points (e.g., the areas where a local His signal is registered or sites where ablation has been performed), and create electrical activation/propagation maps, showing the spatial course of the electrical impulse across the heart, in order to identify sites such as the focus of an ectopic rhythm or a critical isthmus of a reentrant tachycardia (see Figs.10.1 and 10.2). Furthermore, maps created with this systems can be merged with images obtained with other modalities (CT, MRI). Finally, this systems are based on the use of magnetic fields and do not require X-rays, dramatically reducing fluoroscopic exposition with great benefit both for the patient and the operator.

Special considerations are needed about arrhythmia ablation in the particular population of patients with CHD. Complex anatomy requires adequate knowledge of surgical techniques in general and details about the procedure performed in the specific patient (considering the approach variability among different periods and surgeons). Mapping and ablation in the presence of structures like atrial baffles (i.e., after Mustard, Senning, or Fontan operations) can be very challenging, and 3D electroanatomical mapping systems are necessary, better if integrated with other imaging modalities such as CT, MRI, or intracardiac echo [46]. Moreover, structures as the compact node or His bundle can have unusual locations, and this has to be taken in consideration to avoid damage to the normal conduction system during ablation. Similarly, areas target for ablation can have unusual features (e.g., multiple accessory pathways in AVRT) and can be located in positions difficult to reach and/or difficult to ablate because of lack of catheter stability (due to dilatation of the chamber) or a deep location in a hypertrophic cardiac wall. Furthermore, presence of

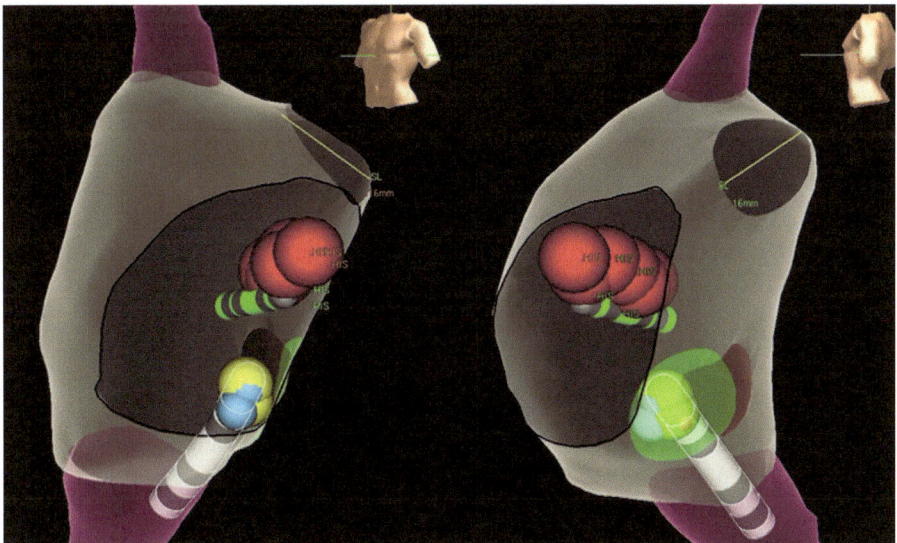

Fig. 10.1 Transcatheter cryoablation of AVNRT in a patient with ostium secundum ASD. Electroanatomical mapping (EnSite Velocity system) shows the defect in the interatrial septum, Hisian region (red dots), and site of ablation (yellow-blue dots) corresponding to the AV nodal slow pathway. *Left* LAO view, *right* LL view

Fig. 10.2 Electroanatomical voltage mapping (CARTO Univu System, LAO view) of a right ventricle of a patient with ToF treated with outflow patch and ventricular arrhythmias. The red area localized in the anterior portion of the RV infundibulum corresponds to low local voltages in the site of surgical scar and patch placement. Reentrant ventricular arrhythmias can arise from such areas. See also the peculiar shape and dilatation of the chamber

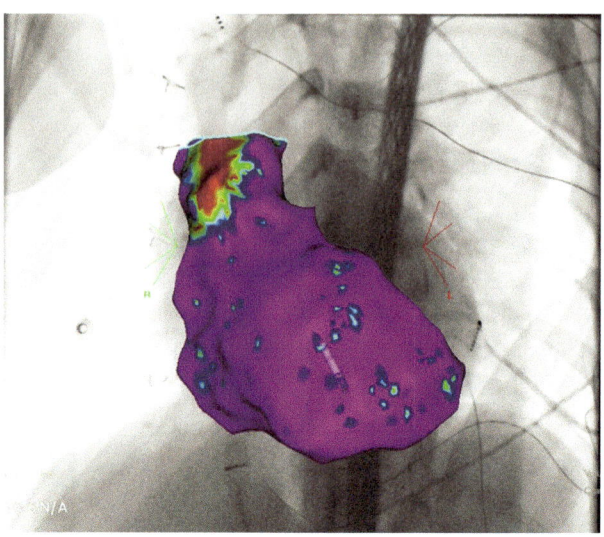

patches or chamber dilatation with thin walls can pose a considerable risk of perforation. Finally, access can be difficult: examples can be the lack of a venous route to the heart as in status post-Fontan operation, the need of a transseptal atrial puncture though a thickened or reconstructed septum, or simply because of challenging femoral approach in patients who have undergone multiple prior catheterizations.

Another therapeutic approach for tachyarrhythmias is represented by implantable cardioverter defibrillators (ICD), capable of detecting a potentially life-threatening tachycardia and interrupting it with a fast anti-tachycardia pacing (ATP) or a shock. Considerations about implantation and technical features are similar to those made for pacemakers, highlighting the higher rate of surgical complications consequent to bigger device and catheter size and intrinsic patients characteristics (usually affected by more complex conditions) [47]. Specific challenges of ICD therapy are posed by inappropriate shocks, especially in patients with complex CHD also associated with SVTs causing high ventricular rate, possibly misinterpreted as a VT/VF by the device. As expressed above, transvenous implantation of endocardial systems is associated with better performances and lower rate of complications but not always feasible [48]. At this purposes, novel approaches have been developed [49], with the entirely subcutaneous ICD representing the most attractive innovating alternative. The principal advantage is the absence of risks connected with transvenous intracardiac or epicardial approach needing thoracotomy and the possibility of implantation regardless of the presence of a venous access. An important disadvantage is the fact that some ECG features such as particularly broad QRS or high T wave compared to the QRS, which are common in CHD, represent a contraindication for excessive risk of inaccurate detection of abnormal rhythms by the device algorithms. At this purpose, patients undergo an ECG screening before being considered eligible for s-ICD implantation. Other disadvantages are the overall higher risk of inappropriate shocks and the lack of pacing function (except a temporary post-shock stimulation). The last limitation can be overcome if the patient is at the same time carrier of an endocardial pacemaker, necessarily with bipolar leads.

Conclusions

Arrhythmias represent a significant cause of morbidity and mortality associated with CHD throughout all the natural history of the disease: they can occur in the fetal or neonatal period, after surgery or during the late follow-up. Awareness about rhythm disturbances is required from all the health professionals dealing with CHD patients. Their non-pharmacological treatment has several peculiarities compared to the general non-CHD population, which must be well-known in order to achieve a good result. Due to the growing number of CHD survivors, consequent to the advances in medical and surgical therapeutic approach, a considerable amount of the current knowledge about them (especially those occurring in adults late after surgical correction) is very recent and in continuous development, representing a very interesting field with rich future perspectives.

References

1. Warnes CA, Liberthson R, Danielson GK, Dore A, Harris L, Hoffman JI, Somerville J, Williams RG, Webb GD. Task force 1: the changing profile of congenital heart disease in adult life. J Am Coll Cardiol. 2001;37(5):1170–5.
2. Harrison DA, Connelly M, Harris L, Luk C, Webb GD, McLaughlin PR. Sudden cardiac death in the adult with congenital heart disease. Can J Cardiol. 1996;12(11):1161–3.
3. Sarubbi B, Pietra S, Somerville J. Sudden death in grown-up congenital heart (GUCH) patients: a 26-year population-based study [abstract]. J Am Coll Cardiol. 1999;33(Suppl A):538.
4. Silka MJ, Hardy BG, Menashe VD, Morris CD. A population-based prospective evaluation of risk of sudden cardiac death after operation for common congenital heart defects. J Am Coll Cardiol. 1998;32(1):245–51.
5. Walsh EP, Cecchin F. Arrhythmias in adult patients with congenital heart disease. Circulation. 2007;115(4):534–45.
6. Keith A, Flack M. The form and nature of the muscular connections between the primary divisions of the vertebrate heart. J Anat Physiol. 1907;41(Pt 3):172–89.
7. Tawara S. Das Reizleitungssystem des Saugetierherzens. Jena: Gustav Fischer; 1906.
8. His W Jr. The story of the atrioventricular bundle with remarks concerning embryonic heart activity. J Hist Med Allied Sci. 1949;4(3):319–33.
9. Purkinje JE. Mikrosckopisch neurologisce Beobachtungen. Archiv Fur Anatomie Physiolgie und Wissenchaftliche Medizin. 1845;12:281.
10. Khairy P, Van Hare GF, Balaji S, Berul CI, Cecchin F, Cohen MI, Daniels CJ, Deal BJ, Dearani JA, Nd G, Dubin AM, Harris L, Janousek J, Kanter RJ, Karpawich PP, Perry JC, Seslar SP, Shah MJ, Silka MJ, Triedman JK, Walsh EP, Warnes CA. PACES/HRS expert consensus statement on the recognition and management of arrhythmias in adult congenital heart disease: developed in partnership between the Pediatric and Congenital Electrophysiology Society (PACES) and the Heart Rhythm Society (HRS). Endorsed by the governing bodies of PACES, HRS, the American College of Cardiology (ACC), the American Heart Association (AHA), the European Heart Rhythm Association (EHRA), the Canadian Heart Rhythm Society (CHRS), and the International Society for Adult Congenital Heart Disease (ISACHD). Heart Rhythm. 2014;11(10):e102–65. https://doi.org/10.1016/j.hrthm.2014.05.009; Epub 2014 May 9.

11. Bink-Boelkens MT, Meuzelaar KJ, Eygelaar A. Arrhythmias after repair of secundum atrial septal defect: the influence of surgical modification. Am Heart J. 1988;115(3):629–33.
12. Gatzoulis MA, Freeman MA, Siu SC, Webb GD, Harris L. Atrial arrhythmia after surgical closure of atrial septal defects in adults. N Engl J Med. 1999;340(11):839–46.
13. Kirsh JA, Walsh EP, Triedman JK. Prevalence of and risk factors for atrial fibrillation and intra-atrial reentrant tachycardia among patients with congenital heart disease. Am J Cardiol. 2002;90(3):338–40.
14. Murphy JG, Gersh BJ, McGoon MD, Mair DD, Porter CJ, Ilstrup DM, McGoon DC, Puga FJ, Kirklin JW, Danielson GK. Long-term outcome after surgical repair of isolated atrial septal defect. N Engl J Med. 1990;323(24):1645–50.
15. Ho SY, Rossi MB, Mehta AV, Hegerty A, Lennox S, Anderson RH. Heart block and atrioventricular septal defect. Thorac Cardiovasc Surg. 1985;33(6):362–5.
16. Godman MJ, Roberts NK, Izukawa T. Late postoperative conduction disturbances after repair of ventricular septal defect and tetralogy of Fallot. Analysis by his bundle recordings. Circulation. 1974;49(2):214–21.
17. Houyel L, Vaksmann G, Fournier A, Davignon A. Ventricular arrhythmias after correction of ventricular septal defects: importance of surgical approach. J Am Coll Cardiol. 1990;16(5):1224–8.
18. Baharati S, Lev M. The myocardium. The conduction system, and general sequelae after surgery for congenital heart disease. In: Engle MA, Perloff JK, editors. Congenital heart disease after surgery: benefits, residua, sequelae: York Medical Books; 1983.
19. Natterson PD, Perloff JK, Klitzner TS, Stevenson WG. Electrophysiologic abnormalities: unoperated occurrence and postoperative residua and sequelae. In: Perloff JK, Child JS, editors. Congenital heart disease in adults. 2nd ed. Philadelphia, PA: WB Saunders; 1998.
20. Karpawich PP, Jackson WL, Cavitt DL, Perry BL. Late-onset unprecedented complete atrioventricular block after tetralogy of Fallot repair: electrophysiologic findings. Am Heart J. 1987;114(3):654–6.
21. Khairy P, Aboulhosn J, Gurvitz MZ, et al. Arrhythmia burden in adults with surgically repaired tetralogy of Fallot: a multi-institutional study. Circulation. 2010;122:868–75.
22. Cuypers JA, Menting ME, Konings EE, et al. Unnatural history of tetralogy of Fallot: prospective follow-up of 40 years after surgical correction. Circulation. 2014;130:1944–53.
23. Drago F, Pazzano V, Di Mambro C, Russo MS, Palmieri R, Silvetti MS, Giannico S, Leonardi B, Amodeo A, Di Ciommo VM. Role of right ventricular three-dimensional electroanatomic voltage mapping for arrhythmic risk stratification of patients with corrected tetralogy of Fallot or other congenital heart disease involving the right ventricular outflow tract. Int J Cardiol. 2016;222:422–9.
24. Daliento L, Corrado D, Buja G, John N, Nava A, Thiene G. Rhythm and conduction disturbances in isolated, congenitally corrected transposition of the great arteries. Am J Cardiol. 1986;58(3):314–8.
25. Wilkinson JL, Smith A, Lincoln C, Anderson RH. Conducting tissues in congenitally corrected transposition with situs inversus. Br Heart J. 1978;40(1):41–8.
26. Rhodes LA, Wernovsky G, Keane JF, Mayer JE Jr, Shuren A, Dindy C, Colan SD, Walsh EP. Arrhythmias and intracardiac conduction after the arterial switch operation. J Thorac Cardiovasc Surg. 1995;109(2):303–10.
27. Cromme-Dijkhuis AH, Hess J, Hählen K, Henkens CM, Bink-Boelkens MT, Eygelaar AA, Bos E. Specific sequelae after Fontan operation at mid- and long-term follow-up. Arrhythmia, liver dysfunction, and coagulation disorders. J Thorac Cardiovasc Surg. 1993;106(6):1126–32.
28. Peters NS, Somerville J. Arrhythmias after the Fontan procedure. Br Heart J. 1992;68(2):199–204.
29. Balaji S, Gewillig M, Bull C, de Leval MR, Deanfield JE. Arrhythmias after the Fontan procedure. Comparison of total cavopulmonary connection and atriopulmonary connection. Circulation. 1991;84(5 Suppl):III162–7.

30. Cecchin F, Johnsrude CL, Perry JC, Friedman RA. Effect of age and surgical technique on symptomatic arrhythmias after the Fontan procedure. Am J Cardiol. 1995;76(5):386–91.

31. Gelatt M, Hamilton RM, McCrindle BW, Gow RM, Williams WG, Trusler GA, Freedom RM. Risk factors for atrial tachyarrhythmias after the Fontan operation. J Am Coll Cardiol. 1994;24(7):1735–41.

32. Attenhofer Jost CH, Connolly HM, Edwards WD, Hayes D, Warnes CA, Danielson GK. Ebstein's anomaly—review of a multifaceted congenital cardiac condition. Swiss Med Wkly. 2005;135(19-20):269–81.

33. Berntsen RF1, Gjesdal KT, Aass H, Platou ES, Hole T, Orning OM. Radiofrequency catheter ablation of two right Mahaïm-like accessory pathways in a patient with Ebstein's anomaly. J Interv Card Electrophysiol. 1998;2(3):293–9.

34. Udink ten Cate F, Breur J, Boramanand N, Crosson J, Friedman A, Brenner J, et al. Endocardial and epicardial steroid lead pacing in the neonatal and paediatric age group. Heart. 2002;88:392–6.

35. Kammeraad JAE, Rosenthal E, Bostock J, Rogers J, Sreeram N. Endocardial pacemaker implantation in infants weighing $\leq$ 10 kilograms. Pacing Clin Electrophysiol. 2004;27:1466–74.

36. Fortescue EB, Berul CI, Cecchin F, Walsh EP, Triedman JK, Alexander ME. Patient, procedural, and hardware factors associated with pacemaker lead failures in pediatrics and congenital heart disease. Heart Rhythm. 2004;1:150–9.

37. Fortescue EB, Berul CI, Cecchin F, Walsh EP, Triedman JK, Alexander ME. Comparison of modern steroid-eluting epicardial and thin transvenous pacemaker leads in pediatric and congenital heart disease patients. J Interv Card Electrophysiol. 2005;14:27–36.

38. Silvetti MS, Drago F, Grutter G, De Santis A, Di Ciommo V, Ravà L. Twenty years of cardiac pacing in paediatric age: 515 pacemakers and 480 leads implanted in 292 patients. Europace. 2006;8:530–6.

39. Silvetti MS, Drago F, Marcora S, Ravà L. Outcome of single-chamber, ventricular pacemakers with transvenous leads implanted in children. Europace. 2007;9:894–9.

40. Silvetti MS, Drago F, De Santis A, Grutter G, Ravà L, Monti L, et al. Single-centre experience on endocardial and epicardial pacemaker system function in neonates and infants. Europace. 2007;9:426–31.

41. Khairy P, Landzberg MJ, Gatzoulis MA, Mercier LA, Fernandes SM, Cotè JM, et al. Transvenous pacing leads and systemic thromboembolism in patients with intracardiac shunts. A multicenter study. Circulation. 2006;113:2391–7.

42. Webster G, Margossian R, Alexander ME, Cecchin F, Triedman JK, Walsh EP, et al. Impact of transvenous ventricular pacing leads on tricuspid regurgitation in pediatric and congenital heart disease patients. J Interv Card Electrophysiol. 2008;21:65–8.

43. Bar-Cohen Y, Berul CI, Alexander ME, Fortescue EB, Walsh EP, Triedman JK, et al. Age, size, and lead factors alone do not predict venous obstruction in children and young adults with transvenous lead systems. J Cardiovasc Electrophysiol. 2006;17:754–9.

44. Karpavich PP. Technical aspects of pacing in adult and pediatric congenital heart disease. Pacing Clin Electrophysiol. 2008;31:S28–31.

45. Gebauer RA, Tomek V, Salameh A, Marek J, Chaloupecky V, Gebauer R, et al. Predictors of left ventricular remodelling and failure in right ventricular pacing in the young. Eur Heart J. 2009;30:1097–104.

46. Alexander ME, Cecchin F, Walsh EP, Triedman JK, Bevilacqua LM, Berul CI. Implications of implantable cardioverter defibrillator therapy in congenital heart disease and pediatrics. J Cardiovasc Electrophysiol. 2004;15:72–6.

47. Sherwin ED1, Triedman JK, Walsh EP. Update on interventional electrophysiology in congenital heart disease: evolving solutions for complex hearts. Circ Arrhythm Electrophysiol. 2013;6(5):1032–40.

48. Atallah J, Erickson CC, Cecchin F, Dubin AM, Law IH, Cohen MI, Lapage MJ, Cannon BC, Chun TU, Freedenberg V, Gierdalski M, Berul CI. Pediatric and Congenital Electrophysiology

Society (PACES). Multi-institutional study of implantable defibrillator lead performance in children and young adults: results of the Pediatric Lead Extractability and Survival Evaluation (PLEASE) study. Circulation. 2013;127(24):2393–402. https://doi.org/10.1161/CIRCULATIONAHA.112.001120; Epub 2013 May 21.

49. Drago F, Fazio G, Silvetti MS, Oricchio G, Michielon G. A successfully novel ICD implantation and medical treatment in a child with LQT syndrome and self-limiting ventricular fibrillation. Int J Cardiol. 2007;118:e108–12.

Nursing Care at the Pediatric Cardiology Ward

11

Mary C. McLellan

Abstract

The pediatric cardiology ward has been evolving in complexity of care and patient acuity. The nurse caring for patients in this environment must have a decreased reliance upon technological monitoring with an increase in nursing assessment compared to other critical care areas. Nursing care on the ward encompasses both postoperative care and medical management of patients. Nurses optimize patient's nutrition goals, pain management and prevention, psychological support, and family support. The ward is a place of transition for acutely ill patients and their families between home, procedural, and intensive care areas with the nurse facilitating successful patient transition by providing education and anticipatory support.

11.1 Introduction

Pediatric cardiology wards continue to evolve with increasing acuity of patients and complexity of care, effectively falling within the term "progressive care" as described by the American Association of Critical Care Nurses (AACN). Pediatric progressive care units (PPCU) may be intermediate care units, direct observation units, step-down units, telemetry units, or transitional care units [1]. The AACN recommends the following core competencies for nurses in PPCUs [1]:

- Arrhythmia monitoring, interpretation, and treatment.
- Basic and advanced life support.

M. C. McLellan, M.P.H., B.S.N., R.N.
The Heart Center, Boston Children's Hospital, Boston, MA, USA
e-mail: mary.mclellan@childrens.harvard.edu

© Springer International Publishing AG, part of Springer Nature 2019
S. F. Flocco et al. (eds.), *Congenital Heart Disease*,
https://doi.org/10.1007/978-3-319-78423-6_11

193

- Drug dosage calculation, continuous medication infusion administration, and monitoring for medication effects.
- Patient monitoring for pre-, intra-, and post-procedures.
- Hemodynamic monitoring and recognition of signs of patient instability.
- Recognition of the signs of cardiopulmonary emergencies and initiation of interventions to stabilize the patient awaiting intensive care unit (ICU) transfer.
- Interpretation of lab values and communication of findings.
- Non-invasive oxygen delivery indications and management.
- Ventilated patient assessment and understanding of long-term mechanical ventilation and weaning.
- Enteral and parental nutrition indications and complications.
- Assessment, monitoring, and management of patients requiring renal therapeutic interventions.
- Recognition and evaluation of the family's need for enhanced involvement in care to facilitate transition to home.

11.2 Patient Assessment

PPCU patients have less requirement for continuous and/or invasive monitoring making the importance of accurate and thorough nursing assessments critical in this environment. Vital signs and pain assessments are typically obtained and assessed a minimum of every 4 h (see Chap. 3 and Sect. 11.3). Vital signs include heart rate, respiratory rate, blood pressure (BP), temperature, and oxygen saturation (see Chap. 3). Some institutions may include assessment of an early warning score when obtaining vital signs (see Chap. 3). Patients with coarctation of the aorta or its recent repair should have daily four extremity blood pressures obtained. Patient with congenital heart disease (CHD) should receive a daily, pre-meal weight to assess fluid balance. The nurse should conduct a systematic physical assessment of the patient every shift and ongoing assessments for symptoms of decreased cardiac output, congestive heart failure (CHF), and/or arrhythmia.

Assessment of cardiac output includes assessment of vital signs, perfusion, and end-organ function (see Chap. 17). Perfusion is assessed by checking capillary refill, skin temperature (cold, cool, warm, hot), skin color (pale, mottled, gray, normal for skin tone), and four extremity pulses (peripheral and central) for strength and quality. End organ perfusion may be assessed using lab values (BUN, creatinine, liver function tests, lactate, and mixed venous saturation) and urine output. Urine output should be assessed at least every 4 h for adequate output.

Cardiovascular assessment for CHF includes observing for presence of diaphoresis (at rest or with exertion), edema (generalized, peripheral, dependant, periorbital), and/or ascites. Respiratory assessment for CHF includes assessing for abnormal breath sounds (rales, crackles, diminished), tachypnea, decreased oxygen saturation, retractions (substernal, intercostal, supraclavicular), grunting, nasal flaring, head bobbing, or shortness of breath with or without exertion. Infants with CHF may be observed to take longer to feed while consuming less, and older children may complain of decreased appetite or nausea.

CHD patients are at risk for arrhythmia from diuretic-related electrolyte imbalances (see Chap. 6), heart dysfunction, congenital abnormalities, and cardiac surgery complications as a primary diagnosis (see Chap. 11) [2, 3]. Children receiving active adjustment to anti-arrhythmic therapy (see Chaps. 5 and 11) typically receive daily 12-lead electrocardiographs (ECG) for formal interpretation. Assessment of the patient's heart rhythm includes a measurement of the patient's PR interval and QTc interval and is compared to the previous ECG. Ongoing assessment of heart rhythm (see Sect. 11.2) should assess for rhythm abnormalities and/or changes from the patient's baseline.

Daily assessment and evaluation of caloric intake should be performed to assess for sufficient calories. The nurse should assess for symptoms of caloric intolerance (i.e., emesis, colic, reflux, loose stools) and necrotizing enterocolitis (NEC) symptoms (blood in the stool, increased abdominal girth, fever, radiologic evidence of free air in the abdomen) in high-risk infants (see Sect. 11.3). Weekly lengths, head circumferences, and daily weights can help to track long-term growth progression.

Hospitalized children with CHD are at risk for pressure ulcer due to edema, hypotension, low cardiac output, history of mechanical ventilation, hypoxia, and device utilization [4, 5]. The Braden Q scale, a validated tool for assessing pressure ulcer risk in pediatric critical care patients, could be used daily to assess patient risk. Nurses should implement preventative measures if pressure ulcer risks are identified.

After cardiac surgery, patients should be assessed for symptoms of surgical complications which include pleural and/or pericardial effusion, atelectasis, pneumothorax, and arrhythmia. The surgical sites, lines, and tubes sites should be assessed for signs of infection. Chest tube output and patency should be assessed every 2–4 h.

11.3 Monitoring Practices

Nurses should be conscientious when determining their patients' alarm parameters and monitors. Inappropriate alarm configuration could lead nurses to not being notified when a valid alarm condition occurs and exposes nurses to an excessive number of false or insignificant clinical alarms [6, 7]. Excessive alarms can desensitize nurses resulting in a phenomenon known as alarm fatigue and is a patient safety risk [8, 9]. PPCU nurses are at risk for alarm fatigue.

PPCU patients are typically monitored from a central location rather than the local monitoring used in procedural areas or intensive care units (ICU). Ideally all alarms in the PPCU should be considered actionable, that is, alarms that require timely intervention [10]. Nurses should set alarm parameters narrow enough to capture actionable alarms while having the alarm parameters wide enough to avoid non-actionable, nuisance alarms [11]. To reduce artifact from ECG monitoring, the patient's skin should be cleaned with soap and water prior to placing ECG leads and the ECG leads changed every 24 h [12, 13].

The American Heart Association (AHA) recommends continuous ECG monitoring for patients at significant risk of an immediate, life-threatening arrhythmia which include: post-cardiac arrest, post-cardiac surgery, pacemaker dependency after lead implantation, external pacing, second-degree or higher atrioventricular block, Wolff-Parkinson-White syndrome, long QT syndrome, acute heart failure, acute pulmonary edema, awaiting transfer to higher level of care, procedural conscious sedation, and unstable arrhythmias [14]. Patients in which monitoring may be beneficial but not essential include patients with chest pain, anti-arrhythmic medication adjustments, subacute heart failure, post-pacemaker or implantable defibrillator placement, syncope evaluation, post-ablation, and/or end-of-life patients where arrhythmia causes discomfort [15]. Cardiac monitoring is not indicated in other patients with such a low risk of a serious event that monitoring has no therapeutic benefit [15].

Pulse oximetry can contribute to the majority of false bedside monitor alarms [9, 16]. There have not been guidelines created for pulse oximetry for pediatric cardiovascular patients. The nurse can use the same clinical judgment on determining what would be actionable alarms regarding pulse oximetry for the patient and whether continuous versus intermittent monitoring would be beneficial. If continuous pulse oximetry is used, it is recommended to rotate probe sites every 8-h to prevent skin breakdown.

11.4   Nutrition and Dietary Considerations

Children with CHD are at risk for malnutrition due to increased metabolic demand, poor caloric intake, and inability to utilize calories effectively (see Chap. 3) [17, 18]. Advancing patients' caloric goals to optimize their nutrition is an important goal for patients in the PPCU. Consultation with a nutritionist can help direct the patient's dietary and nutritional management.

Feeding disorders are common in infants with CHD due to respiratory distress, postoperative complications (i.e., infection, paralyzed vocal cord), poor oral coordination, and gastroesophageal reflux [18]. Speech therapy and occupational therapy can be consulted to assist patients, families, and nurses work on improving the patient's oral coordination (see Chap. 8). To reduce caloric waste and prevent fatigue, the infant should be allowed to oral feed no longer than 30 min per feeding then provide the remainder of the feeding via an enteral tube. This provides the infant an opportunity to work on oral-motor skills and strengths while conserving calories. Another option is to allow the infant or child oral feeds during the day and then supplement with enteral feeds at night. If little or no progress is made with oral feeding skills, long-term enteral feeding would be indicated [19].

Infants with CHD have a ten-fold risk over general newborn populations for developing NEC [20]. Premature birth, hypoplastic left heart syndrome, truncus arteriosus, and episodes of poor systemic perfusion or shock increase the risk for NEC [20]. Vigilance for NEC should be observed in these patients. CHD patients have a high incidence of reflux; preventative measures should be initiated to decrease occurrence [18, 20].

Children with CHF often require a fluid restriction to help maintain their fluid and electrolyte imbalance (see Chaps. 6 and 17). It is better to increase the caloric density of an infant's formula to reduce the amount of volume required for calories rather than fluid restrict in this population. Children should be encouraged to eat food that will decrease the feeling of thirst such as fruits, crispy cold vegetables, and hard candies. Engaging the family to be an active participant in tracking their child's fluid intake can prepare families for home. It is important to make sure the child spaces their fluid intake throughout the day so they do not use up their allotted fluid intake prior to bedtime.

11.5   Postoperative Care

Care after cardiac surgery follows similar principles for other postoperative care practices. Effective pain management (see Sect. 11.6) is essential to enable the patient to participate in the activities needed for postoperative recovery. Early ambulation, cough and deep breathing exercises, incentive spirometry, and chest physiotherapy may reduce and prevent post-operative atelectasis. Oxygen therapy should be titrated as tolerated to achieve the target range of oxygen saturation for the patient.

The patient's diet should be advanced as tolerated. Management of postoperative nausea and vomiting with antiemetics and/or anti-gas medications can help diet progression. A bowel regime to prevent constipation, especially in the setting of possible opioid use and decreased mobility, should be initiated preventively.

The surgical incision may be open to air or covered with a dry sterile dressing for up to 48 h postoperatively depending on surgeon preference. Incisions may be sutured or stapled but more typically have a bonding agent as a skin closure. Sponge baths are recommended for the first week while preventing the surgical site, chest tube locations, or intravenous lines from getting wet. Soap and water is preferred while avoiding lotions, oils, or creams. After the first week, tub bathing or showering may be resumed while trying to avoid soaking the incision for prolonged period of time.

Chest tubes are maintained on low wall suction or waterseal. If clots are observed in the chest tube, the tubing could be stripped or milked by the nurse to advance the clot toward the drainage system. Chest tubes and pacing wire sites should have an occlusive dressing that should be changed at least every 3 days or if the integrity of the dressing is in question. After the chest tube is removed, an occlusive dressing should be placed on the site for 24 h to prevent pneumothorax, and then the site may be open to air or covered with a plastic adhesive bandage. After pacing wire removal, a plastic adhesive bandage can be applied for 24 h and then leave the site open to air.

The child should not be picked up by lifting under the arms until the wound and underlying structures have healed, usually 6 weeks. Patients and parents should be taught to avoid any contact sports after discharge for 6 weeks post-operatively. To avoid strain on the sternotomy, patients should avoid bicycling, active swimming, or driving an automobile for the first 6 weeks postoperatively.

11.6 Medical Care

Patients are admitted to PPCUs for medical management (see Chap. 5), arrhythmia management (see Chap. 11), post-procedure and/or post-cardiac catheterization recovery (see Chap. 14), nutritional interventions (see Chap. 7 and Sect. 11.3), heart failure management (see Chaps. 6, 16, and 17), treatment of comorbidities, treatment of infections, and/or pre-procedure preparation.

The overall goal for medical treatment is to minimize symptoms, optimize heart function, and optimize growth [21]. Medical therapy may include diuretics, digitalis, angiotensin-converting enzyme inhibitors, beta-blockade, anti-arrhythmic therapies, and vasoactive agents (see Chap. 5). The nurse should assess the patient for response to each medication and observe for adverse effects and related lab value changes. The nurse should closely observe for changes in the patient assessment as medication dosages and intervals are changed throughout the hospitalization (see Chap. 5). Some CHD patients may need anticoagulation therapy due to risk for thrombosis [22]. Nurses will need to appropriately time lab specimens and then interpret lab values for therapeutic effect. Nurses should be vigilant for signs of bleeding, venous congestion, or intracranial hemorrhage during anticoagulation and thrombolytic therapy [22]. Education regarding precautions, considerations, and outpatient lab planning should be provided for patients being discharged on anti-coagulant therapy.

Patients with prolonged ICU courses (>5 days) may develop a physical dependence to the sedatives administered in the ICU. Discontinuation or decrease in sedatives may cause withdrawal symptoms including central nervous system irritability, autonomic dysfunction, and gastrointestinal dysfunction [23, 24]. A gradual wean of these medications is recommended to reduce discomfort and stress for the patient and their families. Nurses should assess for withdrawal symptoms and may use a validated withdrawal assessment tool to objectively assess the degree of withdrawal [25].

Infection prevention should always be followed when caring for CHD patients. Proper hand hygiene by clinicians and families prior to handling the patient is highly effective to prevent nosocomial infections. Patients with central venous catheters should receive a daily 2% chlorohexidine bath to prevent central line associated infections [26]. A sterile dressing should be maintained over the central venous catheter and changed every 7 days or sooner if the integrity of the dressing is in question [26].

11.7 Pain Assessment and Management

Acute pain is one of the most common adverse stimuli experienced by hospitalized children and can have adverse effects on the patient's hemodynamic stability, myocardial oxygen consumption, mobility, and ventilation. Pain assessments should be conducted frequently, typically with vital sign activities, before and after a painful procedure and after a pain intervention has been provided. Cultural and language differences or children with developmental disabilities may need additional care when assessing pain [27]. Pain assessment should be multifactorial by using self-report, observation, identification of pain sources, and proxy reporting [28]. Validated behavioral or sensory pain assessments scales will describe pain intensity, and the nurse will need to do additional assessments as to the location and type of pain [28]. It is important when using a pain assessment tool to choose one that is correct for the patient's developmental age or condition.

Effective pain management involves an interdisciplinary therapeutic approach using a combination of pharmacologic, cognitive, behavioral, psychological, and physical treatments. The key to effective pain management is to anticipate predicable painful experiences and assess the patient's condition accordingly [27]. Family members should be active participants in the pain assessment, management choices, and pain management education.

Opioids are indicated for moderate to severe pain. For expected and continuous moderate to severe pain, continuous medication dosing or around-the-clock dosing at fixed intervals is recommended [27]. If immediate relief is needed, intravenous administration is indicated. Older children may prefer the use of patient controlled analgesia to self-administer intravenous pain medication on demand with an optional continuous basal rate. Non-opioid analgesics such as acetaminophen and non-steroidal anti-inflammatory agents can be used in combination with opioids. Enteral administration of pain medications is indicated for mild to moderate pain. Dosages and intervals of pain medication can be adjusted based upon the patient's response. Continuous administration of local anesthetic through a peripheral wound catheter or nerve block catheter provides post-operative pain management while potentially decreasing narcotic utilization and decreased time from procedure to active mobility [29].

11.8 Psychological Support

Staged surgical repairs and interventional catheterizations have increased the number of children who undergo invasive cardiac procedures at various stages in their development. Stressors present for the child during hospitalization include pain, discomfort, separation from parents, dealing with strangers, fear of the unknown, sleep disruption, uncertainty about acceptable behaviors, and loss of autonomy [30, 31]. PPCU patients are typically alert, and aware of themselves and their surroundings compared to other hospital care environments. To help children minimize their stress, the nurse should cluster care together to minimize interruptions. Optimizing the patient's hospital schedule to the child's home schedule (meals, medications, and sleep times) can support normalcy for the patient.

Nurses should prepare children and their caregivers for painful or invasive procedures by assessing the patient's and parent's understanding of the procedure, patient's developmental level and coping styles, information processing preferences, cultural and spiritual practices, support systems, family stressors, and any special communication needs (i.e. language barriers) [31]. Play therapy is an effective technique for providing medical concepts to younger children while exploring their understanding and level of coping about the situation. Child life therapists have expertise in medical play and can assist with desensitizing the child to the hospitalization as well as work with patients toward normal childhood development goals.

Use of anxiolytic agents (i.e., lorazepam, midazolam) and local anesthetics can be administered to patients prior to uncomfortable procedures to reduce stress [32]. Anxiolytic or sedatives used alone do not provide analgesia; pain management should still be utilized [27]. For anticipated severe procedural pain, the use of systemic agents may be required to keep the pain at acceptable levels. Refocusing/distraction techniques may provide conscious redirection of the child's attention from a painful or stressful stimuli to a relaxing or entertaining stimuli such as cartoons, movement toys, bubbles, or books. Cognitive behavioral strategies such as guided imagery, distraction, and relaxation can be used as an adjunct to other pain management modalities. A transitional object (i.e. stuffed animal) can be effective in soothing the patient during the procedure. Infants respond well to a pacifier dipped in concentrated sucrose 24% solution to help self-soothe. Use of positioning or containment, such as bundling or swaddling, can facilitate coping and minimize injury risk during procedures. If possible, minimize painful procedures at the child's bedside to reduce the child's fear by using a treatment room to perform these procedures. Encouraging parents to be present during procedures minimizes parental separation and can help the child cope [33].

11.9 Parental Involvement

Parents are critical in providing emotional support to their child in the PPCU. Parents ongoing active participation and support should be encouraged and supported [34]. Stressors that increase parental anxiety and interfere with their ability to support their child include concern that their child could experience suffering, alterations in their parental role, lack of information, hospital environment, changes in their child, and invasive cardiac procedures [31, 35–37]. Parental transition from the ICU to PPCU may be stressful for families as they experience a change from 1:1 continuous nursing monitoring to higher nurse-to-patient ratios; change in technological monitoring; and new parental role expectations in a less controlled environment [38]. It is helpful for nurses to help parents recognize signs that their child is recovering during this transition period [38].

Education to parents regarding plans, sequences of events, sensory experiences, role expectations, and typical child responses and observing play therapy may help to decrease parental stress [31]. Nurses could invite parents to participate in formal processes, such as rounds or handoff, to increase effective parental communication and comfort levels [33, 34]. Social workers are essential for families of children with CHD and will offer expertise in family assessment, stress management, crisis intervention, advocacy, education, and tangible needs [31]. Parents should be encouraged to room-in, if possible, with their child for 24–48 h to learn the complete care routine of their child [39].

11.10 Patient and Family Education

Education should focus on enabling patients and families to understand [19, 39, 40]:

- Proper feeding techniques and formula preparation.
- Basic infant or child care.
- Infection prevention strategies.
- Infant cardiopulmonary resuscitation and emergency care.
- Early signs and symptoms of illness and disease-specific considerations.
- Safety precautions.
- Safe administration, storage, dosage, timing, effects, and preparation of medications.
- Home equipment operation, maintenance, and problem solving.
- Any special care considerations (i.e., dressing changes, tube changes).
- Dental prophylaxis for high-risk patients.

Parents should prepare and administer medications to their child several times prior to discharge for practice. Teaching families the proper technique on how to prepare, measure, and use an oral syringe will enable safe medication preparation at home. Detailed information, both written and verbal, on each medication's purpose, dose, and side effects should be provided to families. Assisting families with a written medication schedule is helpful, especially for children with multiple medications or complex schedules. During teaching, nurses should request a return demonstration or a teach-back by parents to assess the understanding of the education.

11.11 Discharge Planning

The primary goal for pediatric discharge planning is to enable a smooth transition from the hospital to community-based care [41]. Parental readiness can affect the timing of discharge as well as post-discharge success [41]. A comprehensive discharge plan should include [19]:

- Identification and preparation of in-home caregivers.
- Nutritional plan.
- Safe medication administration.
- Equipment and supply list.
- Identification of, and appointment with, primary care physician and community support services.
- Assessment for adequate physical facilities in the home.
- Emergency care and transport plan.
- Financial resource assessment to ensure home care costs are achievable.

Some pediatric medication may need to be compounded by a pharmacist and may not be immediately available. Compounded medications should be anticipated in advance of discharge. Ideally families should fill the prescriptions and bring them to the hospital for the nurse to double check the dose, concentration, and preparation. Patients being discharged with technologic supports should be assessed for 24-h telephone access, electricity, safe water supply, adequate heating or cooling, and emergency backup plans if there was disruption to any of these systems [19]. Social support should be assessed and appropriate. Individualized intervention plans should be created using available community programs, surveillance, or alternative care placement of the child may be considered [19]. To ensure the continuity of care, children with CHD should have primary care physician and subspecialty clinic appointments coordinated prior to discharge. Community providers should receive a summary of the patient's hospital course and home care plan.

Prior to discharge, a neonate should have received a metabolic screen, hearing screen and baseline neurodevelopmental assessment. Once the infant is stable and approaching discharge, the infant's physiologic stability should be evaluated in their home car seat [19]. If the infant is not stable in their car seat, a car bed may be indicated. Immunizations should be provided prior to discharge if they are due. Parents and families will need to have a clear nutrition plan including access to formula and feeding supplies. Breastfeeding mothers should receive information of breastfeeding support and availability of lactation specialists.

Children with CHD have decreased neurodevelopmental function for a variety for physiological reasons [36]. Nurses should work with discharge planners to facilitate enrollment into early intervention programs, physical therapy, occupational therapy, and/or speech therapy to decrease the impact of neurodevelopmental delay for the child (see Chap. 8). A home visiting nurse can help transition the patient and their families to community-based care after discharge.

Patients with incurable, terminal disease may transition from the hospital to hospice care. Preparation for the child's discharge includes medical follow-up arrangements, home nursing visits, pain and symptom management plan, home oxygen or other equipment and supplies, bereavement support, respite care resources, financial assistance, and a letter for the family alerting emergency services of the child's do-not-resuscitate status [19].

References

1. American Association of Critical Care Nurses. Progressive care fact sheet. 2016. http://www.aacn.org/wd/practice/content/progressivecarefactsheet.pcms?menu=practice. Accessed 14 Oct 2016.
2. Lowry AW, Knudson JD, Cabrera AG, Graves DE, Morales DLS, Rossano JW. Cardiopulmonary resuscitation in hospitalized children with cardiovascular disease: estimated prevalence and outcomes from the Kids' Inpatient Database. Pediatr Crit Care Med. 2013;14(3):248–55. https://doi.org/10.1097/PCC.0b013e3182713329.
3. Ortmann L, Prodhan P, Gossett J, Schexnayder S, Berg R, Nadkarni V, Bhutta A. Outcomes after in-hospital cardiac arrest in children with cardiac disease: a report from get with the guidelines--resuscitation. Circulation. 2011;124(21):2329–37. https://doi.org/10.1161/CIRCULATIONAHA.110.013466.
4. Curley MA, Quigley SM, Lin M. Pressure ulcers in pediatric intensive care: incidence and associated factors. Pediatr Crit Care Med. 2003;4(3):284–90.

5. Tume LN, Siner S, Scott E, Lane S. The prognostic ability of early Braden Q Scores in criti-cally ill children. Nurs Crit Care. 2014;19(2):98–103. https://doi.org/10.1111/nicc.12035.
6. ECRI Institute. Top 10 health technology hazards for 2014 article top 10 health technology hazards for 2014. Health Devices. 2014;42(11):354–80. https://www.ecri.org/Documents/White_papers/Top_10_2015.pdf
7. The Joint Commission. The joint commission announces 2014 National Patient Safety Goal. Jt Comm Perspect. 2013;33(7):1–4. http://www.jointcommission.org/assets/1/18/JCP0713_Announce_New_NSPG.pdf
8. Cvach M, Dang D, Foster J, Irechukwu J. Clinical alarms and the impact on patient safety. Initiat Safe Patient Care. 2009;2:1–8.
9. Lawless S. Crying wolf: false alarms in pediatric intensive care unit. Crit Care Med. 1994;22(6):981–5.
10. Lukasewicz CL, Mattox EA. Understanding clinical alarm safety. Crit Care Nurse. 2015;35(4):45–57. https://doi.org/10.4037/ccn2015113.
11. Karnik A, Bonafide CP. A framework for reducing alarm fatigue on pediatric inpatient units. Hosp Pediatr. 2015;5(3):160–3. https://doi.org/10.1542/hpeds.2014-0123.
12. Cvach MM, Biggs M, Rothwell KJ, Charles-Hudson C. Daily electrode change and effect on cardiac monitor alarms. J Nurs Care Qual. 2013;28(3):265–71.
13. Sendelbach S, Wahl S, Anthony A, Shotts P. Stop the noise: a quality improvement project to decrease electrocardiographic nuisance alarms. Crit Care Nurse. 2015;35(4):15–22.
14. Drew BJ, Califf RM, Funk M, Kaufman ES, Krucoff MW, Laks MM, et al. AHA scien-tific statement: practice standards for electrocardiographic monitoring in hospital settings. J Cardiovasc Nurs. 2005;20:76–106.
15. Drew BJ, Califf RM, Funk M, Kaufman ES, Krucoff MW, Laks MM, et al. Practice standards for electrocardiographic monitoring in hospital settings: an American Heart Association sci-entific statement from the councils on cardiovascular nursing, clinical cardiology, and cardio-vascular disease in the young. Circulation. 2004;110(17):2721–46. https://doi.org/10.1161/01.CIR.0000145144.56673.59.
16. Gross B, Dahl D, Nielsen L. Physiologic monitoring alarm load on medical/surgical floors of a community hospital. Biomed Instrum Tech. 2011;45:29–36. https://doi.org/10.2345/0899-8205-45.s1.29.
17. Cameron J, Rosenthal A, Olson A. Malnutrition in hospitalized children with congenital heart disease. Arch Pediatr Adolesc Med. 1995;149:1098–102.
18. Davis D, Davis S, Cotman K, Worley S, Londrico D, Kenny D, Harrison AM. Feeding difficul-ties and growth delay in children with hypoplastic left heart syndrome versus d-transposition of the great arteries. Pediatr Cardiol. 2008;29(2):328–33. https://doi.org/10.1007/s00246-007-9027-9.
19. American Academy of Pediatrics. Hospital discharge of the high-risk neonate. Pediatrics. 2008;122(5):1119–26. https://doi.org/10.1542/NICU.
20. McElhinney DB, Hedrick HL, Bush DM, Pereira GR, Stafford PW, Gaynor JW, et al. Necrotizing enterocolitis in neonates with congenital heart disease: risk factors and outcomes. Pediatrics. 2000;106(5):1080–7. https://doi.org/10.1542/peds.106.5.1080.
21. Hsu DT, Pearson GD. Heart failure in children part II: diagnosis, treatment, and future directions. Circ Heart Fail. 2009;2(5):490–8. https://doi.org/10.1161/CIRCHEARTFAILURE.109.856229.
22. Giglia TM, Massicotte MP, Tweddell JS, Barst RJ, Bauman M, Erickson CC, et al. Prevention and treatment of thrombosis in pediatric and congenital heart disease a scientific statement from the American Heart Association. Circulation. 2013;128(24):2622–703. https://doi.org/10.1161/01.cir.0000436140.77832.7a.
23. Fisher D, Grap M, Younger J, Ameringer S, Elswick R. Opiod withdrawal signs and symptoms in children: frequency and determinants. Heart Lung J Crit Care. 2013;42(6):407–13. https://doi.org/10.1016/j.hrtlng.2013.07.008.
24. Frank L, Naughton I, Winter I. Opiod and benzodiazepine withdrawal symptoms in paediatric intensive care patients. Instensive Crit Care Nurs. 2004;20:344–51. https://doi.org/10.1016/j.iccn.2004.07.008.

25. Franck LS, Scoppettuolo L, Wypij D, Curley MA. Validity and generalizability of the with-drawal assessment tool-1 (WAT-1) for monitoring iatrogenic withdrawal syndrome in pediatric patients. Pain. 2012;153(1):142–8. https://doi.org/10.1016/j.pain.2011.10.003.

26. O'Grady NP, Alexander M, Dellinger EP, Gerberding JL, Heard SO, Maki DG, et al. Guidelines for the prevention of intravascular catheter-related infections. Am J Infect Control. 2002;30(8):476–89. https://doi.org/10.1067/mic.2002.129427.

27. American Academy of Pediatrics, & American Pain Society. The assessment and management of acute pain in infants, children and adolescents. Pediatrics. 2001;108(3):793–7. https://doi.org/10.1542/peds.108.3.793.

28. Joestlein L. Pain, pain, go away! Evidence-based review of developmentally appropriate pain assessment for children in a postoperative setting. Orthop Nurs. 2015;34(5):252–9. https://doi.org/10.1097/NOR.0000000000000175.

29. Kocabas S, Yedicocuklu D, Yuksel E, Uysallar E, Askar F. Infiltration of the sternotomy wound and the mediastinal tube sites with 0.25% levobupivacaine as adjunctive treatment for postoperative pain after cardiac surgery. Eur J Anaesthesiol. 2008;25(10):842–9. https://doi.org/10.1017/S0265021508004614.

30. Connolly D, McClowry S, Hayman L, Mahony L, Artman M. Posttraumatic stress disorder in children after cardiac surgery. J Pediatr. 2004;144:480–4. https://doi.org/10.1016/j.jpeds.2003.12.048.

31. LeRoy S, Elixson M, Cochair M, O'Brien P, Tong E, Turpin S, Uzark K. Recommendations for preparing children and adolescents for invasive cardiac procedures. A statement from the American Heart Association Pediatric Nursing Subcommittee of the Council on Cardiovascular Nursing in collaboration with the Council on Cardiovascular Diseases of the Young. Circulation. 2003;108:2550–64.

32. Ben-Amitay G, Kosov I, Reiss A, Toren P, Yoran-Hegesh R, Kotler M, Mozes T. Is elective surgery traumatic for children and their parents? J Paediatr Child Health. 2006;42(10):618–24. https://doi.org/10.1111/j.1440-1754.2006.00938.x.

33. Penny DJ, Shekerdemian LS. The American Heart Association's recent scientific statement on cardiac critical care: implications for pediatric practice. Congenit Heart Dis. 2013;8(1):3–19. https://doi.org/10.1111/chd.12028.

34. Rosenbery RE, Rosenfeld P, Silber B, Deng S, Sullivan-Bolyai S. Parents' perspectives on "keeping their children safe" in the hospital. J Nurs Care Qual. 2016;31(4):318–26.

35. Franck LS, McQuillan A, Wray J, Grocott MPW, Goldman A. Parent stress levels during children's hospital recovery after congenital heart surgery. Pediatr Cardiol. 2010;31(7):961–8. https://doi.org/10.1007/s00246-010-9726-5.

36. Menahem S, Poulakis Z, Prior M. Children subjected to cardiac surgery for congenital heart disease. Part 2 - parental emotional experiences. Interact Cardiovasc Thorac Surg. 2008;7(4):605–8. https://doi.org/10.1510/icvts.2007.171066.

37. Utens EM, Bieman HJV, Witsenburg M, Bogers AJJC, Hess J, Verhulst FC. Does age at the time of elective cardiac surgery or catheter intervention in children influence the longitudinal development of psychological distress and styles of coping of parents? Cardiol Young. 2002;12:524–30.

38. Obas KA, Leal JM, Zegray M, Rennick JE. Parental perceptions of transition from intensive care following a child's cardiac surgery. Nurs Crit Care. 2016;21(3):e1–9. https://doi.org/10.1111/nicc.12202.

39. Pye S, Green A. Parent education after newborn congenital heart surgery. Adv Neonatal Care. 2003;3(3):147–56. https://doi.org/10.1016/S1536-0903(03)00075-4.

40. American Heart Association. Prevention of infective (bacterial) endocarditis wallet card. 2016. http://www.heart.org/idc/groups/heart-public/@wcm/@hcm/documents/downloadable/ucm_307644.pdf. Accessed 1 Oct 2016.

41. Weiss M, Johnson NL, Malin S, Jerofke T, Lang C, Sherburne E. Readiness for discharge in parents of hospitalized children. J Pediatr Nurs. 2008;23(4):282–95. https://doi.org/10.1016/j.pedn.2007.10.005.

Nursing Care for Patients with CHD in the Operating Theater

12

Christina Sillman and Marilynne Ngo

Abstract

Congenital heart surgical care has a unique spectrum of patient population ranging from neonatal primary sternotomy to adult re-sternotomy. Surgical goals can range from palliative techniques to corrective techniques depending on disease complexity. The historical complexities in the evolution of surgical techniques add an additional layer of intrigue. Nursing roles within the operating theater are autonomous and diverse and require highly specialized knowledge and skill set. Nursing care must be adaptable and involve high level of critical thinking to ensure patient safety and positive patient outcomes.

12.1 Surgical Operations

The wide spectrum of congenital heart defect type and severity has led to the advancement and development of surgical procedures throughout the history of congenital heart disease. Beginning with the first successful extracardiac surgery on August, 8, 1938, by Dr. Robert Gross [1] at Children's Hospital Boston for PDA closure through the development of cardiopulmonary bypass and to current-day practices, surgical techniques are a history lesson in the evolution of congenital heart care. Surgical techniques may be used as a palliative measure or as therapeutic in restoring typical blood flow patterns, and multiple techniques can be used in

C. Sillman (✉)
The Adult Congenital Heart Program at Stanford, Palo Alto, CA, USA
e-mail: csillman@stanfordhealthcare.org

M. Ngo
Lucile Packard Children's Hospital, Palo Alto, CA, USA

© Springer International Publishing AG, part of Springer Nature 2019
S. F. Flocco et al. (eds.), *Congenital Heart Disease*,
https://doi.org/10.1007/978-3-319-78423-6_12

Table 12.1 Surgical procedures in congenital heart disease

Patent ductus arteriosus repair
Atrial septal defect repair
Ventricular septal defect repair
Partial or total anomalous pulmonary venous return repair
Blalock-Taussig shunt (usually done without CPB)
Waterston shunt
Potts shunt
Mitral valve repair/replace
Tricuspid valve repair/replace
Aortic valve repair/replace
Ross/Konno procedure
Coarctation of aorta repair (sternotomy or thoracotomy, with or without CPB)
Aortic arch repair/reconstruction
Atrioventricular canal repair
Anomalous coronary arteries repair
Double arterial switch
LVOT or RVOT repair
Pulmonary artery band
Pulmonary artery reconstruction
Pulmonary conduit replacement
TOF complete repair
Unifocalization
Rastelli procedure
Mustard/Senning atrial switch
Arterial switch
Double switch
Damus-Kaye-Stansel procedure
Norwood procedure
Classic or bidirectional Glenn shunt (usually done without CPB)
Atriopulmonary Fontan procedure
Lateral tunnel Fontan procedure
Extracardiac Fontan procedure (most often without CPB)
Ventricular assist device placement
Heart transplant

Historical surgical techniques

combination with each other. Table 12.1 lists the various congenital heart surgical techniques commonly performed or historically performed.

12.2   Nursing Roles

The various nursing roles within the operating theater include scrub nurse, circulating nurse, cardiac service lead, and charge nurse. Each role has a unique set of responsibilities focused on patient safety and high-quality perioperative care. Nursing care begins preoperatively and continues through the postoperative recovery handoff. Congenital heart surgical operations typically utilize one scrub nurse and one circulation nurse for all cases. The focus, tasks, and duties of each individual role vary from each other and are unique to the practice of perioperative nursing in congenital heart disease.

12.2.1 Scrub Nurse

Responsibilities include gathering the sterile supplies and instruments needed for the surgical procedure, setup of the table, and assisting the surgeon throughout the case by dispensing instruments and other sterile items to the surgical team.

12.2.2 Circulating Nurse

Responsibilities include the preparation of the operating theater; management of blood products; assisting the anesthesiologist with intubation, IV insertion, and other invasive procedures to prepare the patient for the operation; and assisting the scrub nurse, anesthesiologist, and surgeon who are unable to leave the sterile operating bedside. The circulating nurse assists with the preoperative nursing assessment and transport of the patient to the OR. The circulating nurse constantly assesses for patient safety and high-quality perioperative care.

12.2.3 Cardiac Service Lead Nurse

Responsibilities include organizing and obtaining all equipment and supplies required by the team for the surgical case and serve as a resource nurse for everyone on the cardiac team.

12.2.4 Charge Nurse

Responsibilities include assigning appropriate staff to surgical procedure based on skill set and knowledge base, as well as surgeon request when possible, delegation of tasks to appropriate ancillary staff, and managing meal breaks at appropriate times according to the law mandate.

12.2.5 Education Preparation

Educational preparation for a nursing role in the operating theater varies from region and country regulations. Beyond the basic licensing requirements for nursing, certification in a nursing specialty objectively measures the knowledge base of a registered nurse to certify their qualification to practice in a specialized area of medicine. The CRON credentialing examination provides an elevated level of qualification for the perioperative registered nurse and is a recommended qualification for nurses working with specialized populations such as congenital heart cardiac surgery [2].

12.3   Preoperative Responsibilities

Preparation of the operating theater is an essential part of the nursing role in surgical care of patients with congenital heart disease. Each role has specific responsibilities and tasks and involves autonomous yet collaborative work to avoid duplicate efforts in addition to ensuring upmost patient safety and quality care.

Preoperative responsibilities start with the charge nurse's duty to assess the surgical schedule and assign surgical teams including scrub and circulating nursing staff to particular cases based upon current skill set, expertise, and surgeon preference. A tentative assignment is made well in advanced of the day of surgical cases but remains adaptable as patient cases may be canceled or moved due to unforeseen issues such as illness, abnormal presurgical testing or assessment, or when a more urgent surgical case requires adjustment of the surgical schedule.

Scrub nurse preoperative duties include gathering the sterile supplies for the patient based upon age/size of the patient. Table 12.2 lists the various supplies that are size/weight dependent. The scrub nurse is responsible for the preparation of the

Table 12.2 Size- and weight-dependent surgical supplies

1. Bed
2. Safety belt
3. Chest retractors
4. Vascular clamps
5. Drapes
6. Sutures
7. Blood pressure cuff
8. Electrocardiogram leads
9. External pads
10. Internal paddles
11. Bovie pads
12. Cardiac tourniquets
13. Chest tubes and containment kits
14. Sternal wires
15. Grafts
16. Valves
17. Positioning devices
18. Dressings
19. IV securement devices
20. Heating and cooling mattress and blankets
21. Arterial and venous cannulas for cardiopulmonary bypass

back table and to meet with the surgeon to ensure procurement of proper cardiac implant type and size (valves, grafts, cardiac devices).

Circulating nurse preoperative duties include ensuring appropriately sized surgical bed/table, with positioning supplies ready for patient. The circulating nurse will work with the perfusionist to confirm blood products for the highest level of patient safety utilizing regional blood product verification procedures. The circulating nurse and scrub nurse will work together to count the instruments, sponges, and other intra-op supplies for the first, presurgical, count.

Upon preparation of the operating theater, the circulating nurse will then prepare the patient for transport from preoperative check in to the operating theater. The circulating nurse will receive handoff report from the preoperative nurse, introduce themselves to the patient and family, and systematically perform critical patient verifications. Patient verifications start with patient identity, surgical procedure planned, NPO status, allergies, and current medications and that all consent forms have been understood and signed. The circulation nurse may work with preoperative nurse to place and secure an IV and may draw labs for type and screen with IV placement. Most importantly to the family, the circulating nurse will explain the process for receiving patient updates and approximate timing for surgery completion. The circulating nurse along with anesthesiologist will transport the patient to the OR after sufficient time with the family has been provided.

Nursing empathy and compassion is integral for a positive transfer of patient from family to operating theater team, especially with children. The use of child life specialists or child behavioral specialists is particularly helpful for patients, parents, siblings, and other family members. Preoperative tours of the hospital, patient care units, and operating waiting room are important components of preparing the family for major surgery and are best done prior to the day of surgery.

Upon arrival to the operating theater, the circulating nurse will document time of arrival clearly for patient records and for family updating purposes. The patient is then transferred from the transport gurney to the operating bed with the assistance of the circulating nurse and anesthesiologist. The circulating nurse must secure the patient to the operating bed with a safety strap to avoid accidental injury resulting from a fall.

The circulating nurse will attach the patient to monitors including a 5-lead EKG, pulse oximetry to three extremities, blood pressure cuff to right arm or leg (unless contraindicated), and external defibrillator pads for all patients who have a history of prior surgeries.

The circulating nurse will ensure the patient is comfortable and warm (given a warm blanket) and emotionally comforts the patient throughout the initiation of anesthesia. The circulating nurse will then assist the anesthesiologist and the anesthesia tech with intubation, ensuring the endotracheal tube is well secured prior to leaving the patient's side.

The anesthesia team will then begin placing invasive central venous and arterial lines, and the circulating nurse will remain available for assistance and monitor for adherence to sterile technique and the sterility of the surgical field. After the venous and arterial lines are placed, the circulating nurse will place the urinary catheter

Table 12.3 Surgical positioning techniques

- Ensure the bovie pad is placed on a safe area of the patient's body
- Verify that the patient is not lying on any objects such as syringe, caps, or other items that the anesthesia may have inadvertently left on the bed
- Verify that the draw sheet is not rolled up under the patient that may cause pressure sore later or skin breakdown from the long surgery
- Verify that the patient's spine is aligned in the supine position for median sternotomy incision or lateral position
- Ensure that the knees are flexed and supported with gel roll or rolled up yellow foam. Patient may require compression stocking for deep vein thrombosis precaution if not anticoagulated
- Ensure the heels are supported with yellow foam to prevent foot drop and pressure sore.
- Wrap patients arms up in gel pads and tuck arms in at patient's side to keep them from falling off the OR bed during the surgery when the surgeon required that the patient bed to be rotated from side to side for better exposure of surgical site
- Ensure all IV lines, central line (which is usually an I.J.—internal jugular), and arterial line that have stopcocks connected are well padded so that it will not pressed against the patient's body during the surgery
- The patient's body need to be exposed from the neck to mid-thigh. The groins must be exposed in case the patient condition deteriorates and requires cardiopulmonary bypass emergently before the chest can be opened
- Site preparation of the patient's neck, chest, abdomen, and groins

using sterile technique, insert the rectal temperature probe, and ensure that the temperature probe is properly monitoring the patient's core temperature.

The patient is now ready to be positioned for surgery. The circulating nurse works with the surgical fellow or physician assistant to obtain optimal surgical positioning. Table 12.3 lists the positioning techniques the circulating nurse is responsible for.

After positioning the circulating nurse will then perform site preparation. The various preparation solutions include ChloraPrep, Betadine, or Providine and are usually a two-step process. First, the circulating nurse will scrub to clean the surgical site using sterile 4 × 4 gauze or sponge. Then the circulating nurse will dry the site with sterile paper disposable absorbent towels. Then the circulating nurse will use sterile gauze or sponge to again paint the surgical site with the preparation solution. This solution will stay on the skin until it dries, prior to draping.

The scrub nurse will scrub in for the preparation of the sterile field. Once gowned and gloved using sterile technique, the scrub nurse will then assist the surgical team with their gowning and gloving. The scrub nurse will then work with the surgical physician assistant, surgical fellow, or surgeon to drape the patient and ensure proper exposure of the surgical site.

12.3.1 Patient Verification: Confirming Right Patient, Right Surgery, and Right Site

The World Health Organization Guidelines for Safe Surgery (2009) [3] describes a universal protocol as a standard practice inherently redundant to confirm right patient, site, and procedure. The three steps of the universal protocol include verification, site marking, and time-out.

Verification is communicated to confirm right patient, site, and procedure at every step between the decisions to operate to the beginning of the operation: to be completed with scheduling, preoperative appointments, admission, and all hand-offs or transfers of care. Confirmation of patient identity should be performed using at least two patient identifiers. The patient is involved in the process of verification when awake.

The majority of wrong-site surgery is performed on sites with bilateralism. The second step of the universal protocol involves marking the surgical site with permanent ink while the patient is awake and alert, if possible, to verify surgical site. Each medical institution should have a consistent and clear method of marking surgical sites.

The last step in the universal protocol is the time-out or surgical pause prior to the first incision to do one last thorough verification. The surgical pause contains a set list of checks and confirmations involving the entire surgical team. Patient, procedure, and site is again reviewed along with necessary signed consents, correct patient positioning, and accurate implants or special equipment obtained.

The scrub nurse and circulating nurse are both participating members of the time-out process. The circulating nurse will clearly document the process in the patient's operative report.

12.4 Nursing Care During Surgery

Prior to the first incision, the scrub nurse will pass off the plug-in ends of the internal defibrillator paddle, suction tubing, and bovie cable to the circulating nurse to connect to their respective machinery. The circulating nurse will confirm with the surgeon the desired settings for the bovie machine for cutting and coagulation, as well as the setting for the internal defibrillator pads and the sternal saw to the power source.

The circulating nurse also provides the surgical team with step stools for any team members who need height to allow for proper ergonomics and view of the surgical field.

12.4.1 Circulating Nurse Responsibilities

Throughout the opening of the sternum and dissecting open the chest, the circulating nurse will stay beside the defibrillator to operate the defibrillator as there is a high risk of ventricular dysrhythmia. The circulating nurse will not leave the operating theater until the patient is stable on cardiopulmonary bypass.

Throughout the surgery, the circulating nurse will adjust the bovie setting per the surgeon's request, replace any instruments that are broken or dropped, obtain any provisions needed by the surgical team, open any sutures as needed throughout the surgery, and place dirty sponges in the counter bag to keep track of all sponges. The circulating nurse will also answer the phone and pages of the surgeon or call outside medical team, such as the cardiologist, during surgery. The circulating nurse is responsible for thorough documentation in the patient's medical record.

The primary responsibility of the circulating nurse throughout surgery is to maintain patient safety. The circulating nurse will assess the patient throughout position changes to ensure proper alignment and safety of patient limbs. Patient safety includes close monitoring of vital signs including heart rhythm, oxygen saturation, arterial tracings, and core body temperature. The circulating nurse will also prepare specimens such as blood for lab processing or tissue for pathology or research and report lab results once available. Blood products being received to the OR will be verified by the circulating nurse. Ensuring sterile field is maintained is an important part of patient safety. Ultimately, the circulating nurse must be prepared for the unexpected such as massive bleeding, cardiac arrest, or other emergencies such as fire.

12.4.2 Scrub Nurse Responsibilities

The scrub nurse is within the sterile field and scrubbed in and must remain at the patient's side throughout the surgery. The primary responsibility of the scrub nurse is to arrange and provide instruments for the surgeon. The scrub nurse will work collaboratively with the circulating nurse to communicate sterile supply needs.

12.5   Postoperative Care

Once intracardiac surgery is completed, the circulating nurse will begin preparing for the process of taking the patient off of cardiopulmonary bypass. Tasks involve reheating the patient's body temperature by raising the operating theater temperature and applying warm blankets to the patient's extremities, page the cardiologist to complete a postoperative ECHO to ensure patency of surgical repairs prior to closure of the chest, prepare defibrillator and blood products, and assist the scrub nurse in preparing for closure and chest tube placements.

After the heart is evaluated by the cardiologist with ECHO to ensure surgical repairs and heart function are adequate, the entire team prepares for chest closure. The circulating nurse and scrub nurse will initiate the first count of instruments, sponges, and other surgical items prior to closure of the fascia. The circulating nurse will then prepare thrombin for the scrub nurse to soak the Gelfoam for the physician to provide hemostasis with closure and mix ordered antibiotic with normal saline for the surgeon to use as irrigation of the chest before closure. The circulating nurse will verify surgical procedure documentation with the surgeon prior to the surgeons' exit from the operating theater. All specimens will be verified by the circulating nurse for accurate labeling prior to being transported to pathology.

The circulating nurse will call the cardiovascular intensive care unit (CVICU) the patient is assigned to provide notice for patient transport, usually at an estimated 45 min prior to leaving the operating theater. A standardized handoff from the operating theater to the CVICU helps to provide clear communication regarding the procedure, intubation, medication, ventilator settings, blood loss, and other pertinent items to the CVICU team in order to allow for adequate preparation to receive the patient. A nurse-to-nurse handoff report is also achieved between the circulating nurse and the bedside CVICU nurse who will be receiving the patient.

The circulating nurse and the scrub nurse will then initiate the final count of all instruments, sponges, and other surgical items prior to final closure of the sternum with wire. Once the chest has been closed and the drape is removed, the circulating nurse and the scrub nurse will work together to prepare the patient for transportation to the CVICU.

The scrub nurse will clean the preparation solution off of the patient, apply dressings with date/time, and ensure blood products are available in cooler for transportation. The circulating nurse will place a new patient identification arm band on the patient, ensuring all information is correct, and place any additional bands such as an allergy band. The patient bed will be brought into the room, and the scrub nurse and circulating nurse will work together with the anesthesia team to move the patient to the bed and to attach patient to the transport monitors. The circulating nurse will ensure all access lines have clean dressings, are not actively bleeding, and are prepared for transportation. The Foley catheter containment bag is emptied and hung on the bed for transportation along with the chest tube containment device. The circulating nurse will make a final call to the CVICU to ensure that they are prepared to receive the patient. Prior to leaving the operating theater, the circulating nurse and scrub nurse will ensure that all vital signs, temporary pacing, and invasive measurements (central venous pressure, transthoracic, and arterial waveforms) are being accurately read on the transport monitor and functioning well. Emergency transport supplies are obtained (blood products in cooler, portable oxygen, bag valve mask, portable suction, etc.) for the transportation to the CVICU in case of emergency in route. The scrub nurse typically remains in the operating theater reorganizing the instrumentation and transporting instruments to the decontamination room.

Upon arrival to the CVICU, the circulating nurse will provide the bedside nurse with a final handoff report and be available for any additional questions or concerns. Once the patient is stable in the CVICU, the circulating nurse returns to the operating theater to assist the scrub nurse in processing any remaining specimens, return unused blood to the blood bank, and assist in operating theater cleanup. The circulating nurse will then ensure all required documentation is completed prior to notifying the charge nurse that the surgical case has been completed.

12.5.1 Documentation

Clear and concise documentation is an integral part of the circulating nurse's role in the operating theater. Documentation begins upon meeting the patient in preoperative check in and continues through handoff to the CVICU. Medical charting systems vary from paper and pen to electronic medical records. Some medical record systems will have automatic population of patient information such as vital signs and easy-to-use flow sheets to capture necessary checklist items. The nursing documentation serves as a complimentary documentation to the surgeon's operative note and is most useful for the medical teams caring for the patient in the postoperative period.

Nursing documentation preoperatively must include the patient's "nil per os" (NPO) status describing when the last time they ate food or drank liquids and if any medications were taken by mouth the morning of surgery. The circulating nurse will do a patient assessment preoperatively documenting patient identifiers, neurological status preoperatively, personal items placed in patient bag, mode of arrival (i.e., from home or from inpatient unit), surgical team members' names who will be assisting in transport to the operating theater, name of nurse who provided handoff if patient arrived via inpatient unit, and any other factors deemed clinically important by the circulating nurse with the preoperative assessment.

Intraoperative documentation is integral to maintaining the highest standard for operating theater quality control. Table 12.4 lists some of the common intraoperative nursing documentation components.

Lastly, upon conclusion of surgery, the circulating nurse will debrief with the surgeon prior to leaving the operating theater to verify procedure, implants used, specimens being sent to pathology, and any other pertinent details needed for handoff to the CVICU. Handoff report, nursing staff involved in handoff, and transportation mode, personnel, and transport equipment used for transport from operating theater to CVICU should also be well documented.

Table 12.4 Intraoperative nursing documentation

- Staff (list names of all members involved in the surgical procedure)
- Count (include initial count before patient comes in the room, second count is before closing the fascia, and final count is before the chest is closed with wire)
- Position (include how the patient is positioned, position device used, and who are involved in positioning the patient)
- Pre-incision time-out (include names of all members of surgical team)
- Site prep (always prep from the neck to mid-thigh using ChloraPrep with tint unless patient has allergy to ChloraPrep, and then use Betadine scrub and solution)
- Procedure
- Intra-op medications used
  - Ancef or vancomycin are routinely used to mix with normal saline for irrigation of the chest prior to closing (500 mg in 500 ml NS)
  - Thrombin—prepared in powder form and requires mixing with NS and used to soak Gelfoam for hemostasis
  - Heparin flush—mix 1000 units of heparin in 100 ml NS to get a concentration of 10 units/ml for flushing lines or Gore-Tex shunt on the sterile field
- Lines, drains, and airway includes date, time, name of person placing the line, and location:
  - Urine catheter
  - Double lumen RA line (right atrial, common atrial)—one lumen used for measuring pressure and one lumen used for infusing drips such as dopamine, epinephrine, milrinone, etc.
  - Single lumen LA or PA line (left atrial or pulmonary artery)—*only* used for measuring pressure, never used for drip infusion
  - Intravenous lines
  - Chest tube sites
  - Pacing wires (epicardial—atrial and ventricular leads)
  - Peritoneal drain—drain fluid in the abdomen
- Equipment:
  - Bovie machine—record # assigned
  - Defibrillator machine—record # assigned
  - Slush machine—one side keeps saline warm and one side makes slush and keeps saline cold for use during bypass
- Implant section—document any items that remain inside the patient after the surgery is complete
  - Valves—mechanical or bioprosthetic
  - Homografts—used to replace valve and conduit
  - Bovine pericardium—used as patch
  - Gore-Tex patch
  - Hemashield patch
- Supplies—all supplies used for the surgery
- Specimen—document any specimens to be sent to pathology
- Dressing—type of dressing and location

The circulating nurse must ensure that all nursing documentation is complete and correct as an integral part of the responsibilities of this particular operating theater nursing role. Effective communication is the cornerstone of quality health care, and documentation in the patient's health-care chart is the most efficient way to provide high-quality communication for all team members' reference.

Conclusion

Congenital heart nursing care in the operating theater is a demanding and highly skilled career that offers variety in terms of surgical techniques, patient demographics, and nursing roles. Specialized training, certification, and continuing education are recommended to maintain the highest level of nursing professionalism. Understanding the unique components of the various operating theaters, nursing roles help delineate the autonomous contribution of nursing care for congenital heart patients' undergoing surgery.

References

1. Gross RE, Hubbard JP. Landmark article Feb 25, 1939: surgical ligation of a patent ductus arteriosus. Report of first successful case. JAMA. 1984;251(9):1201–2.
2. Certified perioperative nursing. http://www.cc-institute.org/cnor. Accessed 11 November 2016.
3. World Health Organization. WHO guidelines for safe surgery: safe surgery saves lives. 2009. http://apps.who.int/iris/bitstream/10665/44185/1/9789241598552_eng.pdf. Accessed 10 November 2016.

Nursing Care in Cath Lab

Eliana Zarlenga

Abstract

From 1966 to the present day, paediatric haemodynamics has undergone significant innovation. Over the years interventional cardiology procedures, both haemodynamic and electrophysiological, have become more and more effective and are now the therapy of choice and the most appropriate treatment criterion in many clinical conditions, as surgeons find themselves up against more and more complex lesions. To rise to these challenges, cath labs must necessarily meet very high safety standards and be organised in a way that allows them to deal with the amount of activity and ensures essential care criteria. Many of the important factors for safety are dependent on and must be guaranteed by the members of the nursing team. Nowadays, nurses can count on internationally accredited procedures that are the result of years of research and fine-tuning. In 2008, the World Health Organization published and disseminated guidelines for safety in the operating theatre, called "Guidelines for Safe Surgery". The same WHO guidelines are the basis of the "Manual for safety in the operating theatre: Recommendations and Checklist" published by the Ministry of Labour, Health and Social Policies in October 2009. The checklist is a tool developed with a view to improving safety and quality. It is made up of 20 items that serve as a guide when carrying out checks in the operating theatre. Within the context described above, the activities of the nurse performing duties at a haemodynamic facility are characterised by the need to be able to field a high degree of specialisation. The nurse must know how to relate to others and have the skills needed for performing the process of care, capacity of observation, planning, judgement and decision-taking. Neither should he/she lack the ability to properly interpret information and communicate in a comprehensive way. From the outset, the

E. Zarlenga
Department of Pediatric Cardiac Surgery, Bambino Gesù Children's Hospital
and Research Institute, Rome, Italy
e-mail: eliana.zarlenga@opbg.net

© Springer International Publishing AG, part of Springer Nature 2019
S. F. Flocco et al. (eds.), *Congenital Heart Disease*,
https://doi.org/10.1007/978-3-319-78423-6_13

nurse who is assigned to a cath lab will be supported by a tutor who will follow him/her, step by step, for about 6 months. There is also a practice example of a specific procedure: "Percutaneous transcatheter implantation of Edwards SAPIEN XT pulmonary heart valve". Recovery room (RR) is a place where any patient who needs to have continuous postoperative care is accommodated. The nursing staff attached to the RR must be adequately prepared. Their task is to take continuous and direct care of the patient, and amongst their therapeutic goals, we find establishing pain management, treatment of nausea and vomiting, recovery of normothermia and acid-base and electrolyte equilibrium.

13.1 Introduction

In 1966, Rashkind and Miller [1] were the first ever to describe a technique called Rashkind atrial septostomy, whereby interatrial communication was dilated by literally jerking a balloon across the atrial septum, resulting in a tear, thus giving rise to the age of percutaneous interventional treatment.

Over the years interventional cardiology procedures, both haemodynamic and electrophysiological, have become more and more effective and are now the therapy of choice and the most appropriate treatment criterion in many clinical conditions, as surgeons find themselves up against more and more complex lesions.

From back in 1966 to the present day, paediatric haemodynamics has undergone such significant innovation that the majority of congenital heart disease cases today can be treated percutaneously. We can consider, for example, interatrial and interventricular defects, patent ductus arteriosus, pulmonary valvular stenosis and aortic valvular stenosis.

The main congenital heart diseases that can be treated with haemodynamic interventional procedures are:
- **Rashkind atrial septostomy**
- **Left heart obstruction**
  Aortic stenosis
  Coarctation of the aorta
- **Right heart obstruction**
  Pulmonary valve stenosis
  Pulmonary atresia with intact septum
  Stenosis of the pulmonary arteries
- **Diseases with left-to-right shunt**
  Atrial septal defects
  Ventricular septal defects (muscular and perimembranous)
  Patente ductus arteriosus
- **Hybrid procedures**
  Muscular ventricular septal defect
  Hypoplastic left heart

The scope for intervention does not end here: many other procedures are performed in the catheterisation laboratory, such as embolisation, biopsies and percutaneous pulmonary valve implantation. We could consider the field of electrostimulation: implantation and replacement of single-chamber, dual-chamber and biventricular PMKs and ICDs, as well as single- and dual-chamber temporary PMKs, and as for the field of electrophysiology, TAS, SEF, radio-frequency transcatheter ablations and cryoenergy for almost all types of arrhythmia (e.g., atrial flutter, AF, AVNRT, AVRT, WPW, atrial tachycardia).

For the sake of completeness, we must also add that progress in technology, pharmacology and organisation has in any case enabled optimum results in highly complex patients. In experienced hands, and at dedicated facilities, these procedures can be performed with a high success rate and low associated morbidity and mortality.

These are now high-tech procedures, and while on the one hand they are an increasingly important tool, on the other, they contribute to increasing, if that is possible, the level of complexity.

To rise to these challenges, cath labs must necessarily meet very high safety standards and be organised in a way that allows them to deal with the amount of activity and ensures essential care criteria. Maintaining adequate safety conditions for patients and healthcare professionals is indeed of primary importance, as is ensuring the best use of human and technological resources allocated [2].

For example, it is essential that these laboratories be located within a cardiology and Paediatric surgery medical department, and the operating theatre and cardiac intensive care must be located close by in order to enable intervention in case of an emergency.

The need to continuously improve the quality and safety of the services also means that actions and conduct must be planned and shared as much as possible.

It is therefore necessary to pay special attention and give due importance to communication processes within the team. The nurse cannot and must not work in isolation from the doctor, regardless of whether the latter is a cardiologist, an arhythmologist, a radiologist or an anaesthetist. All the professionals involved in the cath lab must ensure a climate of collaboration and proactively communicate with each other in order to prevent the possibility of accidents.

All this and more will be discussed in more detail and to greater extent in this chapter.

13.2   Safety First

The cath lab is a highly complex environment where many people and professions work together, often with patients in acute conditions who require emergency procedures.

Many of the important factors for safety are dependent on and must be guaranteed by the members of the nursing team; these include, of course, the need for proper control of asepsis in the operative field, for precise identification of the patient and surgical site and for guaranteed presence of all aids required. All of those are critical points which, if not handled properly, can cause complications that could seriously injure the patient.

Nowadays, nurses can count on internationally accredited procedures that are the result of years of research and fine-tuning.

Let us take a closer look at which procedures these are and how they came about.

Solutions to increase safety in the operating theatre have been needed at global level for some time now. The world health assembly which passed a resolution calling upon member states and the World Health Organization to pay the utmost attention to the problem of patient safety was held back in 2002.

Then, in 2008, the World Health Organization published and disseminated guidelines for safety in the operating theatre, called "Guidelines for Safe Surgery".

The same WHO guidelines are the basis of the "Manual for safety in the operating theatre: Recommendations and Checklist" published by the Ministry of Labour, health and social policies in October 2009.

The manual, as already mentioned, takes into account the guidance drawn up by the World Health Organisation under the "Safe Surgery Saves Life" programme and adapts it to Italy. The overall objective is to disseminate recommendations and safety standards and implement the same by using the operating theatre safety checklist.

Sixteen specific targets were advised; the first ten are derived from the WHO guidelines, while the following six were added by the Ministry of Labour, health and social policies.

13.2.1 The 16 Targets for Safety in the Operating Theatre [3]

Target 1	Operate on the correct patient, on the correct surgical site
Target 2	Prevent the retention of foreign material in the surgical site
Target 3	Identify the surgical specimens properly
Target 4	Prepare and position the patient correctly
Target 5	Prevent injury during anaesthesia by ensuring vital functions
Target 6	Manage the airways and breathing
Target 7	Control and manage the risk of bleeding
Target 8	Prevent allergic reactions and adverse events caused by medication
Target 9	Manage recovery and postoperative control properly
Target 10	Prevent postoperative thromboembolism
Target 11	Prevent surgical site infections
Target 12	Promote effective communication in the operating theatre
Target 13	Manage the operative program properly
Target 14	Ensure proper preparation of the surgical report
Target 15	Ensure proper anaesthesia documentation
Target 16	Enable assessment of activities in the operating theatre

13.2.2 Checklist

The checklist is a tool developed with a view to improving safety and quality. It is made up of 20 items that serve as a guide when carrying out checks in the operating theatre. It promotes both changes in individual behaviour and of the system, strengthening the standards for safety and communication processes, thus putting into action valid operations for countering possible failure factors.

Systematic use of the checklist encourages the implementation of safety standards and the prevention of mortality or postoperative complications.

The checklist divides the activity into three phases: Sign in, time out and sign out.

It provides for the sequential performance of 20 controls carried out in the manner described in the summary table attached to the Ministry of Health manual that follows [3].

Phases	The 20 checklist controls
Sign in Before induction of anaesthesia Involvement of all team members is necessary	1. The patient has confirmed identity, surgical site, procedure and consent 2. Confirm marking of surgical site 3. Confirm controls for safety of the anaesthesia 4. Confirm positioning of pulse oximeter and verify proper functioning 5. Identify allergic risks 6. Identify risks related to airway management difficulties or aspiration risk 7. Identify risk of blood loss
Time out After induction of anaesthesia and before surgical incision to confirm that the different controls have been performed Involvement of all team members is necessary	1. All members of the team are present with their name and function 2. The surgeon, anaesthetist and nurse have confirmed the patient's identity—Surgical site, procedure, proper positioning 3. Critical issues—Surgeon 4. Critical issues—Anaesthetist 5. Critical issues—Nurse 6. Confirm antibiotic prophylaxis performed in the last 60 min 7. Display diagnostic images
Sign out Takes place during or immediately after closing of the surgical wound and before the patient leaves the operating theatre Involvement of all team members is necessary	1. Confirm name of procedure carried out and its recording 2. Confirm final count of gauze, scalpels, needles and other surgical instruments 3. Confirm labelling of surgical specimen 4. Confirm issues related to use of medical devices 5. Surgeon, anaesthetist and nurses go over the important aspects and critical elements for postoperative care management 6. Confirm plan for the prophylaxis of venous thromboembolism

The 16 objectives and the checklist are an essential cornerstone for any nurse working in the operating theatre and, therefore, also in a cath lab.

13.3   Cath Lab: Field of Action—Characteristics and Equipment

The cath lab where haemodynamic procedures are performed must have precise characteristics, including logistical, such as the presence of sufficient space to facilitate the movement of the personnel and equipment present.

Its equipment must include:

– Anaesthesia trolley with automatic ventilator fitted with multi-parameter monitor to enable monitoring of invasive and noninvasive blood pressure (NIBP), oxygen saturation (SpO2), electrocardiogram (ECG), temperature (TEMP), central venous pressure (CVP).
– Specific anaesthetic drugs (treatment, analgesics, etc.)
– Drugs for cardiopulmonary resuscitation (adrenaline, adenosine, nitroglycerine, amiodarone, atropine, heparin, etc.)
– Drugs for complications (antiarrhythmics, bronchodilators, corticosteroids, etc.)
– Narcotic drugs (opioids, ketamine, etc.)
– Crystalloid and colloid fluid solutions.
– Material for airway management: face masks, anaesthesia balloons, laryngoscope and blades, endotracheal tubes of various measures (neonatal, paediatric and for adult patients), syringe for cuff inflation, laryngeal masks, oropharyngeal cannulas, spindles, Magill forceps, lubricant, material for local anaesthesia, catheter mounts, bandages, stethoscope.
– Material for finding venous and arterial access.
– Syringes of different sizes.
– Containers for disposal of sharp objects.
– Material for gastric drainage consisting of nasogastric tubes of various sizes and collection bags.
– Bladder catheters of various sizes and urinometer.
– Defibrillator.
– Temporary PMK.
– Docking station and infusion pumps.
– Suction system associated with catheters of different sizes for endotracheobronchial secretions.
– Air body heater and mattresses of various sizes.
– Anti-bedsore devices.
– Apparatus for blood gas analysis and for measurement of clotting time.
– Special mobile cabinets capable of containing all aids (disposable textile kits, needles, guides, angiographic catheters and for angioplasty, prostheses, etc.) with a complete range by types and sizes necessary for diagnostic and surgical procedures.

The theatre must also be provided with radiological equipment suitable for ensuring high performance in terms of quality, use of images and patient and operator safety such as:

- Fixed biplane cardioangiographic unit.
- High-resolution monitor for displaying live images.
- Injector for contrast medium.
- One or more surgical lights.
- Radiological table that is comfortable for the patient but which provides the possibility of access on both sides, suitable for allowing performance of all resuscitation procedures, motorised vertical, longitudinal and transverse movements, with commands for total control of the system.

Legal provisions on radio prevention and protection must be strictly applied to all personnel accessing the theatre.

During procedures, use of the following systems of protection is mandatory: lead apron, thyroid lead collar, anti-RX glasses and dosimeters for measurement of absorbed doses. Mobile barriers that act as a further filter placed between operators and the source of radiation must also be used.

13.4 Characteristics of the Nursing Team and Path of Integration

Within the context described above, the activities of the nurse performing duties at a haemodynamic facility is characterised by the need to be able to field a high degree of specialisation. It is absolutely essential that he/she has bases of knowledge and skills also in the field of intensive care and cardiac resuscitation that are adequate for the high complexity of the diseases and procedures that are treated.

The set of skills should therefore also include good knowledge of anatomy and cardiovascular pathophysiology, working knowledge of electromedical equipment, technical skills and knowledge of electrocardiogram monitoring and other highly specialised techniques.

In addition, the nurse must know how to relate to others and have the skills needed for performing the process of care, capacity of observation, planning, judgement and decision-taking. Neither should he/she lack the ability to properly interpret information and communicate in a comprehensive way.

Continuous updating of the nursing staff is very important in order to constantly increase their professionalism, obviously including constant participation in courses and conferences in order to facilitate cultural and experiential exchange with other situations in Italy and at international level.

From the outset, the nurse who is assigned to a cath lab will be supported by a tutor who will follow him/her, step by step, for about 6 months. At the start, they will be given all the basic information that will serve as the basis for correct behaviour in a room where they will be working with high-risk patients, in a sterile environment, and with the almost constant and continuous presence of ionising radiation. The successive phase of coaching envisages illustration of all equipment, devices and materials needed for procedures and their use.

The objective, at this stage, will be to immediately understand the importance of collaborating with the anaesthetist, particularly in the critical phase of induction of anaesthesia and extubation, and monitoring before, during and after the operation. The theatre nurse is there to help the surgeons; supervises, manages and assists the patient before, during and after surgery; follows the treatment instructions of the anaesthetist and haemodynamic specialist; and records patient- and surgery-related data.

The newly inserted nurses will be helped through their learning process by protocols and departmental procedures. The attentive training and prompt answers of the nurse shadowing them will help them start to become autonomous in the theatre and become key players who can perform the functions of theatre nurse alone and in person. Next, still under the supervision of the tutor nurse, they move up to the next stage, becoming scrub nurses.

The task of the scrub nurse is to assist and help the haemodynamic cardiologist perform the procedure and manage materials. The scrub nurse must be motivated and specialised, ready to face any eventuality and to be able to juggle all the various stages of the intervention according to clinical protocols.

The activities in this phase are to prepare and equip the field and keep it sterile, prepare the injector with the contrast medium according to the patient's weight, prepare two pressure lines (kit of transducers with related washing bags composed of saline solution and heparin), adequately cleanse diagnostic catheters and guide wire to be passed to the surgeon, prepare the inflation device of catheters for angioplasty and dilute drugs. Scrub nurses must be able to anticipate any impromptu needs based on their adequate knowledge of the techniques already acquired.

In the early days, during activities in the theatre, newly inserted nurses will be assisted by the tutor nurses; next, they will autonomously perform their first simple diagnostic procedures. Lastly, they will become autonomous in performing haemodynamic interventional procedures.

At the end of the period needed, usually 6 or more months, the tutor will draft a written report of the training path of the newly inserted nurse, providing details of the skills acquired.

At this point, the nurses can even be inserted in on-call shifts, as they are now able to perform all activities in total autonomy.

Their training will have ensured that they are able to:

- Perform daily checks of the availability and proper operation of the equipment and aids required to plan operations.
- Implement all procedures required to ensure asepsis in their own operative field and in that of all surgeons in the room, according to the protocol of conduct.

- Prepare the equipment and all aids in the cath lab and organize the activities of collaborators according to the surgery to be performed.
- Check all the instruments and materials used for surgery, as the surgery progresses and on completion.
- Assess and monitor the patient before, during and after surgery, follow the treatment instructions of the anaesthesiologist and haemodynamic specialist and record patient- and surgery-related data.

13.5 Daily Organisation and Description of Activities

We now enter into the details of activities.

At the beginning of the day, after viewing the daily operating session schedule and using the theatre checklist, where all findings are documented, the cath nurse completes the necessary controls, from checking the proper operation of vital sign monitors, by making sure the relative cables for measuring the signs are present, to checking the presence and proper operation of the laryngoscope and making sure there are drugs for anaesthesia, cardiopulmonary resuscitation and any complications.

Other checks needed involve making sure all material, disposable and not, is present; setting up the automatic fan; checking the proper operation of the suction device, the pressure alarms of medical gases and the connection to the system for outlet of anaesthetic gases, the proper functioning of the X-ray table, the surgical light and the thermal heater; carrying out the test operation of the defibrillator; and making sure the large and small plates, cables, the electrically conductive gel and disposable plates for defibrillation are all present and function properly.

Lastly, the cath nurse prepares the fluid therapy and whatever is needed to position one or more peripheral venous routes.

Once the theatre has been inspected and prepared according to the age, weight and type of procedure, the nurse, together with the anaesthetist, is ready to welcome the patient and his or her parents. Once the patient has been identified with the help of the ID bracelet and parents if the child is not yet able to express himself or herself, the nurse reads the nursing records, checks the patient's pre-procedure checklist, makes sure the informed consent forms for invasive haemodynamic and anaesthesia procedures are present and that health records are complete and checks that the patient has fasted and is clean, which involves presurgical washing, a trichotomy if necessary and appropriate clean clothing.

Along with the haemodynamic specialist, the nurse plans the activities needed for the operation and checks that all materials and aids are present, as well as the varied range of prostheses to be implanted.

The patient's parents are in the meantime seated in comfortable waiting rooms where, throughout the procedure, they will be informed of the progress of the procedure and reassured by the nursing coordinator or a delegate of the same. At the end of the procedure, they will have an interview with the surgeon who performed the operation in which they will be given all the details.

The patient is then accompanied into the theatre and moved onto the X-ray table where the oximeter, ECG electrodes, pressure cuff and thermometer will be positioned on him or her. At this point, the anaesthetist may start inducing anaesthesia. The nurse, at this stage, helps the anaesthetist position the tubes in the patient, connecting the fluid solutions to peripheral routes, program infusion pumps and the patient in the correct position according to the procedure to be performed.

Below is a description of a specific procedure.

13.6 Percutaneous Transcatheter Implantation of Edwards SAPIEN XT Pulmonary Heart Valve: Procedure

The Edwards SAPIEN XT pulmonary heart valve is implanted in all patients with right outflow tract stenosis who have previously requested the implantation of a duct.

The valve in question is composed of a stainless steel stent and a bovine pericardial bioprosthetic valve. The SAPIEN XT valve is available in three sizes: 23, 26, and 29 mm.

In most cases, implantation of the valve is preceded, usually 3 months before, by the placement of a stent in the right outflow duct, so that the valve will be more stable.

The patient undergoes general anaesthesia and is laid down on the X-ray table, facing upwards, completely disrobed and with their arms above their head, because the procedure requires the use of latero-lateral projections.

We place two femoral venous accesses, one femoral arterial access, one in the radial artery for monitoring bloody pressure and a bladder catheter, and antibiotic prophylaxis is started.

After putting on anti-X-ray protection, the scrub nurse and haemodynamicist begin with surgical hand washing, while the theatre nurse prepares the arena by dressing the operators in sterile gowns and the materials by preparing the sterile field.

Materials required:

The haemodynamic kit consisting of drapes, gowns, gauze, bowls, machinery covers and sterile bulkhead covers; surgical gloves; bags of sterile physiological solution; ChloraPrep and heparin syringes of various sizes; contrast medium; needles, guide introducers and catheters of various types suited to the patient's weight.

After placing the introducer, you proceed to push the catheter through the femoral vein until it reaches the pulmonary artery, pressures are measured, and angiography is performed to evaluate the size of the valve; then, through the femoral artery with a catheter, an angiograph is run to calculate the distance between the coronary arteries and the site of the valve to be implanted. At this point, we bring in the always aseptic mother's table, which has four large bowls, one small capsule, bags of saline solution, a luer lock syringe, contrast media, an inflation device, gauzes, heparin, scalpels, anatomic forceps and an Edwards valve—A device for clamping and delivery.

A capsule is prepared with a mixture of contrast and saline to 15%, which will be used for inflating the catheter. After defining the extent of the valve to be implanted, we proceed to progressive washing of the same using three different containers of saline and heparin solution.

The valve is shaped and mounted for delivery on NOVAFLEX which has previously been washed and both lumens rinsed. Meantime, in the femoral vein, we perform various steps to gradually increase blood in the vessel using a dilator washed with saline and heparin solutions. The valve is positioned, and we then proceed with the appropriate device to inflate and release it.

After the procedure, before removing the introducer from the patient, we perform a tobacco bag, and apply a pressure dressing.

The patient is awakened, restabilised and accompanied to the recovery room.

13.7 Recovery Room (RR)

The recovery room, also referred to as the awakening area, is a place that is intended to accommodate any patients who need to have continuous postoperative care, and as we have to consider the obvious need to minimise the duration of the patient transportation, this has to be located close to the haemodynamic rooms.

The RR must be a quiet and not a noisy place, in which the temperature should be maintained between 21 and 22 °C and the humidity between 40 and 50%. Air exchange must ensure adequate extraction of residual anaesthetic gases, which patients who have undergone general anaesthesia exhale. The room's lighting must be pleasantly constant, uniform and indirect. The environments in question must always be free of unnecessary equipment and in clean and rigorously hygienic condition.

For each bed, there must be a correspondingly adequate number of UPS electrical outlets, an oxygen supply, compressed air and suction, oxygen therapy systems (humidifiers and flow metres), face masks, an air heater fitted to mattresses of various sizes, a defibrillator, a temporary pacemaker, a multi-parametric monitor for measuring blood pressures and oxygen saturations (SpO2) invasively and noninvasively (NIBP), electrocardiograms (ECG), temperatures (TEMP), a manual ventilation system, a mechanical ventilation system, intake systems, a laryngoscope, endotracheal tubes and tubes of various sizes, and for parenteral infusions, a syringe pumps with electronic operations and a compliant systems for accurate analgesia, the medications needed for cardiopulmonary resuscitation, antiemetics and analgesic therapies.

Under normal conditions, the stays of patients in the RR is limited to the time required to achieve stabilisation of vital signs, with special attention to consciousness and control of respiratory, cardiovascular, neuromuscular, metabolic and renal functions. The nursing staff attached to the RR must be adequately prepared. Their task is to take continuous and direct care of the patient, and amongst their therapeutic goals, we find establishing pain management, treatment of nausea and vomiting, recovery of normothermia and acid-base and electrolyte equilibrium.

On the arrival of the patient, the nurse must necessarily be aware of their clinical history and know about any problems related to the intraoperative course; in this context, the handover between the cath nurse and the anaesthesiologist is very important. Clinical documentation, including the anaesthetic chart, follows the patient into the RR.

Once out of this initial phase, we switch to monitoring, at intervals, the established vital signs: heart rate, respiratory rate, temperature and blood pressure; they administer the therapy prescribed by the anaesthetist; monitor urine output, the patient's state of consciousness, nausea and vomiting; and assess pain. The latter must be monitored using scoring scales like the Visual Analogue Scale (VAS) and Pain Neonatal Scale (PIPP, CRIES and NIPS).

All activities carried out by the nurse are transcribed on the nursing sheets or anaesthesia chart.

Once the vital functions and the state of consciousness have been restored, the nurse prepares the patient for transfer. Discharge can only be effected when specifically ordered by the anaesthetist, who, for his/her assessments, will use the Aldrete Score System tool, which has been in use since 1970, and uses the following scale:

13.7.1 Aldrete Scale

Respiration	2	1	0
	Able to cough and take deep breathes	Dyspnea /shallow breathing	Apnoea
O2 saturation	2	1	0
	Maintains >92% on room air	Needs 02 inhalation to maintain 02 saturation >90%	Saturation <90% even with supplemental 02
Consciousness	2	1	0
	Fully awake	Can be aroused on calling	Not responding
Circulation	2	1	0
	BP ± 20 mmHg pre-op	BP ± 20–50 mmHg pre-op	BP ± 50 mmHg pre-op
Activity	2	1	0
	Able to move four extremities voluntarily or on command	Able to move two extremities voluntarily or on command	Able to move 0 extremities voluntarily or on command

BP Blood Pressure.

References

1. Rashind WJ, Millere WW. Creation or an atrial septal defect without thoracotomy. A palliative approach to complete transposition of the great arteries. JAMA. 1966;196:991–2.
2. Standards and guidelines for diagnostic laboratories and invasive cardiovascular therapy. Ital J Cardiol. 2008;9(9):643–51.
3. Ministry of Labour, Health and social policies—manual for safety in the operating room. Recommendations and check list—October 2009.

Nursing Care in ICU

14

Michele Sannino and Giulia P. Pisani

Abstract

At a cardiac intensive care unit, working as a team is very important to guarantee the best possible outcome for the patient. Nowadays nurses are one of the most important members of this team. They have to interact with all healthcare professional who are in charge of taking care of the patient. They have to know the basics of anatomy, physiopathology and surgery of patients with congenital heart disease in order to make the best choices and collaborate actively with the care team. Nurses take part in planning patient care together with the intensivist in both the preoperative and the postoperative period. One of the most important duties of nurses is to be able to assist the intensivist and cardiac surgeon in case of emergency. They are required to have a good understanding of the technologies used to sustain vital functions. The nurse must participate actively in the handover of patients from the operating room after surgery and be able to react appropriately to any problem that may occur and have the best passage of information. A correct nutrition is very important for patients with CHD in both the preoperative and the postoperative period. Choosing the correct type of nutrition and the correct administration is the duty of the nurse. A correct nutritional scheme a correct nutritional scheme is important to guarantee the right calorie intake, which helps achieve a better outcome.

M. Sannino (✉) · G. P. Pisani
Department of Cardiothoracic and Vascular Anesthesia and ICU,
IRCCS Policlinico San Donato, Milan, Italy
e-mail: michele.sannino@grupposandonato.it

© Springer International Publishing AG, part of Springer Nature 2019
S. F. Flocco et al. (eds.), *Congenital Heart Disease*,
https://doi.org/10.1007/978-3-319-78423-6_14

14.1 The Importance of a Nurse at the Cardiac Intensive Care Unit

At a postoperative cardiac intensive care unit (CICU), the nurse plays a crucial role in ensuring the patient receives complete and optimal care. In this setting, the nurse has to pay special attention towards any kind of actual or potential problem that may occur. The nurse, performing a comprehensive assessment of patient's medical history, has to identify every patient's needs and carry out correct and specific interventions.

In the past, the nurse was relegated to a marginal role; nowadays they have an active role at the CICU. Their cultural background is greater, and because of this, they are more independent and can identify and deal with any kind of problem and with every aspect of patient care, contributing to achieving the best possible outcome [1].

The progresses in medicine enables better-quality patient assistance in all medical settings and have highlighted the increasing importance of nursing care [2].

14.2 Working as a Team

In critical care medicine, such as at CICUs, doctors and nurses have to act as a team; their roles are interdependent to face every actual or potential emergency or urgency. Working as a team is important to react rapidly and effectively in order to choose the best intervention based on their clinical expertise and competence.

Emergency and urgency are two different terms used to denote two different situations:

- Emergency: a situation in which there is an impairment of vital parameters and the need for an immediate intervention to stabilize them. It is a life-threatening situation.
- Urgency: a situation in which there is an alteration of vital parameters and the risk of subsequent impairment, and intervention is needed to prevent this.

The therapeutic options available for patients with congenital heart disease (CHD) have changed and improved exponentially over the past two decades. Thanks to better prenatal diagnosis of CHD, preoperative evaluation of patients has led to a better stratification of risk, improvement of surgical techniques, innovation in cardiopulmonary bypass and in anaesthesiological management, as well as in postoperative care.

The emergence of multidisciplinary teams composed of paediatric cardiologists, electrophysiologists, cardiac surgeons, anaesthesiologists, critical care physicians, perfusionists, psychologists, physiotherapists and nurses did improved all aspects of patient assistance. At CICUs, this team can guarantee better pain management and better pharmacologic, haemodynamic, ventilatory, and nutritional support using new technologies and competences, in the context of evidence-based medicine.

All these innovations have led to better medical and surgical management of patients with CHD, and, as a consequence, their survival rate has grown rapidly, and a new population of adult patients known as GUCH, grown-up congenital heart disease, is born [2].

14.3 The Need for Preoperative Evaluation

Preoperative evaluation of patients with CHD is crucial, and it has to be conducted considering every detail of their medical history to stratify the intra- and perioperative risk.

An accurate preoperative evaluation must include physical examination (comprehensive of airways evaluation) and routinary diagnostic exams, such as biochemical blood exams, complete blood count, infectious disease screening according to local protocols, ECG, thoracic radiologic evaluation and echocardiography. In selected cases, cardiac catheterization and angiography could be done to complete the data available [3].

The clinical evaluation has to take into account every aspect and detail that may negatively influence the clinical conditions of the patient, with the aim of reaching the day of surgery in the best clinical condition possible, i.e., good haemodynamic parameters, oxygen saturation and diuresis, compatibly with the cardiac pathophysiology and age of the patient.

In the majority of cases, surgery is planned, so cardiologists and anaesthesiologists have already completed a preoperative evaluation and discussed the best surgical approach together with the cardiac surgeons. In these situations, when the patient arrives at the CICU from the operating theatre, the intensivist can evaluate the patient considering actual clinical conditions, intraoperative course of surgery and preoperative clinical evaluation and diagnostic exams, having a complete picture of the patient's clinical status. Based on this knowledge, the intensivist establishes a clinical plan by collaborating with the nurse as well.

In contrary, in case of emergency surgery, a patient can be admitted directly to the CICU, and not to the ward, and so the intensivist and also the nurse have to actively participate in the preoperative evaluation together with cardiologists, surgeons and anaesthesiologists choosing both a preoperative and a postoperative plan of care [2].

14.4 Postoperative Care

After surgery, the patient is transferred from the operating theatre to the postoperative CICU. The CICU is situated near the operating room to limit transportation time an to guarantee a rapid intervention in case of emergency.

14.4.1 The Handover

Upon arrival at the CICU, the operating room (OR) team, composed of anaesthesiologist, surgeon, perfusionist and nurse, hand over the patient to the CICU team composed of intensivist and a nurse.

The OR team describes the surgery and gives all the information about the intra-operative course of surgery [4]:

- Operation performed
- Duration of cardiopulmonary bypass and aortic cross-clamp
- Types of cardioplegic solution used
- Airway management and ventilation, paying attention to whether the intubation was difficult or not
- Vascular access available and if there were any problems
- Drugs used, in particular the need for inotropic agents encountered to support haemodynamics
- Blood transfusions, if applicable
- Description of vital parameters during the procedure: heart rate and rhythm, blood pressure, central venous pressure, oxygen saturation, left atrial pressure, cerebral saturation and diuresis
- ECG and its alterations
- Intraoperative echocardiogram evaluation
- Any concerns regarding anatomy or repair (coronary anatomy, size of shunts, residual valvular regurgitation, etc.)
- Intraoperative problems: during induction, pacemaker use, problems in weaning from cardiopulmonary bypass, bleeding and how it was managed

The first step in taking care of a patient with CHD after surgery is plan the assistance taking into account the local protocols and the local and international guidelines. These actions can help in assuring the best standards in terms of quality of care.

The initial assessment must focus on cardiovascular stability, adequate ventilation and analgesia.

After the handover, the nurse and the intensivist proceed with monitoring the patient [4, 5].

14.4.2 Monitoring the Patient

Monitoring refers to the continuous measurement and registration in real time of the vital parameters of patients. Monitoring a patient means not only connecting them to measuring instruments and register vital parameters but also to have a complete picture of their clinical status.

A measuring instrument becomes a monitor when it is capable of delivering a warning when the variable being measured falls outside a preset limit [3].

The aims of monitoring are:

- Providing thorough information of the patient's clinical status
- Early warning of onset of pathological events
- Providing information that could help in choosing the best therapeutic option
- Providing data which permit to verify the efficacy of a therapy

Duties of the nurse are:

- To have knowledge of all the equipment they use to monitor the patient
- Be able to correlate the data measured with the clinical conditions of the patient
- Interpret the data and confirm if they are reliable
- Detect any problems with the instrumentations and know how to solve them
- Decide how frequent the data have to be registered basing the decision on the patient's conditions

The kind of monitoring system to be applied has to respect the protocol of the institution and the international guidelines and to be tailored to the needs of the patient: age, pathology and kind of surgery, in order to obtain the most useful data possible.

At the CICU, the monitoring apparatuses most often used consist of [2, 6]:

- ECG in continuous: derivation dII; 12 derivation if necessary
- Blood pressure with invasive or noninvasive method
- Arterial oxygen saturation
- Central venous oxygen saturation
- Central venous pressure
- Core and peripheral temperature
- Diuresis
- Quantity and quality of liquids from drainage
- Neurological monitoring

14.4.2.1 Electrocardiography Continuous Monitoring

Continuous ECG monitoring permits to visualize in real time the electrical activity of the heart. This is done by positioning electrodes on the patient's chest surface and limbs and connecting them to an electrocardiograph by electric leads. This permits to evaluate the electrocardiogram, heart rate and rhythm.

The derivation most commonly used on the multiparametric monitor is standard lead II of 12-lead ECG. Three leads are applied:

- Red: to the right shoulder
- Yellow: to the left shoulder
- Black: to right lower chest

If the nurse notices some alterations on the ECG monitor, first of all they have to check the patient's condition; then verify the reliability of the alterations (electrodes can be disconnected or lead damaged) correlating them with other data on the multiparameter monitor, such as blood pressure; call the doctor; and perform a 12-lead ECG [7].

All patients undergoing cardiac surgery, adults and children, have temporary epicardial pacing wires, which are positioned during surgery and used to stimulate the heart if necessary, connecting them to external pacemakers. The intensivist chooses the better modality of stimulation to treat any kind of hypokinetic or hyperkinetic arrhythmia which can occur in the postoperative period, in order to guarantee haemodynamic stability [8].

14.4.2.2 Continuous Monitoring of Blood Pressure

Continuous monitoring of blood pressure (BP) can be done using an invasive or noninvasive method.

In the postoperative period, blood pressure is always monitored invasively. This is very important because the haemodynamics may not be stable, and the use of inotropic drugs or vasodilator agents or IV fluid resuscitation can influence BP. The arterial vascular access is also used to perform blood samples for blood gases analysis, which are very important to understand the respiratory and metabolic status of the patient and guide diagnosis and therapies. Invasive BP monitoring gives the most accurate and reliable measurements [9, 10].

The invasive method consists in inserting a catheter in an artery using an aseptic technique, either by percutaneous catheterization or rarely by direct arterial cutdown. The radial artery is the most frequently used site; other sites commonly used are femoral, axillary and humeral arteries.

The catheter is connected to a transducer system. The transducer is connected to an amplifier, and an oscilloscope in turn relays the information to the monitoring equipment. A continuous slow (1 mL/h) arterial infusion of heparinized or non-heparinized saline is required to maintain patency of the artery and to prevent the migration of blood into the tubing and transducer.

Before connecting the circuit to the patient, it has to be washed and primed with saline solution, checking that there are no air bubbles, which can cause arrhythmias and cardiac arrest.

As the column of saline moves back and forth with arterial pulsation, a pressure wave is generated, resulting in an arterial pressure waveform [9].

The presence of an arterial waveform on the monitor confirms the correct insertion of the catheter in the artery.

When the arterial line is connected to the transducer, it is necessary to calibrate the system. The static calibration is obtained by zeroing the transducer; the pressure is registered putting the transducer in communication with the ambient air; this corresponds to the atmospheric pressure assumed as a referral point of 0 mmHg, which is called zero point [10].

This operation is necessary to find a referral point between the atmospheric pressure, which is a constant, and the blood pressure, which is variable, and is obtained by placing the transducer at heart level; mid-axillary line is right atrial level if supine.

To do this:

- Place the transducer at the level of the fourth intercostal space, at the median axillary line.
- Put the transducer in line with ambient air.
- The step where you level out the measurement, by resetting the measurement to the value zero. From this point on you are able to measure the pressure accordingly.
- Close the communication between the transducer and ambient air.

This operation must be repeated every time the patient changes position, because if the transducer moves over or under the heart level, the pressures registered by the system will not reflect the real blood pressure values.

The monitoring system automatically registers [7]:

- Systolic pressure: associated with the peak of pressure wave
- Diastolic pressure: associated with the nadir of pressure wave
- Mean blood pressure: derived by an algorithm which considers systolic and diastolic pressures, area under the curve and time of cardiac cycle

Complication deriving from arterial catheterization may occur, and they are [4]:

- Ischemia can occur in the anatomical region haemodynamically supplied by the artery which is used for this measurement.
- Vascular insufficiency/occlusion.
- Thrombus formation.
- Emboli.
- Infections.
- Haematoma.
- Haemorrhage secondary to accidental disconnection of the catheter from the line. To prevent this, it is important to check that all the connections sites are firmly fixed.

14.4.2.3   Central Venous Pressure Monitoring

The monitoring of central venous pressure (CVP) is very important in patients at the CICU, because significant information about cardiovascular function can be obtained.

A central venous line is useful for [9]:
- Measurement of central venous pressure
- Secure and reliable IV access
- Administration of hypertonic solutions or drugs which require central administration such as inotropes or total parenteral nutrition (TNP)
- Measurement of central venous oxygen saturation (SvO_2) and acid-base balance
- Transvenous cardiac pacing, if epicardial wires are not in place

The CVP measures blood pressure in the terminal tract of the superior vena cava and estimates the right atrial pressure and the right ventricular end-diastolic pressure in patients who have a normal tricuspid valve [9]. So it is an indirect index of the volemic status of the right ventricle and so of the preload.

CVP uses the same electromechanical pressure transducers as arterial pressure monitors and it's normal values are in the interval between 4 and 12 mmHg. The most common sites of insertion of the catheter are a jugular vein and a femoral vein.

The catheter is inserted with the Seldinger technique in which the vein is entered with a needle, then a flexible guidewire is advanced with no resistance and the needle is removed. A dilator is passed over the guidewire to enable the passage of the catheter, widening the site of insertion. The catheter is then inserted over the guidewire and the guide removed.

Generally a multi-lumen catheter is inserted in order to use the line also for infusions. The distal lumen is connected to the pressure transducer.

Absolute figures, which are rarely of use in CVP interpretation, are more useful to evaluate the trend either up or down. CVP varies with intrathoracic pressure and so with ventilation:

- Normal spontaneous inspiration produces a fall in CVP.
- Mechanical positive pressure ventilation causes a rise in mean CVP.
- Positive end-expiratory pressure (PEEP) may increase CVP.

Thus CVP is better measured at the end of expiration.
High CVP values indicate:

- Hypervolemia
- Right heart failure
- High pulmonary resistance
- Elevate pulmonary artery pressure (i.e., severe acute lung injury), which can mask hypovolemia
- Increase in venous tone, which can mask hypovolemia
- Cardiac tamponade and pericardial constriction, in association with low BP

Low CVP values indicate:

- Hypovolemia
- Venous vasodilatation

Cannon waves on CVP are large "a" waves associated with atrioventricular asynchrony or junctional rhythm when the atrium contracts against a closed tricuspid valve [7, 9, 11].

14.4.2.4   Respiratory Monitoring

To evaluate the efficacy of respiratory gas exchange, two methods can be used:

- Pulse oximetry, which is a noninvasive method
- Blood gas analysis, in which an arterial blood sample is required

Both methods allow obtaining the arterial oxygen saturation value, which can be defined as the haemoglobin saturation calculated as the percentage of the fraction of oxygen-saturated haemoglobin relative to total haemoglobin (unsaturated and saturated) in the blood.

Pulse oximetry is monitored by placing the oximeter's sensors on the fingertip, nose and earlobe or, in the case of neonates, on the hand or foot. The pulse oximeter's function is based on spectrophotometry principles because it detects the differences in light absorption by oxygenated and deoxygenated haemoglobin. A pulse oximeter transmits two different light wavelengths (660 and 940 nm), both of which have different absorption spectra for oxygenated and deoxygenated haemoglobin. A light-intermittent diode transmits the light through an arterial bed, and a microprocessor compares the absorption of the two waveforms to determine the saturation ratio [9].

Pulse oximeter displays a waveform, pulse rate and oxygen saturation percentage. The value obtained by pulse oximeter is not always reliable, because it is influenced by many factors can modify the peripheral perfusion, such as systemic hypoperfusion, hypotension, vasoactive drugs and hypothermia. In addition, the patient's movement and sensor displacement can alter the reliability of the value. The observation of alteration in waveform on the monitor helps in detecting which values are reliable.

Arterial blood gases analysis is considered the gold standard to evaluate the efficacy of respiratory exchange [10]. It provides measurement of partial pressure of oxygen (PaO_2), partial pressure of carbon dioxide ($PaCO_2$), oxygen saturation pH, bicarbonates and other data such as haematocrit, electrolytes, glucose and lactate, thereby providing information about the metabolic and respiratory status.

Venous blood gases analysis reflects the values of partial pressure of oxygen and carbon dioxide at the tissue level (PvO_2 and $PvCO_2$). There are differences between the values of PaO_2 and PvO_2 because PvO_2 is influenced by distribution and consumption of oxygen, instead of PaO_2, which is influenced by pulmonary function (taking into account cardiopulmonary interaction, especially in CHD patients). Because of this, PvO_2 must not be used in substitution of PaO_2 [10].

Blood gases analysis is very important to evaluate the alteration of acid-base balance due to respiratory or metabolic alterations.

In CHD patients, when considering blood gases analysis values, it is important to take into account the pathophysiology of each patient because the presence of right-to-left shunts or palliative surgery which led to systemic desaturation can alter the values.

It is very important to pay attention to the PaO_2 value, in order to correct it in case of *hypoxaemia* to avoid rapid worsening. Causes of a fall of PaO_2 and saturation could be hypoventilation, right-to-left shunt, parenchymal lung disease, pulmonary oedema, atelectasis, pneumonia and intrapulmonary haemorrhage [4].

Values considered as the normal range are:

- pH: 7.35–7.45
- PaO_2: > 60 mmHg
- $PaCO_2$: 35–45 mmHg
- HCO_3^-: 22–26 mEq/L
- SpO_2: 95%

PaO_2 value has to be related to the fraction of inspired oxygen (FiO_2), which is the percentage of oxygen the patient is inspiring. To better understand this concept, three examples can be considered:

- Patient 1: spontaneous breathing with valid respiratory mechanic, eupneic, quiet, PaO_2 85 mmHg, no alteration of peripheral perfusion
- Patient 2: oxygen mask FiO_2 35%, not quiet, feverish, tachypneic, PaO_2 85 mmHg, no good peripheral perfusion
- Patient 3: sedated, intubated on mechanical ventilation FiO_2 85%, PaO_2 85 mmHg, first day post-surgery

First of all it is important to evaluate the patient clinically and then to evaluate the differences in PaO_2 between the patients considering the PaO_2/FiO_2 ratio. In patients with CHD it is important to consider that this ratio can be applied only if the patient has a completely corrected pathology and no cause of systemic desaturation, such as palliative procedure. Considering also that in this population we cannot strictly apply the criteria of the Berlin definition of ARDS (2011) [12], the following can be considered:

- $PaO_2/FiO_2 > 300$ normal
- PaO_2/FiO_2 200–300 mild respiratory distress
- $PaO_2/FiO_2 < 200$ severe respiratory failure

Evaluating the example patients [7]:

- Patient 1: PaO_2 85 mmHg breathing ambient air FiO_2 21% so the ratio PaO_2/FiO_2 is 404 standing for normal
- Patient 2: PaO_2 85 mmHg breathing in mask FiO_2 35% so the ratio PaO_2/FiO_2 is 242 standing for mild respiratory distress
- Patient 3: PaO_2 85 mmHg on mechanical ventilation FiO_2 85% so the ratio PaO_2/FiO_2 is 100 standing for severe respiratory failure

14.4.2.5 Acid-Base Balance Monitoring

Blood gases analysis is important to detect rapidly acid-base disorders and find out the cause. It is important to interpret the data derived from the blood gases analysis taking into account the clinical conditions of the patient, paying particular attention to cardiovascular, pulmonary and metabolic disorders and drugs used [13].

The body regulates the pH in a range between 7.35 and 7.45; if the pH is lower than 7.35, acidosis occurs; if is higher than 7.45, alkalosis occurs.

Acids can be divided into respiratory acids and metabolic acids; respiratory acids are represented by CO_2 excreted via lungs, and metabolic acids, known also as fixed organic acids (because not excreted by lungs), dissociate into anions (A^-) and H^+ ions and are excreted in the urine. They form lactates through carbohydrate metabolism, ketoacids (acetoacetate and β-hydroxybutyrate) through fat metabolism and phosphates and sulphates through protein metabolism [9].

The regulatory mechanism has three components [9, 14]:

- Immediate buffering: the main buffers are bicarbonates, plasma proteins, haemoglobin and phosphates.
- Immediate respiratory response: H^+ ions stimulate chemoreceptors to increase ventilation, and more CO_2 is excreted, lowering $PaCO_2$.
- Slow renal response: the kidney reabsorbs filtered bicarbonate ions, raising plasma HCO_3^-, and excretes fixed acids in response to respiratory acidosis. This response anywhere between 12 h and up to several days.

Acid-base disorders are acidosis (respiratory and metabolic) and alkalosis (respiratory and metabolic), which are identified by evaluating pH, HCO_3^- and $PaCO_2$ in arterial blood sample.

Normal values in an arterial blood sample are considered to be:

- pH 7.35–7.45
- $PaCO_2$ 35–45 mmHg
- PaO_2 90–100 mmHg
- SpO_2 95–98%
- Base excess: −2 mEq/L
- HCO_3^- 22–26 mEq/L
- K^+ 3–4.5 mEq/L
- Na^+ 135–148 mEq/L
- Lactate <2 mmol/L

In acidosis, pH is <7.35:

- Respiratory acidosis: $PaCO_2$ > 45 mmHg, metabolic compensation through renal bicarbonate retention (HCO_3^- high).
- Metabolic acidosis: Low HCO_3^-, in compensation $PaCO_2$ < 35 mmHg,

In alkalosis, pH is >7.45:

- Respiratory alkalosis: $PaCO_2$ < 35 mmHg, normal HCO_3^-.
- Metabolic alkalosis: high HCO_3^-, in compensation $PaCO_2$ > 45 mmHg.

14.4.2.6 Diuresis Monitoring

The diuresis monitoring is done via urinary bladder catheterization. The urinary catheter is placed in the operating room before the surgical procedure takes place. The catheter is made of silicone and has a probe to continuously measure the internal temperature. The catheter is connected to a closed collection system which allows hourly evaluation of the quality and quantity of urine [9].

There is a correlation between kidney function, volume of circulating blood and blood pressure. In case of reduction of blood volume and blood pressure, the renal perfusion will fall and so will the production of urine, causing oliguria (urine output in adults <400 mL/24 h, in children <0.5 mL/kg/h, in neonates <1 mL/kg/h). In this case, it is necessary to act in order to evaluate the causes of the reduction of urinary output and intervene to correct them. If urine output falls abruptly when catheterized, always check if the catheter is blocked, flushing it with saline [2, 9, 15].

14.4.2.7   Body Temperature Monitoring

Body temperature reflects the thermoregulatory ability of the body.

After surgery it is important to monitor the core temperature of the patients. During surgery, the OR's low temperature, no clothing, perspiration, large infusions of liquid and administration of anaesthetic agents delay the body's own regulatory mechanisms, contributing to altering the core temperature.

In particular, during cardiac surgery, the active cooling in cardiopulmonary bypass circuit results in the cooling of the patient's core and so in a reduction of his metabolic rate, allowing a reduction of cardiac output.

Some surgery to correct complex CHD may be done in circulatory arrest with profound hypothermia (until 24 °C) to reduce even more the metabolic rate and to decrease the risk of cerebral damage deriving from prolonged hypoxemia [16].

So every cardiac surgery patient experiences some degree of hypothermia which has implications on the entire organism (i.e., alteration of heart rhythm, glycaemic control, coagulation).

Monitoring temperature could appear very simple, but it is necessary to pay attention in doing it. The temperature must be measured at the arrival of the patient from the OR, and if possible monitored continuously.

It can be measured as:
- External temperature: axillary or inguinal
- Internal temperature: rectal, tympanic, urinary bladder

In the CICU, it is also important to monitor the peripheral temperature, measured at a body extremity such as the foot and associated with the detection of a peripheral pulse (i.e., pedal or tibial) because it allows to evaluate the peripheral perfusion [7].

14.4.2.8   Neurological Status Monitoring

Neurological monitoring is one of the most important duties of the nurse in the CICU, who is taking care of patients with neurological lesions. In these cases, every activity should be aimed at preventing secondary damage which can cause worsening of the patient's conditions.

It is prudent to always consider Monroe and Kellie's hypothesis, which states that the cranium is a closed system in which there are three elements in equilibrium: blood, cerebrospinal fluid and brain tissue. The increase in volume or quantity of one of these causes a reduction in free space for the other two elements. This results in compression of the entire system, a rise in the intracranial pressure (ICP) and a reduction of cerebral perfusion pressure (CPP) and so of the oxygen delivered to the brain. CPP is defined as the difference between the mean arterial pressure (MAP) and intracranial pressure (CPP = MAP − ICP) [17].

Neurological monitoring is implemented through the assessment of parameters that permits to understand the clinical status of the patient. There are a lot of neurological scales elaborated to evaluate the neurological status; the most popular is the Glasgow Coma Scale (GCS).

The GCS is used to describe the general level of consciousness in patients with traumatic brain injury (TBI) and to define broad categories of head injury. The GCS is divided into three categories, eye opening (E), verbal response (V) and motor response (M). The score is determined by the sum of the score in each of the three categories, with a maximum score of 15 and a minimum score of 3, as follows:

GCS score = E + V+ M

- E—eye opening
  - Spontaneous (4 points)
  - To sound (3 points)
  - To pain (2 points)
  - None (1 point)
- V—verbal response
  - Orientated (5 points)
  - Confused (4 points)
  - Inappropriate words (3 points)
  - Incomprehensible sounds (2 points)
  - None (1 point)
- M—motor response
  - Obeys commands (6 points)
  - Localizes pain (5 points)
  - Flexion withdrawal (4 points)
  - Abnormal flexion (decorticate) (3 points)
  - Extension (decerebrate) (2 points)
  - None (1 point)

Other neurological status information could be obtained by observing patient's pupils. Pupil size (in mm) should be assessed in both light and dark, by shining a light obliquely from below the patient's face directly into the pupil [18, 19]. Pupil documentation should include the millimetre size of the pupils in light, the size in dark and the light and dark reactivity of the pupils:

- Isocoria, equality of size of the pupil
- Anisocoria, unequal pupil size [20]
- Pupil equal and round or not
- Miosis, constriction of the pupil
- Mydriasis, dilation of the pupil

It is also necessary to check the presence of reflexes:

- Photomotor reflex: pointing a light at one eye provokes miosis of both the eye at which light is pointed and of the other eye (consensual response).
- Accommodation reflex: in response to focusing on a near object, then looking at a distant object (and vice versa), comprising coordinated changes in vergence, lens shape and pupil size.
- Convergence: the simultaneous inward movement of both eyes toward each other, usually in an effort to maintain single binocular vision when viewing an object approaching, for example a fingertip that is approaching the nose of the patients, indicating the presence of miosis.
- Mydriasis in response to a pain stimulus in any parts of the body [21].

14.4.3 Nutrition

Correct nutrition is very important in CHD patients both in the preoperative and the postoperative period.

Nutrition support can be administered via enteral nutrition or parenteral nutrition.

Enteral nutrition has always been preferred when the gastroenteric tract is not compromised because it is safer, easier and less expensive and also because it prevents the atrophy of intestinal villi and so the risk of bacterial transmigration.

Studies conducted on children who have received an adequate enteral nutrition have underlined a reduction in the duration of hospitalization and a lower rate of infectious complications. Furthermore, studies conducted in children in postoperative period after cardiac surgery have a better outcome if the nutrition allows a good growth rate.

In the CICU, total parental nutrition supports is necessary in patients with complex CHD requiring long stay in the Intensive Care Unit in order to achieve an optimal caloric intake in the immediate postoperative period, but also it is necessary to take into account the possibility of complications that can occur from this kind of therapy, such as infections.

Gastrointestinal tract motility and peristalsis can be drastically reduced in patients receiving opiates and narcotics; furthermore critically ill patients can have problems in deglutition or gastroesophageal reflux; all of these conditions could compromise and slow down the passage to enteral nutrition [22].

14.4.3.1 Enteral Nutrition

Enteral nutrition is administered via a nasogastric tube, which is a radiopaque silicone catheter inserted via the nasal cavity, pharynx and then oesophagus, stomach and up to duodenum or jejunum.

The nasogastric tube is usually inserted in the OR with careful attention: it is important to choose the correct diameter of tube, measure the correct length and, after positioning, check if it has reached the right place. Every time before the administration of the nutrition, it is important to check the nasogastric tube position, because it could have been displaced.

The nutrition administered should be of low density to prevent the occlusion of the tube.

In enteral nutrition exists the risk of gastroesophageal reflux and *ab ingestis* pneumonia due to aspiration or passage of aliments in the respiratory tract via airways, for example, in comatose patient the normal cough reflex is reduced.

In choosing the gastroenteric tract of administration, it is important to allow it to work by placing the tip of the tube as proximally as possible. In comatose patients, the normal cough reflex is reduced so placing the tube in the duodenum or jejunum is safer than in the stomach, reducing the risk of aspiration and *ab ingestis* pneumonia. In this case, the tube is positioned nasoduodenal or nasojejunal beyond the pylorus, which acts against the reflux [23].

The nutritional support administration can be intermittent or continuous.

In intermittent nutrition, the administration is performed giving a bolus every 3 or 4 h.

In case of complications such as vomit, diarrhoea and gastric stagnation, a continuous administration could be the best choice. In this kind of administration, a pump specifically made for nutritional infusion is used, allowing a constant flow. The constancy of flow reduces the number and intensity of peristaltic contractions, prolonging bowel transit time, reducing the osmotic load, preventing diarrhoea and facilitating digestion and adsorption.

This continuous administration can be given cyclically for 8 or 12 h a day or for 24 h.

Duties of the nurse are:

- Wash and change the infusion tubing every 24 h
- Wash the tube with warm water every time the nutrition is started or stopped
- Check periodically and before each meal for the presence of gastric stagnation
- Mark with a pen the entry point of the tube in the nostril to allow detection of displacement [24–26]

14.4.3.2 Total Parenteral Nutrition

The parenteral nutrition consists of the administration of nutrients via a vein excluding the gastroenteric tract [27].

This kind of nutrition is useful in those patients in which oral nutrition or enteral nutrition are not possible or not recommended.

In total parenteral nutrition, all the nutrients, amino acids, lipids, glucose, vitamins, electrolytes and oligo elements are administered directly in the blood stream in a quantity sufficient to overcome the nutritional and caloric necessary for a prolonged time.

The vascular access could be central or peripheral; the central vein permits the administration of solution at high caloric content. The use of hyperosmolar glucose solutions enables achieving an adequate caloric intake, introducing a modest volume of liquid.

The peripheral administration is done with the infusion of nutritive mixtures in superficial arms veins, and so hypertonic solutions cannot be used. This via permits to overcome the caloric needs for 2 weeks. For longer administration, it is better to choose a central vein catheter, and it is better to choose the total parental nutrition which can last for more than 2 or 3 months.

If possible, it is better to associate a parenteral nutrition with administration of food via the gastroenteric tract in a partial parenteral nutrition to allow fast passage to normal food intake.

The complications deriving from parenteral nutrition could be infections, such as central catheter infection, or metabolic, such as hyperglycaemia, also in nondiabetic patients [28–30].

References

1. Justice L, Ellis M, St George-Hyslop C, Donnellan A, Trauth A, Drouillard B, Watt C, Callow L. Utilizing the PCICS nursing guidelines in managing the CICU patient. World J Pediatr Congenit Heart Surg. 2015;6(4):604–15. https://doi.org/10.1177/2150135115593131.
2. Ofori-Amanfo G, Cheifetz IM. Pediatric postoperative cardiac care. Crit Care Clin. 2013;29:185–202. https://doi.org/10.1016/j.ccc.2013.01.003.
3. Gwinnutt G. Lecture notes clinical anaesthesia. 2nd ed. Oxford: Blackwell Publishing; 2004.
4. Anders M. PICU cardiac guide pediatric cardiac critical care book. 5th ed. 2014. http://picu-doctor.org/PICU/. Accessed 2 Jan 2017.
5. Karakaya A, Moerman AT, Peperstraete H, Francois K, Wouters PF, de Hert SG. Implementation of a structured information transfer checklist improves postoperative data transfer after congenital cardiac surgery. Eur J Anaesthesiol. 2013;30:764–9. https://doi.org/10.1097/EJA.0b013e328361d3bb.
6. Carl M, Alms A, Braun J, Dongas A, Erb J, Goetz A, Goepfert M, Gogarten W, Grosse J, Heller AR, Heringlake M, Kastrup M, Kroener A, Loer SA, Marggraf G, Markewitz A, Reuter D, Schmitt DV, Schirmer U, Wiesenack C, Zwissler B, Spies C. S3 guidelines for intensive care in cardiac surgery patients: hemodynamic monitoring and cardiocirculary system. Ger Med Sci. 2010;8:Doc12. https://doi.org/10.3205/000101.
7. Sanzo T. Manuale per l'infermiere in terapia intensiva e cardiochirurgia pediatrica. Edizioni del Faro; 2014.
8. Payne L, Zeigler VL, Gillette PC. Acute cardiac arrhythmias following surgery for congenital heart disease: mechanisms, diagnostic tools, and management. Crit Care Nurs Clin North Am. 2011;23:255–72. https://doi.org/10.1016/j.ccell.2011.04.001.
9. Barry P, Morris K, Ali T. Oxford specialist handbooks in paediatrics. Paediatric intensive care. Oxford: Oxford University Press; 2010.
10. Bigatello LM. Manuale di terapia intensiva del Massachusetts General Hospital. Italian 1st ed. Springer; 2015.
11. Ricci A, Tomasone F. Techniques for detection of the central venous pressure (pvc) and reliability of the measurements. Scenario. 2011;28(2):31–3.
12. ARDS Definition Task Force, Ranieri VM, Rubenfeld GD, Thompson BT, Ferguson ND, Caldwell E, Fan E, Camporota L, Slutsky AS. Acute respiratory distress syndrome: the Berlin definition. JAMA. 2012;307(23):2526–33. https://doi.org/10.1001/jama.2012.5669.
13. Andreoni B, Chiara O, Coen D, Vesconi S. Diagnosi e trattamento delle emergenze medico-chirurgiche. Milan: Elsevier Masson; 2009.
14. Hamm LL, Nakhoul N, Hering-Smith KS. Acid-base homeostasis. Clin J Am Soc Nephrol. 2015;10(12):2232–42. https://doi.org/10.2215/CJN.07400715.

15. Koo J, Baxter C, Kellogg K, Mize J, Riley C, Callow L. Guidelines for the general principles of postoperative care: the neonatal and pediatric cardiac surgery patient what the pediatric critical care nurse needs to know. In: The Pediatric Cardiac Intensive Care Society, guidelines. http://www.pcics.org/wp-content/uploads/2014/12/Neo_Pedia_Guidelines_Postoperative_Care.pdf. Accessed 12 Dec 2016.
16. Stark FJ, de Leval MR, Tsang VT. Surgery for congenital heart defects. 3rd ed. Chichester: Wiley; 2006.
17. Kim DJ, Czosnyka Z, Kasprowicz M, Smieleweski P, Baledent O, Guerguerian AM, Pickard JD, Czosnyka M. Continuous monitoring of the Monro-Kellie doctrine: is it possible? J Neurotrauma. 2012;29:1354–63. https://doi.org/10.1089/neu.2011.2018.
18. Teasdale G. Institute of Neurological Sciences NHS Greater Glasgow and Clyde. Glasgow Coma Scale: do it this way. 2015. http://www.glasgowcomascale.org/. Accessed 24 Nov 2016.
19. Christensen B. Adult Glasgow coma scale. 2014. http://emedicine.medscape.com/article/2172603-overview. Accessed 24 Nov 2016.
20. Eggenberger ER. Anisocoria clinical presentation. 2016. http://emedicine.medscape.com/article/1158571-clinical#b4. Accessed 13 Dec 2016.
21. Mutani R, Lopiano L, Durelli L, Mauro A, Chiò A. Il Bergamini di Neurologia. Edizioni libreria Cortina di Torino; 2012.
22. DeSena HC, Nelson DP, Cooper DS. Cardiac intensive care for the neonate and child after cardiac surgery. Curr Opin Cardiol. 2015;30:81–8. https://doi.org/10.1097/HCO.0000000000000127.
23. McClave SA, Taylor BE, Martindale RG, Warren MM, Johnson DR, Braunschweig C, McCarthy MS, Davanos E, Rice TW, Cresci GA, Gervasio JM, Sacks GS, Roberts PR, Compher C, Society of Critical Care Medicine, American Society for Parenteral and Enteral Nutrition. Guidelines for the provision and assessment of nutrition support therapy in the adult critically ill patient: Society of Critical Care Medicine (SCCM) and American Society for Parenteral and Enteral Nutrition (A.S.P.E.N.). JPEN J Parenter Enteral Nutr. 2016;40(2):159–211. https://doi.org/10.1177/0148607115621863.
24. Bankhead R, Boullata J, Brantley S, Corkins M, Guenter P, Krenitsky J, Lyman B, Metheny NA, Mueller C, Robbins S, Wessel J, A.S.P.E.N. Board of Directors. Enteral nutrition practice recommendations. JPEN J Parenter Enteral Nutr. 2009;33(2):122–67. https://doi.org/10.1177/0148607108330314.
25. Thomas DR. Enteral tube nutrition. In: MSD manual professional version. 2015. http://www.msdmanuals.com/professional/nutritional-disorders/nutritional-support/enteral-tube-nutrition. Accessed 20 Nov 2016.
26. Braegger C, Decsi T, Dias JA, Hartman C, Kolacek S, Koletzko B, Koletzko S, Mihatsch W, Moreno L, Puntis J, Shamir R, Szajewska H, Turck D, van Goudoever J, ESPGHAN Committee on Nutrition. Practical approach to paediatric enteral nutrition: a comment by the ESPGHAN committee on nutrition. J Pediatr Gastroenterol Nutr. 2010;51(1):110–22. https://doi.org/10.1097/MPG.0b013e3181d336d2.
27. American Society for Parenteral and Enteral Nutrition (ASPEN). What is parenteral nutrition. 2016. http://www.nutritioncare.org/about_clinical_nutrition/what_is_parenteral_nutrition/. Accessed 20 Nov 2016.
28. Thomas DR. Total parenteral nutrition (TPN). In: MSD manual professional version. 2015. http://www.msdmanuals.com/professional/nutritional-disorders/nutritional-support/total-parenteral-nutrition-tpn. Accessed 20 Nov 2016.
29. Boullata JI, Gilbert K, Sacks G, Labossiere RJ, Crill C, Goday P, Kumpf VJ, Mattox TW, Plogsted S, Holcombe B, American Society for Parenteral and Enteral Nutrition. A.S.P.E.N. clinical guidelines: parenteral nutrition ordering, order review, compounding, labeling, and dispensing. JPEN J Parenter Enteral Nutr. 2014;38(3):334–77. https://doi.org/10.1177/0148607114521833.
30. American Society for Parenteral and Enteral Nutrition (ASPEN). Aspen practice tools: critical care toolkit. Algorithms. 2016. http://www.nutritioncare.org/Guidelines_and_Clinical_Resources/Toolkits/Critical_Care_Toolkit/Practice_Tools/. Accessed 12 Dec 2016.

Nursing Care for Patient with Heart Failure

15

Mauro Cotza and Giovanni Carboni

Abstract

Heart failure (HF) in congenital heart disease (CHD) can affect patients either as an evolution of the primary pathology or as a complication after corrective or palliative heart surgery. Extracorporeal life support (ECLS) is a strategy that substitute whole-body circulation when refractory heart failure cannot be further treated with conventional therapies. Extracorporeal membrane oxygenation (ECMO) can be instituted as a short-term support to take time to recovery or to bridge patients to other assistance devices or heart transplantation. Ventricular assist devices (VAD), conversely, can be used for a long-term support, when recovery is unlike to be achieved in a short time and months are the target bridging time. ECMO and VAD are special topics that require a multidisciplinary team with a specific training, assuring a daily service in intensive care unit (ICU) for ECMO and in the ward or at home for VAD.

15.1 Introduction

Patients affected by CHD who suffer HF could benefit from medical and surgical treatment but, when end-stage HF arises, heart transplantation or mechanical circulatory support becomes the only option available.

Organ donor's shortage is much more evident in those affected by CHD [1], and only a very small cohort of patients can benefit of heart transplantation because of unfavorable listing criteria.

M. Cotza (✉) · G. Carboni
ECMO/ECLS Unit, IRCCS Policlinico San Donato, Milan, Italy

© Springer International Publishing AG, part of Springer Nature 2019
S. F. Flocco et al. (eds.), *Congenital Heart Disease*,
https://doi.org/10.1007/978-3-319-78423-6_15

Heart transplantation, in reality, is often a faraway possibility for these patients that, even if they appeared to be good candidates, can die on waiting list.

In this scenario, extracorporeal life support (ECLS) represents a valuable alternative to keep patients with CHD and afflicted with end-stage HF alive or improve their illness condition when chronic HF led to a multi-organ deterioration, precluding the enrollment in transplantation waiting list.

Several devices are available for mechanical circulatory support, but patients affected by CHD present some peculiar characteristics:

1. Their body size vary from small neonates to large adults.
2. Heart chambers can be hypoplastic and restrictive, with flow obstruction.
3. The heart may present septal defects with left-to-right or right-to-left shunts.
4. Pulmonary circulation may depend directly from systemic venous blood return, without ventricular pump (cavo-pulmonary connections).
5. Pulmonary flow may depend from systemic arterial circulation due to congenital abnormalities (MAPCAs) or staged palliation (aortopulmonary shunts).
6. They can present isomerism with abnormal systemic venous return and heart apex position (meso- or dextrocardia).
7. They underwent multiple heart surgeries for staged palliation or relapsing pathology with blood sensitization.

Furthermore, HF at age of presentation can appear as acute decompensation that requires a promptly intervention (i.e., lifesaving treatment) or as a chronic condition that progressively worsens and cannot further be treated with conventional therapy.

According to the expected time and the urgency of support, we currently have the venous-arterial extracorporeal membrane oxygenation (V-A ECMO, ECMO as follows) for short-term support and in case of urgent implantation; conversely, ventricular assist devices (VAD) represent the optimal strategy when longer support time are expected and patient can be implanted in a near-to-elective condition.

ECMO assisted both heart and lung function, while VAD assists one or both ventricles but does not provide any respiratory support; Table 15.1 reported the characteristics of both ECLS systems.

ECLS strategies are limited by particular indications and exclusion criteria that can be summarized in:

- Acute or chronic heart decompensation
- Not further medical therapy
- Reversible condition ("bridge to recovery")
- Benefit from a longer time of circulatory support ("bridge to bridge")
- Eligible to heart transplantation ("bridge to transplant")
- Absence of absolute contraindications (end-stage not reversible organs failure, concurrent neoplastic disease with poor life expectancy, major or end-stage neurological impairment, severe pulmonary or aortic regurgitation),
- Questionable relative contraindications (age, body size, psychosocial attitudes)

Table 15.1 ECLS characteristics

	ECMO	VAD
Devices (indication to support)	ECMO system (BTR, BTB, BTT)	• Para-corporeal centrifugal pump (BTR) • Para-corporeal pneumatic pump (BTB, BTT) • Full implantable centrifugal/axial pump (BTT, DT) • Total artificial heart (BTT)
Time to support	Short term (>30 days)	• SHORT (<30 days) • MEDIUM (weeks, months) • LONG TERM (months, years, destination therapy)
Cannulation site	• Central: RA-AO, LA (if needed) • Peripheral: ICA-RJV, FA-FV, AXA (rarely)	• R-VAD: RA-PA, RV free wall-PA • L-VAD: LA-AO, LV apex-AO • Bi-VAD: RA-PA, LV apex-AO
Circulatory support	Centrifugal pump, continuous flow	• Centrifugal pump, continuous flow • Pneumatic pump, pulsatile flow • Axial pump, continuous flow
Ventilation support	Hollow fiber polymethylpentene oxygenators	None
Temperature management	Integrated heat exchanger	None
Patient management	ICU stay: sedation, paralysis, intubation (ICU high care)	ICU stay: sedation, paralysis, intubation (ICU high care) Ward: cannulas/driveline daily care, pump parameters caregivers education Home: driveline daily care, pump parameters

ECMO extracorporeal membrane oxygenation, *VAD* ventricular assist devices, *BTR* bridge to recovery, *BTB* bridge to bridge, *BTT* bridge to transplant, *DT* destination therapy, *RA* right atrium, *AO* aorta, *LA* left atrium, *ICA* internal carotid artery, *RJV* right jugular vein, *FA* femoral artery, *FV* femoral vein, *AXA* axillary artery, *R-VAD* right ventricular assist device, *PA* pulmonary artery, *RV* right ventricle, *L-VAD* left ventricular assist device, *LV* left ventricle, *Bi-VAD* biventricular assist device, *ICU* intensive care unit

These topics are highly detailed in Extracorporeal Life Support Organization (ELSO) Guidelines [2] and reported in ELSO Red Book [3] and in International Society of Heart and Lung Transplantation (ISHLT) Guidelines [4].

All data coming from the ELSO Registry and from the International Registry of Mechanically Assisted Circulatory Support (INTERMACS) and from its pediatric domain (PEDIMACS) for VAD are used to update these guidelines, implementing the tools for clinicians.

In this scenario, nursing care doesn't look just an approach of the patient on ECLS (similar to a critical care patient and discussed in a specific chapter) but rather investigates the "ECLS-Patient" conjugate, the physiological relationship between the device and the man.

Several caregivers are involved in ECLS, but ECMO and VAD specialist spent the most of their time bedside the CHD patient.

According to the ELSO definition [5], either physicians, nurses, respiratory therapists, and perfusionist [6] can be defined "ECMO Specialist": they must receive a specific training for elective and urgent ECLS [7] and should take care of this particular cohort of patients, depending upon background academic education, clinical experience, and institutional policy. The same is for VAD.

Below we will see in a glance the two ECLS strategies, emphasizing how they work, in search of parameters to take care of, and providing some tips to solve difficult situations.

15.2 ECMO

15.2.1 ECMO Circuit

During ECMO, cardiocirculatory support is achieved by an external device that reduces cardiac work while providing flow to the patient.

The blood is diverted from the systemic venous circulation to a pump (Fig. 15.1) that generates the suction and the propelling force. An external drive unit, controlled by a console (Fig. 15.2), drives the pump that pushes blood inside a membrane oxygenator.

Centrifugal pumps are the most widely employed: they are preload and afterload dependent as native heart, they act in a self-controlled mode, and they have been implemented in the easy-to-use and easy-to-transport characteristics.

Membrane oxygenator (Fig. 15.3) is an artificial lung made of micro-fenestrated hollow fibers: blood flows outside the fibers while, inside, an air mixture allows gas exchange. Blood is enriched of oxygen and removed by carbon dioxide (moved by a partial pressure gradient) as normally happens inside alveolar-capillary membrane.

Ventilation setting is quite easy: an air blender modifies air-to-blood flow ratio ("sweep gas") and FiO_2. No respiratory rate or ventilator pressures are present or other different ventilation modes.

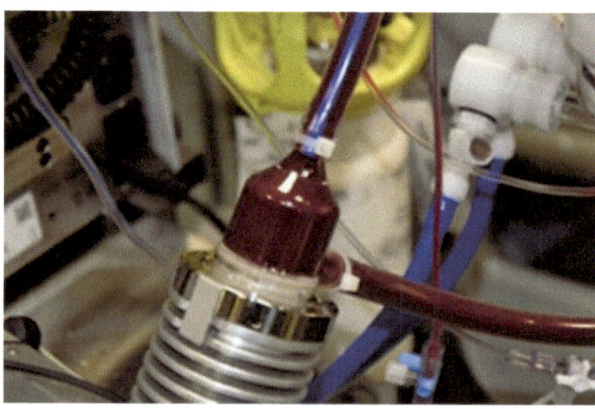

Fig. 15.1 Centrifugal diagonal ECMO pump, pump inlet and outlet

Fig. 15.2 ECMO console

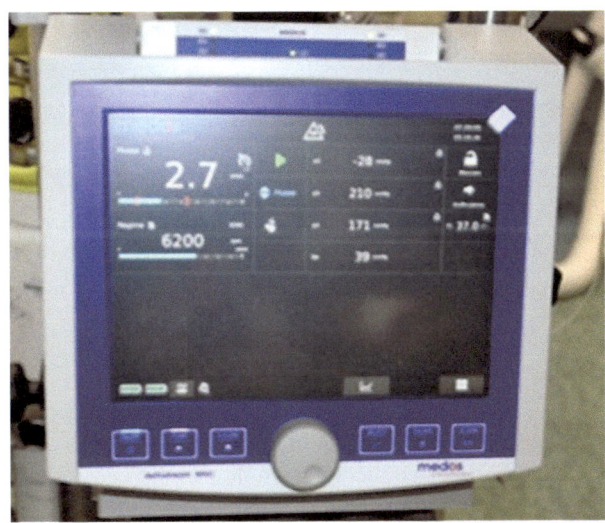

Fig. 15.3 Hollow fiber polymethylpentene membrane oxygenator with flow transducer

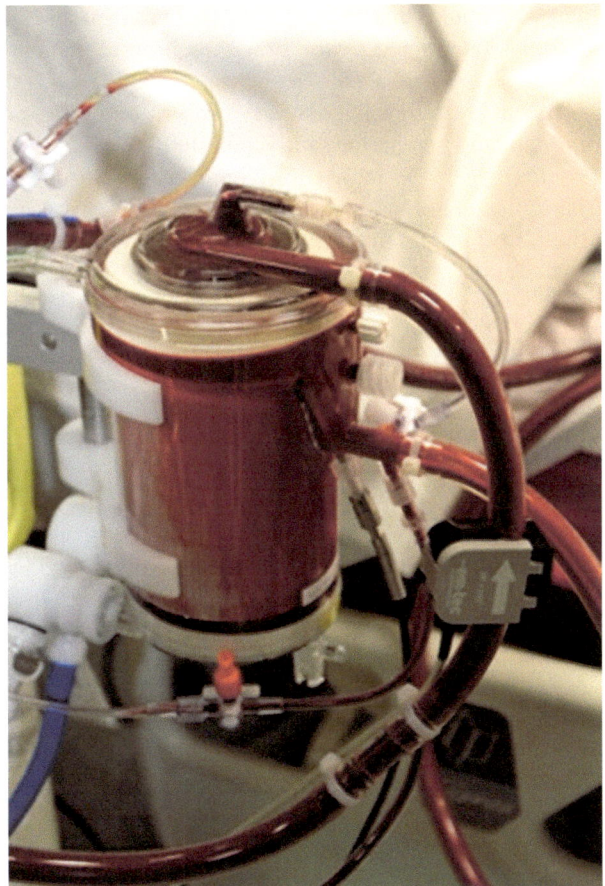

Fig. 15.4 Venous and arterial ECMO cannulas

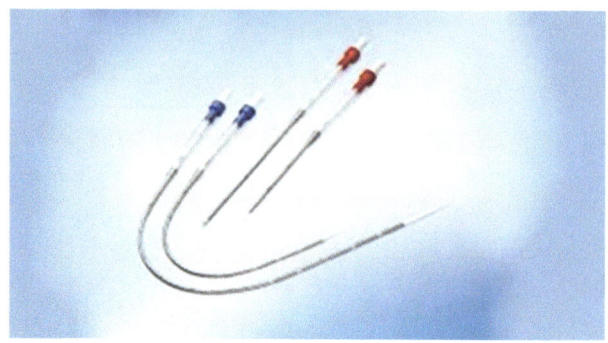

A heat exchanger is generally integrated to keep warm the patient or cool to provide protective hypothermia.

Plastic tubes connect the single parts to each other and connect the patient to the ECMO system too.

Finally, the "arterialized" blood is returned to the patient via special wire reinforced cannulas that connect the patient to the ECMO circuit (Fig. 15.4). Shape and size are determined by the flow they have to guarantee and depend from the cannulation site.

Surface coating is generally present along the circuit tip-to-tip, to minimize inflammatory reaction and coagulation cascade activation: different heparin coatings (Rheoparin, Medos Xenios-AG®; Bioline, Maquet Getinge® GMBH) or phosphorylcholine coatings (P.H.I.S.I.O., Sorin LivaNova®) mimic vessel endothelium but cannot inhibit completely autonomic recognition of foreign surfaces.

15.2.2 Modality of Support and Cannulation

Heart failure must be only treated with a V-A ECMO: heart and circulation are bypassed, and cardiac output is ECMO dependent. The residual cardiac function plays the biggest role.

If acute HF occurs (cardiac arrest, cardiogenic shock, or failed weaning from cardiopulmonary bypass, CPB), ECMO fully supports circulation, particularly in the early hours when hemodynamic shock is present.

In chronic HF, the heart function slowly worsens: the primary aim is to prevent further deterioration, and ECMO works in parallel to the native circulation. Flow can be assessed to let heart beat, with pulse pressure that seems to be beneficial to the microcirculatory system integrity and heart diastolic function, and prevent thrombus formation in heart chambers due to an inadequate washout.

ECMO cannulation can be achieved through a central (Fig. 15.5) or a peripheral approach (Fig. 15.6).

Central approach requires median sternotomy and has to be done in the operating room (OR), in sterile conditions, but it is not mandatory in case of emergency: ICU

Fig. 15.5 Central
cannulation on children

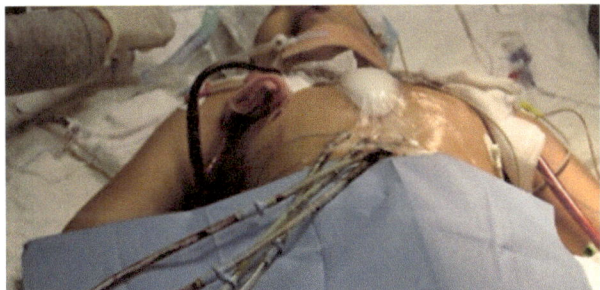

Fig. 15.6 Peripheral
cannulation in neonate

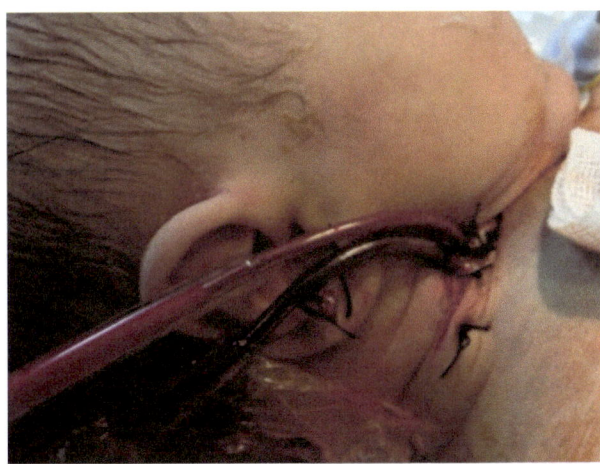

personnel should have a specific protocol to set up a sterile surgical area for that purpose. It's the choice of preference after cardiac surgery (the same cannulas can be left in place), in the early postoperative course, when left ventricular drainage ("venting") is necessary or in case of any other contraindication to peripheral cannulation.

Cannulation is accomplished directly through the aorta and the right atrium, so that larger cannulas can be easily inserted and no vessel is totally occluded, preventing the risk of distal ischemia.

This approach obliges to keep the chest open: a spacer is fixed at the sternal sides to leave the cannulas coming out from the mediastinum (Fig. 15.7), and a Gore-Tex® membrane is sutured along the skin borders and around cannulas, to protect the pericardial space. A dressing flat completes the procedure.

Major risks are bleeding, infections, and cannula dislocation: daily nursing practice includes standard care of the membrane and the cannulas (cleansing, disinfection, application of sterile gauze, coverage with plaster), avoiding unnecessary mobilization.

Alternatively, dedicated transthoracic cannulas (EXCOR®, Berlin Heart GmbH; CentriMag®, Thoratec Corp) can be used: generally employed in VAD for medium- and long-term support, they are equipped with suture flange or a vascular graft to be

Fig. 15.7 Open chest:
bleeding complications and
tamponade

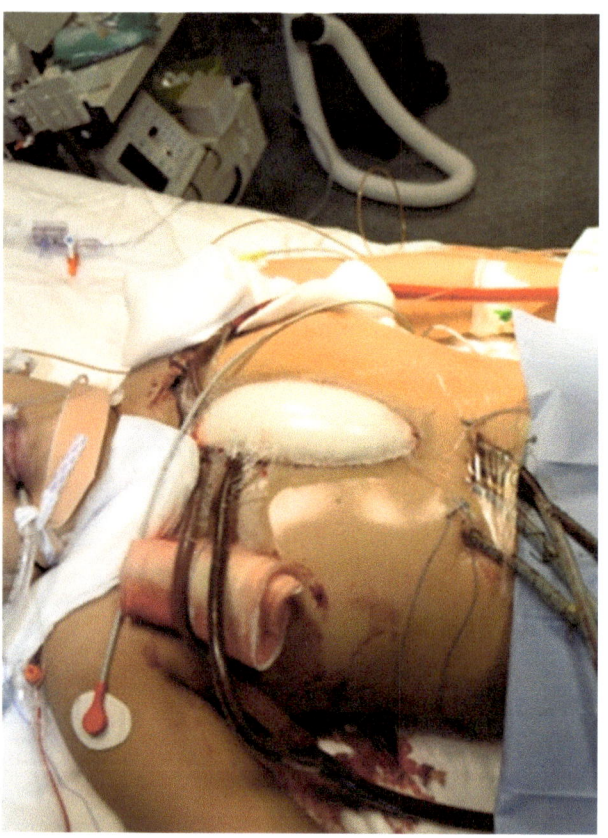

secured permanently. Once they are passed out through a subcostal incision, the sternum is approached and the skin closed. Their use on ECMO is very infrequent (cost) and dedicated to specific situations (bridge-to-bridge/bridge-to-transplant).

Transthoracic echo (TTE) is routinely performed around the membrane: a sterile gel should be used and promptly removed and cleansed. The TTE probe can also be inserted in a sterile sheath (even a glove) filled with ultrasound gel or eco-reflecting lubricant. Cannulas position, gauzes color, and system pressures must be checked before and after the exam, to confirm neither dislocation nor bleeding. ICU physician or perfusionist should be alerted, and a pair of clamps must be available to stop ECMO in case of emergency or to verify vent drainage, if present.

Peripheral approach consists in the cannulation of neck vessels below 15–18 kg of weight (right internal jugular vein, IJV, and right carotid artery, CA; Fig. 15.8) and groin vessels in case of larger children and adults (femoral vein and artery; Fig. 15.9). Axillary artery is used rarely.

Some surgical palliations can be detrimental for peripheral ECMO course: cavo-pulmonary bidirectional Glenn or Fontan impair completes systemic venous drainage. A double-site peripheral cannulation can be required and adequately planned [8].

Fig. 15.8 Neck
cannulation

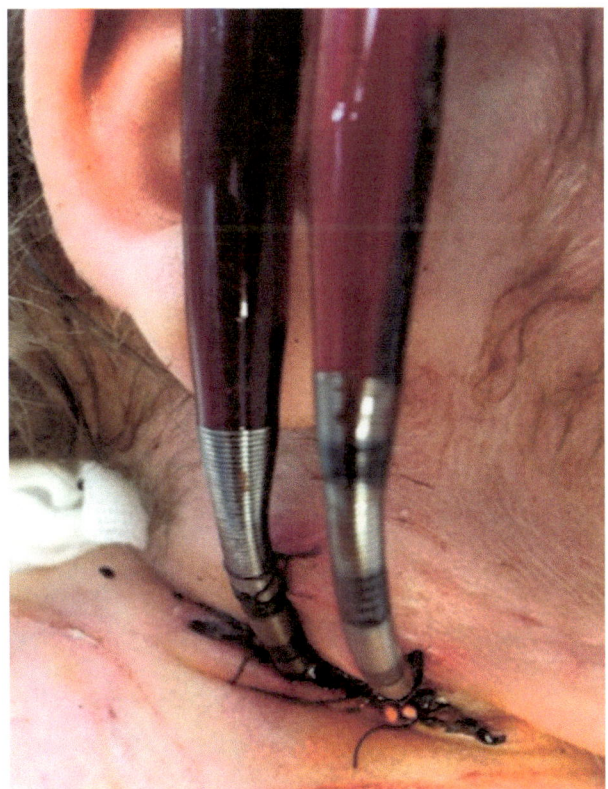

Fig. 15.9 Groin
cannulation with distal
reperfusion line

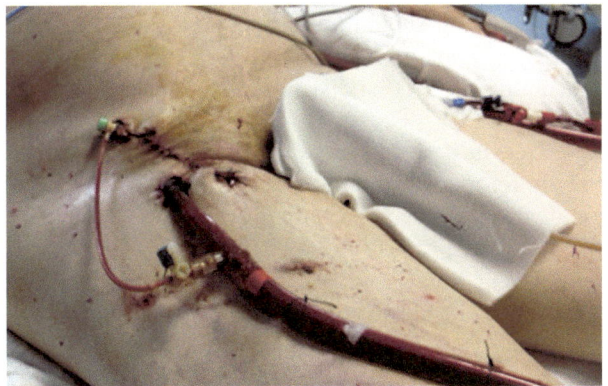

The same considerations should be done in case of known aortic arch interruption, hypoplasia, and aortic coarctation or bovine trunk in neonates (Fig. 15.10): cannulation of carotid artery or femoral artery could result not effective or obstructive for the bloodstream to the brain. A central or multisite cannulation may be more indicated.

Fig. 15.10 Bovine arterial trunk

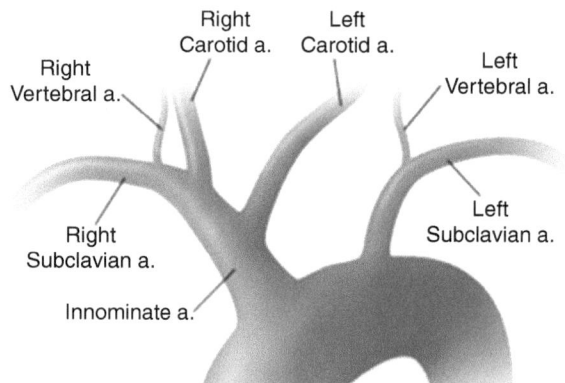

A careful assessment should be done prior to cannulation: bedside eco-Doppler investigation requires short time to be done and gives strong information about cannula placement. Pediatric cardiologist should be alerted in time, and eco-machine has to be ready for a TTE or a TEE evaluation shortly before cannulation.

If "blinded" cannulation has been already performed, TTE can confirm cannula position and flow adequacy. Transcranial Doppler (TCD) gives information on cerebral perfusion with near-infrared spectroscopy (NIRS).

NIRS is useful to early detect pathological variation of regional cerebral and visceral flow patterns, either during cannulation (iatrogenic anatomical obstruction) or during the ECMO run [9, 10]. Pads should be applied early to obtain the baseline to refer shortly after.

A multiport invasive arterial pressure strategy (brachial and femoral) also allows to discriminate any under or no-perfuse area too.

Everything should be ready before cannulation, unless ECMO is deployed in emergency condition or as E-CPR: ECMO specialist is required to be aware of the incoming process, and specific flow charts are useful to limit waste of time and resources.

Even in case of percutaneous cannulation, it is strongly recommended to be ready for a conversion to surgical cutdown: a dedicated surgical instrument and a skilled team have to back up the procedure.

15.2.3 ECMO Flow Modifiers

ECMO flow is calculated as for CPB (Table 15.2).

Nevertheless the "calculated" flow is referred to normal cardiac output: the ECMO system works in parallel to native circulation, and a full support is often redundant. Rarely, it could be ineffective, requiring higher flows.

The Fick equation does not consider that the patient native flow must be added to that of ECMO, and this could result in under- or over-perfusion.

Table 15.2 ECMO flow indexed

Weight (kg)	Indexed ECMO flow
0–10	120–150 mL/kg; BSA × 3.0
10–20	BSA × 2.8
20–30	BSA × 2.6
>30	BSA × 2.4

BSA body surface area

Fig. 15.11 SVO$_2$ patient monitoring Edward Lifesciences PediaSat (courtesy of Edwards Lifesciences)

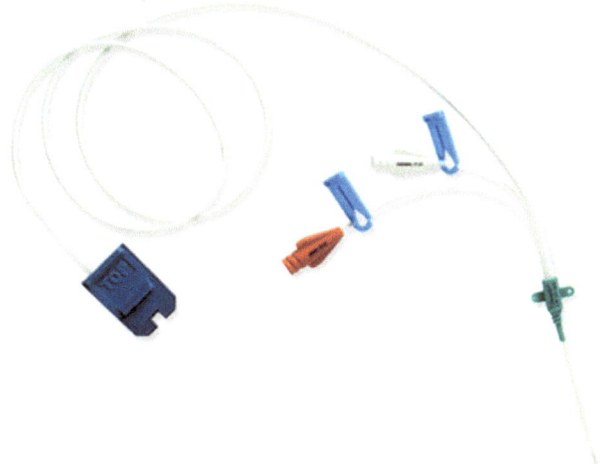

Further, concomitant surgical palliation or congenital abnormalities of the pulmonary circulation may lead to wrong evaluation, and ECMO specialist should be aware of it.

Triggers should be identified to obtain the optimal result: oxygen supply (DO$_2$) must be related to oxygen consumption (VO$_2$), but the ratio DO$_2$/VO$_2$ is just part of the information you need.

A central venous oxygen saturation (SVO$_2$) over 70% remains a gold standard, but, in CHD, values depend on left-to-right atrial shunts: if ECMO venous cannula drains both systemic and pulmonary venous return (atrial septal defects, partial or total anomalous pulmonary venous return), samples can show higher SVO$_2$.

CHD patients with aortopulmonary shunts live in a constant low cardiac output: this condition is compounded by ECMO, which drain the heart chambers and increased the gradient between the aorta and lungs, despite apparent higher SVO$_2$ values.

So even absolutely useful in normal condition, devices (Figs. 15.11 and 15.12) addressed to constantly monitoring SVO$_2$, either on the patient (PediaSat® Oximetry Catheter, Edwards Lifesciences) or on ECMO (CardioHelp, Maquet Getinge group; Data Master® and BCare5®, Sorin LivaNova), can deceive clinicians leading to a false optimistic interpretation.

Fig. 15.12 SVO₂ ECMO monitoring on Maquet CardioHelp (courtesy of Maquet)

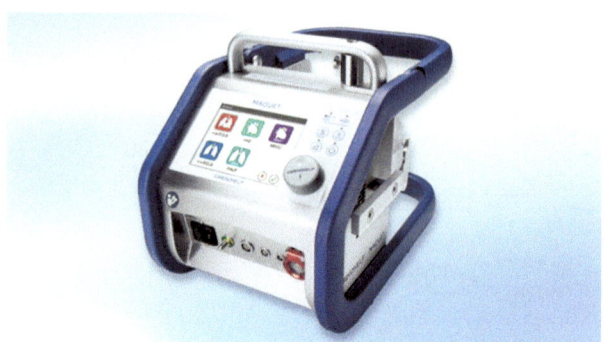

NIRS has been used to investigate both cerebral and visceral perfusion [7], but the conflicting results suggest using it as a perfusion trend tool rather than evaluating the absolute number on the device.

Lactates seem to positively correlate to perfusion adequacy and clinical outcome on ECMO [11, 12]: blood samples should be repeated frequently to assess the trend. Peak serum concentration and trend upon time seem to be most valuable indicators.

Urine output is an easy method to evaluate perfusion: 1–5 mL/kg/h is generally considerately an acceptable result even on ECMO. Unfortunately clinicians often stress urine output with diuretics which could be not a reliable indicator.

Further, if low mean arterial pressure on ECMO (microcirculatory shock after long-lasting CPB, cardiogenic shock, or cardiac arrest) and high systemic venous pressure (inadequate venous drainage or fluid overload) occur, glomerular ultrafiltration is reduced or totally absent, even at full flow, and urine output can mislead.

Carbon dioxide production (VCO_2), measured by exhaled CO_2 from the oxygenator, is an expression of tissue oxygen consumption (VO_2): CO_2 cell production by capnography has been validated on CPB and its part of a so-called goal-directed perfusion [13]. The same concept can be translated to ECMO, given the limitations previously explained.

Some of the most sophisticated online blood gas analyzer (M4, Spectrum Medical®) integrated a capnometer to be added online to ECMO: once calibrated, it shows O_2- and CO_2-derived parameters besides hemoglobin content, flow, and temperature, even in a graphical mode, to identify trends (Fig. 15.13).

Nursing becomes a complex interpretation of different information, sometimes misleading, aimed to optimize the flow of ECMO: data should be crossed each other, and any decision processes must be shared with ECMO team to determine and eliminate confounders, particularly during the weaning course.

15.2.4 Fluid Management

The ECMO paradox is maintaining an adequate intravascular volume to preload the ECMO system and preventing fluid overload (FO) because it is associated with increased mortality if FO > 10%, particularly in the pediatric population [14].

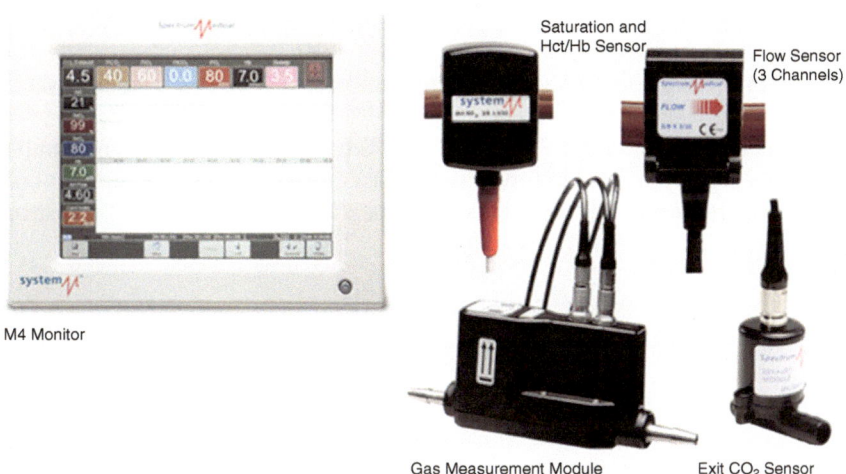

Fig. 15.13 Spectrum Medical M4 gas-analyzer and capnometer (courtesy of Spectrum Medical)

Given that corrections are not associated with improved survival, early interventions may be more clinically effective than attempting fluid removal after significant FO has developed.

ECMO patients may suffer renal failure because of the underlying chronic condition or because exacerbated by CPB, by fluoroscopy during cath lab, or by an acute cardiac failure.

A restrictive policy should be considered, but ECMO often obliges to replace volume, particularly after surgery: ECMO requires anticoagulation, CHD patients are sometimes staged palliation with several previous surgeries, coagulation factors and platelets are largely consumed, and bleeding is a common phenomenon. Severe bleeding (>2 mL/kg/day or hemoglobin fall 2 g/dL in 24 h) should be treated immediately [15].

If medical bleeding is the major issue, fresh frozen plasma (FFP) and platelets are generally infused at 10–30 mL/kg (I.N.R. > 1.5–2) and 10 mL/kg (count<80,000 cells/mm^3), respectively.

This can result in iatrogenic anemia, particularly in smaller children: red blood cells (RBC) administration could be necessary (10 mL/kg) to keep hematocrit above 30–35% but institutional transfusion triggers which often oblige to transfuse RBC a time at which the patient did not appear to be oxygen delivery dependent according to global measures of tissue oxygenation [16].

If urine output is not adequate, continuous renal replacement therapy (CRRT) may be applied to prevent FO, but some concerns could arise upon the risk of puncture in an anticoagulated patient and the use of CRRT catheters in neonates and small children.

Circuit ports used for ECMO system pressures can be usefully connected to the CRRT devices.

CRRT are generally not validated for use with ECMO and often oblige to override pressure limits.

Some clinicians suggest connecting CRRT inlet to pre-membrane and CRRT outlet to pre-pump port: positive pressure of pre-membrane port is compensated by negative suction of CRRT and vice versa.

The major complaint to CRRT on ECMO is the connection to the pre-pump port where active suction can lead to massive air embolism, particularly if no bubble detector is present: ECMO specialist must be aware of this potential catastrophic event and should be trained to manage it.

15.2.5 ECMO Ventilation

V-A ECMO provides both cardiac and lung function so that native ventilation must be adjusted to trans-pulmonary flow: protective ventilation (4–6 mL/kg) could be safely used, preventing ventilator-induced lung injury (VILI).

In peripheral cannulation lung function is crucial: the mixing area between native and ECMO flow can be located in the ascending aorta (cannulation of neck vessels) or in the thoracic/abdominal aorta (femoral cannulation).

If lungs are affected by respiratory distress syndrome (RDS), desaturated blood "feeds" the ascending aorta and the arch (coronaries and carotids artery) in what is called "Harlequin syndrome" ("blue" upper part of the body, "red" lower part). NIRS, pulse-oximetry, and blood gas of the right arm (unless "lusoria artery") help to discriminate and suggest for alternative strategies: increasing ECMO flow, decreasing fluid overload, adjusting ventilation titrated to Et-CO_2 and NIRS, and converting ECMO to hybrid cannulation (VV-A ECMO) or patient pronation. Cyanotic patient better tolerate this condition.

Baseline of CHD patients should be considered: in cyanotic patient normal ventilation is not appropriated, resulting in possible cellular damage due to free radicals of oxygen.

As carbon dioxide management strongly influenced brain and lung flow, hyper- or hypocapnia must be closely monitored to keep normal lung to brain ratio.

Patients presenting aortopulmonary shunts are at higher risk because of redundant ventilation: in some cases sweep gas must be kept switched off or minimally active.

Again, ET-CO_2 can be useful to assess correct perfusion/ventilation ratio of the lungs: the targeted value should be around 35–45 mmHg, with a CO_2 gap to arterial patient blood gas of 5–8 mmHg.

Online gas analyzers (CDI 500, Terumo®; M4, Spectrum Medical®) are helpful to promptly modify ECMO ventilation and may prevent frequent phlebotomies, particularly in neonates.

15.2.6 ECMO Anticoagulation

ECMO requires anticoagulation, and bleeding and thrombosis are both faces of the same coin. Balancing these two aspects is large part of the ECMO job.

Hemostatic activation by ECMO results in platelet adhesion to the circuit, with shape changing and platelet release of granuli and mediators that lead to platelet activation in a positive feedback loop.

Platelet receptors are expressed and induce aggregation through fibrinogen bridging and further platelet activation. Fibrinogen adsorption to the circuit facilitates platelet adhesion and ECMO transmembrane gradient could increase, alerting about possible oxygenator thrombosis with ventilation impairment.

Thrombin is moderately generated on ECMO by contact activation pathway (material dependent), and, if surgery is concomitant, even tissue factors pathway contributes to coagulation cascade generating larger amount. Hyperfibrinolysis occurs in case of clot formation within the circuit or the patient.

Preventing ECMO circuit thrombosis motivates anticoagulation, but it's not just a matter of ECMO: when HF impairs ventricle ejection, heart chamber stagnation ("smoke like effect") will result in an increased risk of clots, and embolic spray may occur, with neurological impairment.

Patients with CHD further suffer from coagulation disorder mainly for liver dysfunction secondary to right heart pressure or volume overload. Coagulation and anticoagulation factors are both poorly represented, and hemostasis becomes a tricky balancing act.

Unfractioned heparin (UFH) is the most widely used anticoagulant: empowering antithrombin (AT) activity, it slows thrombin formation. After a bolus for cannulation (50–100 UI/kg), a correct anticoagulation is generally obtained with an infusion rate of 5–20 UI/kg/hr but can largely vary from zero (in case of severe bleeding) up to 50–70 UI/kg/hr (when patients are refractory to anticoagulation). UHF overdosage should be never reverted with protamine sulfate: infusion rate reduction or temporary suspension is much more indicated.

Heparin is contraindicated in suspected or ascertained immune heparin-induced thrombocytopenia (HIT II). This event may occurs on ECMO but could be early detected in respect to normal platelets consumption.

As HIT II is a mixed laboratory test and clinical findings definition, thrombocytopenia and multisite thrombosis should suggest further investigation with ELISA-based immunoassay: it's sensitive but not specific so that functional assay should be used to confirm or not and prevent withholding UHF when it can be safely administered. Any clinical sign of thrombosis deserves an eco-evaluation.

Direct thrombin inhibitors (DTI) are coming in the routine use but in very skilled centers: either Argatroban® [17] (0.5–1 µg/kg/min infusion) or Bivalirudin® [18] (0.05–0.5 mg/kg bolus followed by 0.03–0.1 mg/kg/h infusion) has been safely used on ECMO and VAD in children.

DTI have some potential advantages over UHF [19]: they bind thrombin directly, independently of AT levels and its fluctuations, seem to provide a more predictable dosing regimen, inhibit both clot-bound and circulating thrombin and, finally, do not cause HIT II.

DTI are not provided of any antidote: anyway short halved time allows (about 20 min) a rapid reversal, but drug excretion is dependent on organ function (liver for Argatroban®, kidney for Bivalirudin®). An accurate evaluation about drug choice must consider this aspect.

Anticoagulation monitoring is the key point (Table 15.3).

Table 15.3 Coagulation parameters during ECLS (from "ECMO-Extracorporeal Life Support in Adults", Sangalli et al., Ch. 7)

	ACT (s)	TEG K (R TIME, min)	FibTEM (mm)	LAB (A-PTT, PTT ratio)	INR	Platelets (10³/nL)	AT3 (%)	D-dimers (ng/L)	Fibrinogen (mg/L)
L-VAD	>150	10–12	>10	45–60, 1.5–1.8	1.3–1.5	>80,000 (bleeding) >45,000	70–80	<300	>100
R-VAD	>150	10–12	>10	45–60, 1.5–1.8	1.3–1.5	>80,000 (bleeding) >45,000	70–80	<300	>100
BI-VAD	>150	10–12	>10	45–60, 1.5–1.8	1.3–1.5	>80,000 (bleeding) >45,000	70–80	<300	>100
ECMO V-A	180–220	16–25	>10	50–80, 1.5–2.0	1.3–1.5	>80,000 (bleeding) >45,000	70–80	<300	>100

ACT activated clotting time, *TEG K* kaolin activated thromboelastography, *FibTEM* fibrinogen thromboelastometry, *A-PTT* activated prothrombin time, *PTT ratio* prothrombin time ratio, *INR* international normalized ratio, *AT3* antithrombin 3

Rapid response tests allow to promptly modify anticoagulant infusion, whenever thrombotic or bleeding event occurs: point-of-care tests (POCT) are actually extensively used in most of the ECMO programs, but it has not reached a consensus opinion on what is the most suitable [20].

Activated clotting time (ACT) is still the most widely used POCT to investigate whole blood response to anticoagulation: it's low cost, fully available in most centers, but it's affected by several confounders and does not provide information about specific hemostatic disorders. An ACT of 180–200 s is generally considered the optimal target for a safe ECMO run.

Anti-factor Xa activity level (Anti-Xa) measure ex vivo UFH activity: it is not affected by coagulation disorders, but it's influenced by AT levels, hyperbilirubinemia, and high plasma free hemoglobin. Unfortunately these occurrences can be common on ECMO. Normal values are considered between 0.3 and 0.7 U.I/mL.

Thrombo-elastogram (TEG®) and rotational thrombo-elastometry (ROTEM®) POCT investigate the viscoelastic properties of whole blood from the time of fibrin formation to clot lysis, including platelet contribution, and provide information about native coagulation in presence of UNFH, pairing samples with and without heparinase. Fibrinogen function and hyperfibrinolysis can be also detected with dedicated tests. As for ACT, a time to gel point (R time, CFT) of 1.5 times to the baseline can be considered a safe value for running an ECMO.

Conventional laboratory tests for ECMO include activated partial thromboplastin time (a-PTT) or ratio (a-PTT ratio), prothrombin time (PT) or international normalized ratio (INR), AT, fibrinogen, D-dimers, and platelet count: the routine checks should be performed every 6–8 h or more frequently in case of severe bleeding or suspected thrombosis.

Fibrinogen and platelet depletion with D-dimers increase is suggestive for ongoing ECMO thrombosis: membrane and pump inspection are mandatory as transmembrane gradient evaluation. Anticoagulation must be increased, and a possible ECMO replacement can be scheduled.

Rather than evaluating the singles tests, it's arguable if a multifactorial approach could be more useful, integrating POCT and conventional laboratory tests [21].

15.3 VAD

If you expect that MCS is going to be protracted for longer time and lung function integrity is guaranteed, a ventricular assist devices are reasonably the best choice.

In the overall pediatric population, nearly 20% of patients receive MCS prior to transplantation [22].

Once ventricular function has been assessed, VAD is implanted via a medium sternotomy, and one or both ventricles can be assisted.

Right or left atrium and pulmonary artery or aorta can be cannulated for VAD, but ventricular apex guarantees the best drainage and overcomes mitral or tricuspid

Fig. 15.14 Para-corporeal
VAD cannulation

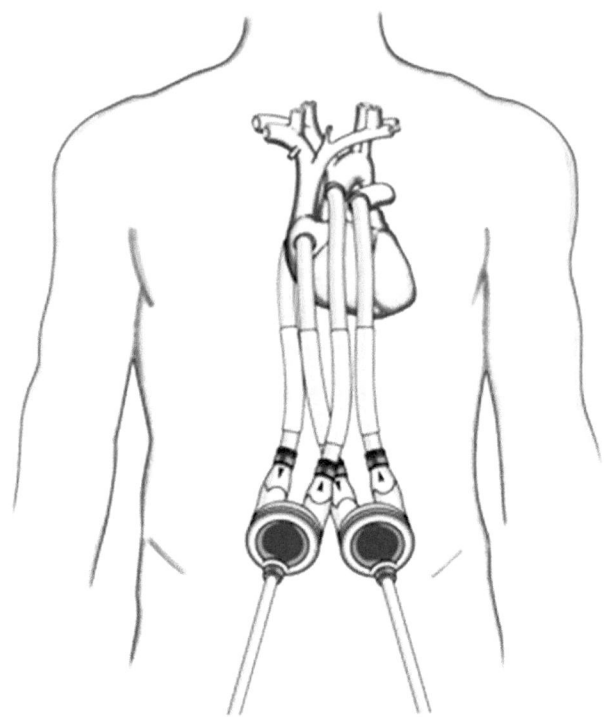

regurgitation (Fig. 15.14). Aortic and pulmonary regurgitation, even slight, has to be carefully evaluated because on long-term support, they generally worsen.

Septal defects are common in CHD and are generally a limitation: left-to-right shunt in a R-VAD may result in systemic low cardiac output, while right-to-left shunt in a L-VAD may result in severe cyanosis.

Single-ventricle physiology has a miscellaneous of variables that makes VAD implantation a real challenge: heart failure in a failing Fontan has to be consider not only as a ventricular dysfunction but rather as a complex disease in which VAD preloading could be ineffective because of innappropriate filling due to capillary leak syndrome, pulmonary barrage or unfavorable allignment of the inlet cannula within the systemic ventricle.

Secondary to the indication (bridge to transplant, bridge to bridge, bridge to recovery, destination therapy), VAD are divided in short-, medium-, and long-term (Table 15.1).

CentriMag® and PediVAS® (Thoratec SJM) are maglev centrifugal pump certified up to 30 days of continuous use, but some clinicians reported an off-label extension of time [23, 24]. Pump is placed bedside and connected with a dedicated circuit in a para-corporeal way: cannulas exit from subcostal spaces. Patient can be awake and weaned from ventilators, but it's not recommended in the youngest or when patient compliance is not guaranteed. Parent's collaborations are a valuable resource. Magnetic levitation, without any shaft/bearing, is compatible with lower anticoagulation protocol.

Fig. 15.15 Berlin
EXCOR (courtesy of
Berlin Heart)

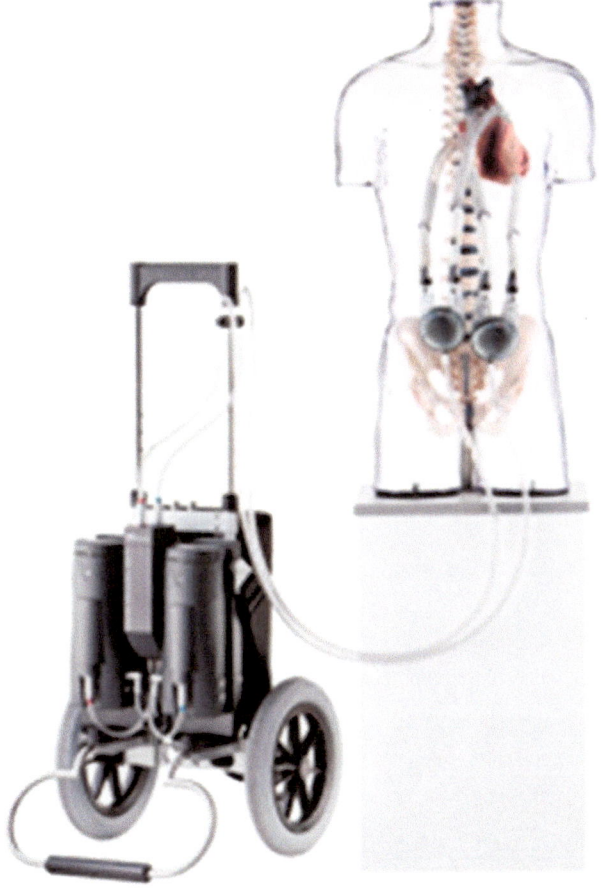

Even if already quite diffused in Europe, the FDA approval of the Berlin Heart EXCOR (Fig. 15.15) for pediatric MCS provided a major option for children and infants who experienced poor results with devices designed for adults [25].

The para-corporeal pulsatile Berlin Heart EXCOR is actually the primary device applicable to infants and small children. It's a pulsatile device, pneumatically driven by an external console (Figs.15.15 and 15.16) that allows moving the patient to the ward, waiting for listing/transplant. Dedicated transthoracic cannulas are directly sutured to the atria or ventricles and great vessels and fixed to the mediastinal wall, so that patient could be safely mobilized.

Support for up to a year is possible, but a limitation is the important incidence of strokes that has been reported in 25–30% of patients [26, 27]. Nursing care comprehends a close inspection of Excor ventricles and valves to exclude thrombosis (Fig. 15.17) and transthoracic ports and cannulas cleansing (Betadine®; Chlorhexidine 0.015%, Farvicett®) and antimicrobial medication (Kendall sponge 0.5% PHMB, AMD™) to prevent infection occurrence.

Fig. 15.16 IKUS console
(courtesy of Berlin Heart)

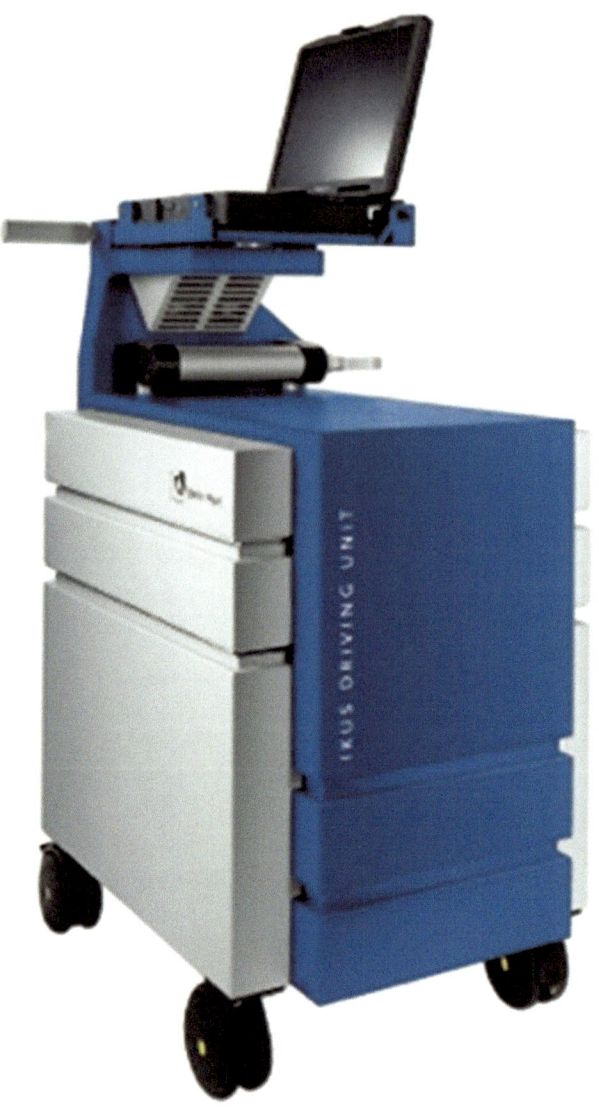

Another limitation of mechanical support is HLA sensitization, which has been observed in up to 60% of pediatric patients [28].

The high mortality with attempted ECMO support to transplantation compared to the Berlin Heart EXCOR has refined the basic therapeutic algorithm [29], so that most patients requiring ECMO are transitioned to a Berlin Heart or other durable device before transplantation. Among patients with cardiomyopathy, successful bridging to transplantation occurs in about 80% of patients supported with the Berlin EXCOR [29, 30].

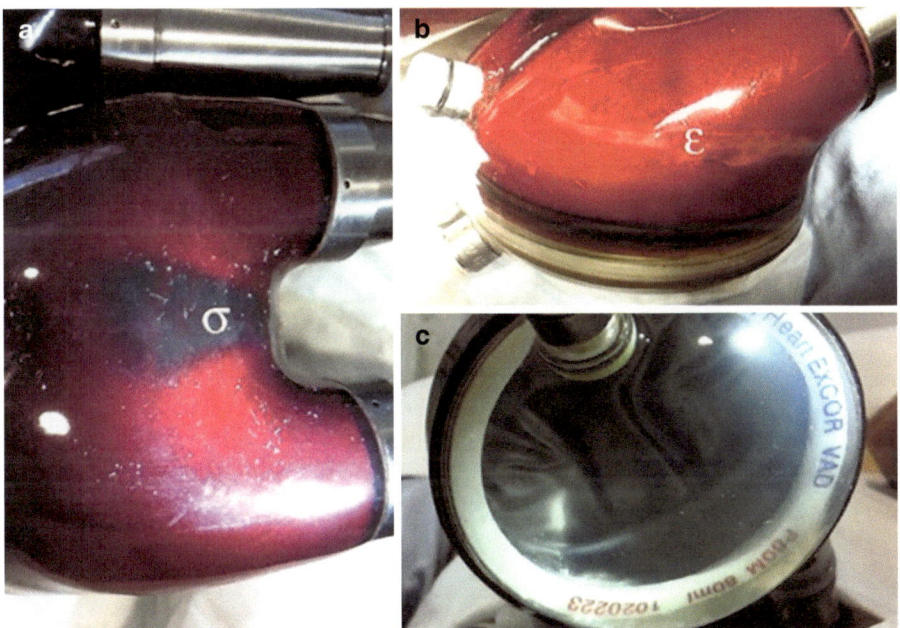

Fig. 15.17 EXCOR thrombosis

However, the results are less good among patients with CHD, particularly those with single ventricle, and CHD accounts for less than 20% of VAD implants in pediatric patients [31].

The overall mortality for functional single-ventricle patients supported with the EXCOR exceeds 40% [26] and is particularly high in the first 3 months of life, where the mortality exceeds 90% for single-ventricle patients [30, 32].

Patients and parents counseling is part of the VAD course: psychological and social compliance should be maximized.

The third-generation full implantable devices are employed among older children and adolescents, and even if the inferior limit is generally defined in 0.7 m^2 BSA, some author's reported their use in smaller patient.

HVAD (HeartWare, Framingham, MA) continuous-flow pump is the most often utilized [33], but CHD patients receiving VADs represent a quite almost anecdotic population, and single-ventricle physiology seems to be the worst candidate to be supported, while systemic right ventricle could be the best one. Other systems like Jarvik 2000 VAD (Jarvik Heart, Manhattan, NY), Heartmate3 (SJM Thoratec, Pleasanton, CA) and HeartAssist5 (Reliant Heart, Houston, TX) (Figs. 15.18 and 15.19) have been successfully reported in CHD patients [33].

Miniaturized investigational continuous-flow devices, including the MVAD (HeartWare) and the Infant Jarvik 2000 VAD, offer promise for the future. The

Fig. 15.18 HeartWare HVAD (courtesy of HeartWare)

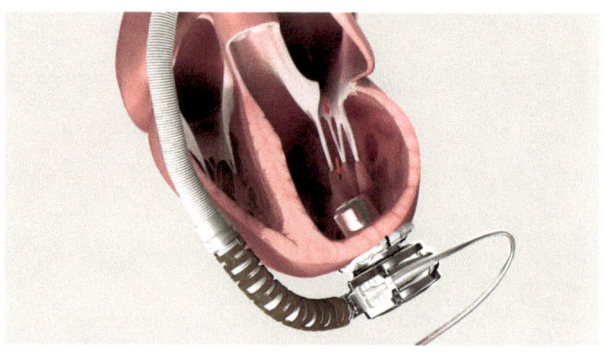

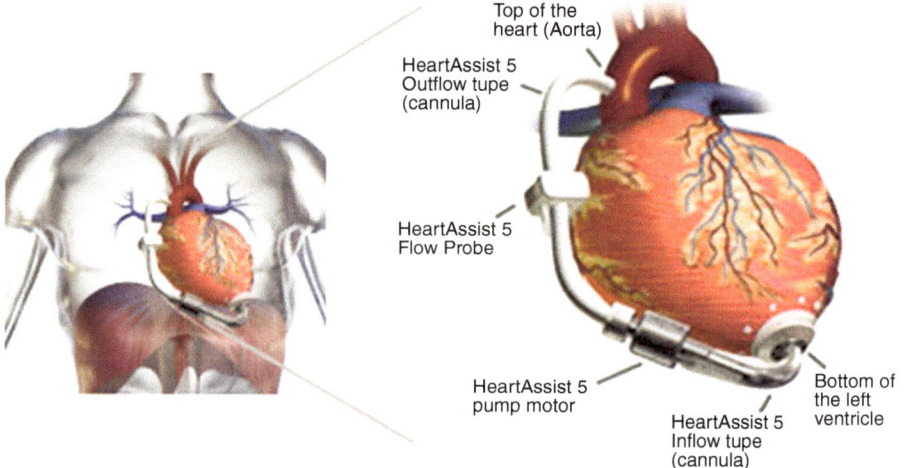

Fig. 15.19 ReliantHeart HeartAssist5 (courtesy of Reliant Heart)

PumpKIN trial sponsored by the National Heart, Lung, and Blood Institute is looking to the Infant Jarvik 2000 among small pediatric patients.

The 50 cc SynCardia total artificial heart (SynCardia Systems, Inc., Tucson, AZ) is currently undergoing clinical trials for older adolescents who need biventricular support [34].

References

1. Ross HJ, Law Y, Book WM, Broberg CS, Burchill L, Cecchin F, Chen JM, Delgado D, Dimopoulos K, Everitt MD, Gatzoulis M, Harris L, Hsu DT, Kuvin JT, Martin CM, Murphy AM, Singh G, Spray TL, Stout KK, American Heart Association Adults With Congenital Heart Disease Committee of the Council on Clinical Cardiology and Council on Cardiovascular Disease in the Young, the Council on Cardiovascular Radiology and Intervention, and the Council on Functional Genomics and Translational Biology. Transplantation and mechanical

circulatory support in congenital heart disease: a scientific statement from the American Heart Association. Circulation. 2016;133(8):802–20.

2. https://www.elso.org/Resources/Guidelines.aspx
3. Annich G, Lynch W, MacLaren G, Wilson J, Bartlett R. ECMO: extracorporeal cardiopulmonary support in critical care. Red Book. 4th ed. Extracorporeal life support.
4. Feldman D, Pamboukian SV, Teuteberg JJ, Birks E, Lietz K, Moore SA, Morgan JA, Arabia F, Bauman ME, Buchholz HW, Deng M, Dickstein ML, El-Banayosy A, Elliot T, Goldstein DJ, Grady KL, Jones K, Hryniewicz K, John R, Kaan A, Kusne S, Loebe M, Massicotte MP, Moazami N, Mohacsi P, Mooney M, Nelson T, Pagani F, Perry W, Potapov EV, Eduardo Rame J, Russell SD, Sorensen EN, Sun B, Strueber M, Mangi AA, Petty MG, Rogers J, International Society for Heart and Lung Transplantation. The 2013 International Society for Heart and Lung Transplantation guidelines for mechanical circulatory support: executive summary. J Heart Lung Transplant. 2013;32(2):157–87.
5. https://www.elso.org/Portals/0/IGD/Archive/FileManager/97000963d6cusersshyer documentselsoguidelinesfortrainingandcontinuingeducationofecmospecialists.pdf
6. https://healthmanagement.org/c/icu/issuearticle/european-perfusionists-in-ecls-ecmo-roles-responsibilities
7. Duncan BW, Ibrahim AE, Hraska V, del Nido PJ, Laussen PC, Wessel DL, Mayer JE Jr, Bower LK, Jonas RA. Use of rapid- deployment extracorporeal membrane oxygenation for the resuscitation of pediatric patients with heart disease after cardiac arrest. J Thorac Cardiovasc Surg. 1998;116(2):305–11.
8. Booth KL, Roth SJ, Thiagarajan RR, Almodovar MC, del Nido PJ, Laussen PC. Extracorporeal membrane oxygenation support of the Fontan and bidirectional Glenn circulations. Ann Thorac Surg. 2004;77(4):1341–8.
9. Caicedo A, Papademetriou MD, Elwell CE, Hoskote A, Elliott MJ, Van Huffel S, Tachtsidis I. Canonical correlation analysis in the study of cerebral and peripheral haemodynamics interrelations with systemic variables in neonates supported on ECMO. Adv Exp Med Biol. 2013;765:23–9.
10. Maldonado Y, Singh S, Taylor MA. Cerebral near-infrared spectroscopy in perioperative management of left ventricular assist device and extracorporeal membrane oxygenation patients. Curr Opin Anaesthesiol. 2014;27(1):81–8.
11. Buijs EA, Houmes RJ, Rizopoulos D, Wildschut ED, Reiss IK, Ince C, Tibboel D. Arterial lactate for predicting mortality in children requiring extracorporeal membrane oxygenation. Minerva Anestesiol. 2014;80(12):1282–93.
12. Park SJ, Kim SP, Kim JB, Jung SH, Choo SJ, Chung CH, Lee JW. Blood lactate level during extracorporeal life support as a surrogate marker for survival. J Thorac Cardiovasc Surg. 2014;148(2):714–20.
13. Ranucci M, Carboni G, Cotza M, de Somer F. Carbon dioxide production during cardiopulmonary bypass: pathophysiology, measure and clinical relevance. Perfusion. 2017;32(1):4–12.
14. Selewski DT, Cornell TT, Blatt NB, Han YY, Mottes T, Kommareddi M, Gaies MG, Annich GM, Kershaw DB, Shanley TP, Heung M. Fluid overload and fluid removal in pediatric patients on extracorporeal membrane oxygenation requiring continuous renal replacement therapy. Crit Care Med. 2012;40(9):2694–9.
15. Kumar TK, Zurakowski D, Dalton H, et al. Extracorporeal membrane oxygenation in postcardiotomy patients: factors influencing outcome. Thorac Cardiovasc Surg. 2010;140:330–6.
16. Fiser RT, Irby K, Ward RM, Tang X, McKamie W, Prodhan P, Corwin HL. RBC transfusion in pediatric patients supported with extracorporeal membrane oxygenation: is there an impact on tissue oxygenation? Pediatr Crit Care Med. 2014;15(9):806–13.
17. Young G, Boshkov LK, Sullivan JE, Raffini LJ, et al. Argatroban therapy in pediatric patients requiring nonheparin anticoagulation: an open-label, safety, efficacy, and pharmacokinetic study. Pediatr Blood Cancer. 2011;56:1103–9.
18. Young G. New anticoagulants in children. Hematology. 2008:245–50.
19. Ranucci M, Ballotta A, Kandil H, et al. Bivalirudin-based vs. conventional heparin anticoagulation for postcardiotomy extracorporeal membrane oxygenation. Crit Care. 2011;15:R275.

20. Bembea MM, Annich G, Rycus P, et al. Variability in anticoagulation management of patients on extracorporeal membrane oxygenation: an international survey. Pediatr Crit Care Med. 2013;14(2):e77–84.
21. Ranucci M, Baryshnikova E, Cotza M, Carboni G, Isgrò G, Carlucci C, Ballotta A. Group for the Surgical and Clinical Outcome Research (SCORE). Coagulation monitoring in postcardiotomy ECMO: conventional tests, point-of-care, or both? Minerva Anestesiol. 2016;82(8):858–66.
22. Blume ED, Naftel DC, Bastardi HJ, Duncan BW, Kirklin JK, Webber SA, Pediatric Heart Transplant Study Investigators. Outcomes of children bridged to heart transplantation with ventricular assist devices: a multi-institutional study. Circulation. 2006;113(19):2313–9.
23. Sung SY, Hsu PS, Chen JL, Tsai CS, Tsai YT, Lin CY, Lee CY, Ke HY, Lin YC. Prolonged use of levitronix left ventricular assist device as a bridge to heart transplantation. Acta Cardiol Sin. 2015;31(3):249–52.
24. Zafar F, Castleberry C, Khan MS, et al. Pediatric heart transplant waiting list mortality in the era of ventricular assist devices. J Heart Lung Transplant. 2015;34(1):82–8.
25. Almond CS, Bucholz H, Massicott P, et al. Berlin Heart EXCOR pediatric ventricular assist device Investigational Device Exemption Study: study design and rationale. Am Heart J. 2011;162(3):425–35.
26. Weinstein S, Bello R, Pizarro C, et al. The use of the Berlin Heart EXCOR in patients with functional single ventricle. J Thorac Cardiovasc Surg. 2014;147(2):697–705.
27. Massad MG, Cook DJ, Schmitt SK, et al. Factors influencing HLA sensitization in implantable LVAD recipients. Ann Thorac Surg. 1997;64(4):1120–5.
28. Davies RR, Haldeman S, McCulloch MA, Pizarro C. Ventricular assist devices as a bridge-to-transplant improve early posttransplant outcomes in children. J Heart Lung Transplant. 2014;33(7):704–12.
29. Rossano JW, Woods RK, Berger S, et al. Mechanical support as failure intervention in patients with cavopulmonary shunts (MFICS): rationale and aims of a new registry of mechanical circulatory support in single ventricle patients. Congenit Heart Dis. 2013;8(3):182–6.
30. Rossano JW, Goldberg DJ, Fuller S, et al. Successful use of the total artificial heart in the failing Fontan circulation. Ann Thorac Surg. 2014;97(4):1483–40.
31. Pearce FB, Kirklin JK, Holman WL, Barrett CS, Romp RL, Lau YR. Successful cardiac transplant after Berlin Heart bridge in a single ventricle heart: use of aortopulmonary shunt as a supplementary source of pulmonary blood flow. J Thorac Cardiovasc Surg. 2009;137(1):e40–2.
32. Blume ED, Rosenthal DN, Rossano JW, et al. Outcomes of children implanted with ventricular assist devices in the United States: first analysis of the Pediatric Interagency Registry for Mechanical Circulatory Support (PediMACS). J Heart Lung Transplant. 2016;35(5):578–84.
33. Strueber M, Schmitto JD, Kutschka I, Haverich A. Placement of 2 implantable centrifugal pumps to serve as a total artificial heart after cardiectomy. J Thorac Cardiovasc Surg. 2012;143:507–9.
34. Ryan TD, Jefferies JL, Zafar F, et al. The evolving role of the total artificial heart in the management of end-stage congenital heart disease and adolescents. ASAIO J. 2015;61(1):8–1.

Nursing Care for Patients with Congenital Heart Disease During Follow-Up: Transfer and Transition

16

Serena Francesca Flocco and Eva Goossens

Abstract

The developmental transition from childhood to adulthood is a complex process in the life of every youngster. This developmental process appears to be, however, more challenging and complex for children who are born with a congenital heart disease (CHD), because they not only have to deal with dynamics, changes, and difficulties characterizing adolescence, but also the consequences of their chronic condition and the need to adhere to lifelong follow-up care. Adolescence, with its prominent physical, biological, hormonal, psychological, and behavioral changes, is considered the most critical transitional phase of life. During this stage of life, patients with CHD, as compared to "healthy" adolescents, should learn how to integrate their medical condition with their identity and future lifestyle.

Hence, accompanying an adolescent afflicted with CHD from adolescence toward adulthood requires focused attention not solely to their medical needs but also to existential needs and academic and vocational pursuits, getting ready for the job market, having meaningful recreational activities and/or sports, and establishing a family when desired. Over the past decades, attention from healthcare professionals shifted from ensuring survival during the first years of life towards achievement of an acceptable quality of life for patients with CHD in the longer run.

S. F. Flocco
Pediatric and Adult Congenital Heart Disease Center, IRCCS Policlinico San Donato University Hospital, San Donato Milanese (MI), Italy

E. Goossens (✉)
Department of Public Health and Primary Care, Academic Center for Nursing and Midwifery, KU Leuven, Leuven, Belgium

Research Foundation Flanders (FWO), Brussels, Belgium
e-mail: eva.goossens@kuleuven.be

© Springer International Publishing AG, part of Springer Nature 2019
S. F. Flocco et al. (eds.), *Congenital Heart Disease*,
https://doi.org/10.1007/978-3-319-78423-6_16

271

Over the past decades, various national and international specialized heart centers developed clinical care pathways dedicated to these specific transitional needs of adolescents suffering from a congenital heart defect. Such programs create a bridge between the worlds of the child who grows into a teenager and that of the (emerging) adult.

16.1   Introduction

This chapter will address issues related to the transition from adolescence to adulthood of children born with a congenital heart defect (CHD). Adolescence is a particular developmental period for every person, an age period often defined in terms of crisis and distress, characterized by intense and sudden emotional, social, and psychological changes, associated with physical changes as a result of pubertal development [1]. These changes are described as variable, occurring over a short period of time and involving different aspects of life (e.g., morphological, sexual, psychological changes) leading the adolescent to engage in a process of control, containment, and attribution of meaning to what is happening [2]. These changes become more pronounced by the state of morbidity and the impact of CHD on the person's overall well-being. This developmental path is indeed more complex for adolescents born with CHD, as they do not only face the dynamics, changes, and difficulties characterizing adolescence, but are furthermore subjected to lifelong follow-up care keeping them aware of their heart defect.

16.2   Health and Psychosocial Challenges in Adolescents with CHD

Adolescence is a challenging period of life, characterized by significant changes affecting one's body (i.e., biological maturation), mind (i.e., cognitive development), and behavior (i.e., social values and establishment of relationships). During this developmental phase, adolescents might elaborate grief toward their old self-image to build a new one [3]. Many developmental tasks are to be achieved by adolescents: establishing new and mature relationships with peers, gaining a feminine or male social role, accepting their bodies, achieving emotional independence from parents and other adults, developing intellectual knowledge and proficiencies, developing a set of personal values and an ethical consciousness as a guide for their own behaviors, and directing themselves toward both personal and professional independence [4].

By establishing cognitive competences (i.e., hypothetical deductive thinking), adolescents are supposed to gain insight into aspects of health and disease. In the first phase (i.e., physiological phase), adolescents describe disease as the not-functioning or anomalous functioning of organisms or internal processes that cause a gradual sequence of events which culminate in pathological situations. In the following phase (i.e., psychophysiological phase), the disease is still described as internal physiological processes, but adolescents are also aware that thoughts and feelings can affect organic processes [5].

The heart defect can influence the quality of patients' lives in a permeating way, interfering with many of their developmental tasks [6] resulting in loss of existential continuity (due to frequent medical check-ups or to new illness episodes), isolation or necessity to give up social and life experiences (e.g., the impossibility to share physical activities), and their body image marked by scars or other signs. These are all factors affecting the self-image of adolescents who might struggle to accept themselves with their growing bodies, to be in relationships with peers, and to test and know themselves [7, 8]. Because of these struggles, young people with CHD are susceptible to feelings of surrender, depression, anxiety, passivity, or addiction.

As in line with other complex chronic conditions, CHD generates a strong and long-lasting emotional strain [9]. When a physical dysfunction, related to the disease, appears to be permanent, this might produce a great psychological burden for patients, adding to the feeling of dependence from medical care, which might affect the patient's psychological development and personality formation. The condition, interfering with other life experiences, influences their self-image [6]. During this developmental period, it is essential for adolescents to show their ability to handle different situations and to gain independence. Unfortunately, some adolescents try to overcome this internal conflict, through denial of their disease, resulting in therapy non-adherence and risky health behaviors [9].

Family context appears to be essential during the developmental process of transition toward adulthood and adult care. Apprehensive, suffocating, and overprotective parenting styles are found to increase difficulties experienced by adolescents [9]. Parents, who have trouble in allowing their children with CHD to grow toward independence, are found to substitute their children, avoiding them to gain responsibility for their own pathological situation. It is common that many adolescents appear to have increased feelings of being different, with feelings of inferiority and frustration [10].

Taking care of adolescents with CHD entails, therefore, a comprehensive awareness of the complex nature of adolescence, as a compulsory transitional phase during one's life course. In this professional attitude, it is important not to limit the attention to the biopsychosocial characteristics but to achieve integration between medical, ethical, and psycho-educational aspects [2]. Considering the abovementioned findings, it is evident how the concept (and consequently the practical aspect) of transition is important, meant as the adolescent's passage from pediatrics to adult healthcare, with the consequent passage of competences and responsibilities from the pediatric care *team* to the adult care *team*.

16.3   Transition and Transfer: Conceptual Definitions

The developmental process affecting adolescents with CHD becoming young adults is a process consisting of two different components: the developmental transition process and the event of transfer of care. Often these terms are improperly used interchangeably although they are two well-distinct entities.

There are various definitions for the concept of "transition" to be found in literature. Differences between such definitions can be found in the focus they have on specific and differentiated aspects. Transition is often defined as "the process by which adolescents and young adults who have chronic childhood illnesses are prepared to take charge of their lives and their health in adulthood" [11]. The definition published by the Society for Adolescent Medicine (1993), however, defined transition as "the purposeful, planned movement of adolescent and young adults with chronic physical and medical conditions from child-centered to adult-oriented health care systems" [12]. The key factors in this definition appear to be intentionality and planning of the passage or transfer from pediatric cardiology toward ACHD care [13].

Scal et al. [14], however, defined the transition as "the process by which the youth with chronic conditions develop the skills and secure the resources to assure that their health care needs are met as they transition from adolescence to adulthood." Clearly, in this case, greater prominence is given to the role of young people as an active, rather than a passive, subject of the transition process. As part of the transition process, adolescents are supposed to acquire the appropriate set of skills and secure the necessary resources in order to ensure that their specific needs are met.

Davies et al. [15] focused in their definition of transition, rather on to the fact that transition should start at an early age and emphasize the mandatory action of the multidisciplinary team. The transition process should address not only the direct healthcare needs of the young adult, but also the needs and concerns of the parents who are involved as prominent guides during that developmental process.

Transfer, on the other hand, is defined as "an event or series of events through which the adolescents and young adults with chronic physical and medical conditions move their care from a pediatric toward an adult-oriented health care setting" [11]. In contrast to the phase of transition, transfer of care appears to be a specific event, representing the passage at which adolescents are physically and practically moved from a Pediatric Congenital Heart Center to an Adult Congenital Heart Center (ACHD), often called as GUCH Unit (Grown-up Congenital Heart Unit) or an ACHD Unit (Adult Congenital Heart Disease Unit) [16–18].

All these definitions emphasize that a transition process is deemed essential to prepare teenagers and their parents to the passage from adolescence to adulthood, including the evolvement to increased patient self-management and independence. Hence, transition does not solely entail the practical transfer from child-focused to adult-oriented services but includes a preparatory process aimed to meet medical, psychosocial, educational, and vocational needs of young people with chronic conditions, such as CHD. During transition, the patient has to face the delicate transformations related to this developmental stage and the problems related to their disease [19–25]. It is therefore essential to describe transition as a wider process, a passage from dependency as a child to autonomy as an adult, through the construction of a sense of identity and self-image. Furthermore, it is utmost important to ensure continuity of care for the patient allowing him/her to cope with the occurring changes in care but guaranteeing the best patient-related outcomes.

This transition requires a gradual adaptation of the patient and the family to the new system of adult care. In order to move toward a successful transition process, it is important to take into account the needs and experiences of the patient and his family at this particular developmental stage, monitoring their fragility but, above all, their resources in the autonomous management of the disease. It is also crucial to remember that the adult service relies on autonomous and responsible patients, so the task of pediatric services is also to train their patients in gaining a sense of autonomy, dedicating their time and attention to discuss their concerns, and monitoring "self-administration" [26]. The know-how level of the healthcare professionals and the attention and collaboration between pediatric and adult team members can affect the success of the transition process. Switching to adult services means actually to interrupt an established care relationship and to start a new one: to know the new staff and the functioning of the adult service. Being aware of a collaboration between the two services can help to increase the sense of patient's personal safety during the transition phase [27].

The paper of the American Heart Association [28] subdivided the entire transition process into three consecutive phases, which act as guiding principles:

- *Pre-transition phase*: It is a family's process, since the family should be supported and encouraged to develop positive expectations about the ability of children to become autonomous and independent in managing their medical care from an early age.
- *Transition phase*: In this phase, the young patients should be helped to understand their diagnosis and medical history, to gain knowledge of anatomy and physiology of the cardiovascular system, in order to grasp the impact of their heart defect on their health and well-being. They should also be taught to recognize all indicative signs and symptoms of a deteriorating health condition, as well as to acquire skills which enable them to move into the adult healthcare system.
- *Transfer toward adult-focused cardiac care*: The actual transfer of care is essential for both the management of the patient and his pathology. The transfer is related to the different models of care in different health systems worldwide. There are countries where GUCH/ACHD units are recognized and well organized and countries where assistance is provided within pediatric or adult cardiology centers. As early as 2014, the European Society of Cardiology has defined the need and usefulness of having dedicated support structures for the adult with CHD in order to optimize care [29].

16.4   Timing of Transition and Transfer of Care

The process of transition should be individualized according to each patient's medical and developmental condition. Congenital heart defects and other complex chronic illnesses have an impact on the developmental milestones of each patient, and this should be strongly considered when transitioning care [30]. Physical and emotional maturity is the primary requirement defining the timing to start initiating the transition process as well as the transfer to adult care environments. There exists no single "right" timing or predefined age for transfers nor a rigid age limit defining child versus adult services. The ongoing process of transition might begin at the time of diagnosis and end following the transfer to an adult care facility [27]. However, the process of transitioning, which means preparing young patients for successful transfer to an adult healthcare provider at a later time, is recommended to start early at the age of 12 years [31, 32]. A gradual process toward establishing autonomy, understanding one's cardiac anatomy and health status, and becoming aware of relevant lifestyle issues are key elements to assure the patient is ready for the actual handing off to adulthood [7]. "Envisioning a future" has been identified as an important first step in the transition process for individuals with special healthcare needs or disabilities recommended "starting early" [33], which can be assisted with the creation of a written healthcare transition plan [34].

Although the age of initiating transition and/or transfer is mandated in some countries, ideally, the timing of transfer should be flexible and depend on a patient's chronological age, medical and developmental status, adherence to therapy, maturity and independence, the preparation and readiness of both patient and family, and the availability of appropriate adult healthcare providers [33]. Adolescents and young adults with CHD and their parents prefer the transition process to be individualized to each adolescent [35]. Transition and education regarding self-management should not culminate with transfer to adult care but should continue through the period of emerging adulthood to face the ongoing changes. Poor knowledge among ACHD patients regarding birth control, pregnancy, and genetic counseling, as well as the continued need for vocational and employment advice, highlight the importance of ongoing education during adulthood [36, 37].

16.5   Organizing a Transition Program

The question how to approach this problem may be different in several distinct countries, because the way of approaching adolescents might be different. Centers that care for adolescents and young adults with CHD need to develop structured plans for the transfer of care from the department of pediatric cardiology to that of adult congenital cardiology. A comprehensive program with a progressive approach, beginning in childhood and adolescence, is assumed to achieve better results than programs that focus solely on the transfer to the adult care at a specified age.

Currently, sufficient empirical data are not available to support the identification of "best practices" regarding transition in patients with CHD or other complex chronic conditions. However, descriptive and qualitative studies have indicated that key elements of an effective transition program include the following steps [32]:

1. A policy on timing of transfer to adult care (age 18 years or when leaving school is recommended by many, although with flexibility).
2. A preparation period and education program that focus on a set of skills enabling young people and their families to function in an adult clinic (e.g., understanding the disease, treatment rationale, and source of symptoms; recognizing deterioration and taking appropriate action; learning how to seek help from health professionals and how to operate within the medical system).
3. A coordinated transfer process including a detailed written plan and pretransfer visit to the adult clinic, with an introduction to the adult provider and with a designated coordinator such as a clinic nurse.
4. An interested and capable ACHD regional center that is at least equivalent in quality to that of the pediatric source the patient is leaving (see subsequent discussion).
5. Administrative support.
6. Primary care involvement.

Transitional care appears to be more successful in healthcare settings characterized by the following conditions (39):

1. The preparation for transition begins before adolescence, and transition is seen as an essential component of high-quality healthcare.
2. There is a formal transition program.
3. Young people are not transferred to adult services until they have the necessary skills to function in an adult service and have finished growth and puberty.
4. There is an identified person in both the pediatric and adult teams who has responsibility for transition arrangements (usually nurse specialists or transition coordinator).
5. Management links are developed between the pediatric and adult systems, and financial and contracting issues are worked out in detail and put in writing.
6. The evaluation of transition arrangements is undertaken as part of a continuous quality improvement process.
7. Transfer is planned and carried out during a period of the medical stability.
8. After transfer, there should be an ongoing consultation with the referring pediatric cardiologist.

Therefore, a formal program of transition should consist in providing a continuous health assistance, centered on the patient, appropriate for his/her age and development phase, comprehensive and with the mandatory flexibility. Such a program should include contents that are educational and informative about medical conditions of CHD; should promote in every person communicative abilities, self-care, and self-advocacy; and should stimulate the decision process. It also should encourage more personal and medical independence and more control system of one's health; in this way, it could support self-sufficiency and responsibility. The final target should focus on optimizing the young patients' quality of life, encouraging positive expectations about life and realistic points of view toward future professional productivity.

Conclusions

Because increasing numbers of young people who have complex congenital conditions are surviving into adulthood, there is an urgent need for programs designed to facilitate a smooth passage from pediatric to adult healthcare environments and from childhood over adolescence to adulthood. Pediatric cardiology providers should establish transition and transfer policies and offer transition program to all adolescents with CHD. Individualized one-on-one education is an effective method of improving adolescents' knowledge of their CHD and improving their self-management skills. Best practices in transitional care for adolescents with congenital heart disease remain largely based upon expert opinion rather than being evidence based, given the paucity of rigorous studies evaluating transition practices. How to support and educate parents through the transition process has also not yet been evaluated nor has the role and impact of transition coordinators in congenital heart disease been studied comprehensively.

However, recent literature has described the outcome of programs focused on improving knowledge among adolescents of their CHD. Significant research opportunities remain in this important field. Providing transitional care should be considered as a complex intervention. In order to deliver a successful transition service, this needs to be a service that can be developed and will evolve over time, based on the insights gained longitudinally. All the components of a transition service need to work together and are therefore interrelated.

References

1. Simonelli C. La formazione alla salute nell'età evolutiva: gli adolescenti e il rischio da HIV. Rivista di Sessuologia Clinica. 2000;VII(1):5–9.
2. Bertelloni S. Adolescentologia. Percorsi medici e socio-educativi. Milano: Tecniche nuove; 2010.
3. Camaioni L, Di Blasio P. Psicologia dello sviluppo, Bologna. 2nd ed: Il Mulino; 2007.
4. Havighurst R. Social and psychological needs of the aging. Ann Am Acad Pol Soc Sci. 1952;279(1):11–7.
5. De Carlo N, Senatori Pilleri R. Le malattie croniche nel ciclo di vita. Aspetti psicologici, comunicativi e di organizzazione sanitaria. Milano: Franco Angeli; 2012.
6. Birks Y, Sloper P, Lewin R, Parsons J. Exploring health-related experiences of children and young people with congenital heart disease. Health Expect. 2007;10(1):16–29.
7. Berghammer M, Dellborg M, Ekman I. Young adults experiences of living with congenital heart disease. Int J Cardiol. 2006;110(3):340–7.
8. Moons P. The importance of methodological rigour in quality-of-life studies. Eur J Cardiothorac Surg. 2010;37(1):246–7.
9. Chiang Y-T, Chen C-W, Su W-J, Wang J-K, Lu C-W, Li Y-F, et al. Between invisible defects and visible impact: the life experiences of adolescents and young adults with congenital heart disease. J Adv Nurs. 2015;71(3):599–608.

10. Claessens P, Moons P, de Casterlé BD, Cannaerts N, Budts W, Gewillig M. What does it mean to live with a congenital heart disease? A qualitative study on the lived experiences of adult patients. Eur J Cardiovasc Nurs. 2005;4(1):3–10.
11. Knauth A, Verstappen A, Reiss J, Webb GD. Transition and transfer from pediatric to adult care of the young adult with complex congenital heart disease. Cardiol Clin. 2006;24(4):619–29, vi
12. Viner R. Transition from paediatric to adult care. Bridging the gaps or passing the buck? Arch Dis Child. 1999;81(3):271–5.
13. Heery E, Sheehan AM, While AE, Coyne I. Experiences and outcomes of transition from pediatric to adult health care services for young people with congenital heart disease: a systematic review. Congenit Heart Dis. 2015 Sep;10(5):413–27.
14. Scal P, Horvath K, Garwick A. Preparing for adulthood: health care transition counseling for youth with arthritis. Arthritis Rheum. 2009;61(1):52–7.
15. Davies H, Rennick J, Majnemer A. Transition from pediatric to adult health care for young adults with neurological disorders: parental perspectives. Can J. 2011;33(2):32–9.
16. Dore A, Guise P de, Mercier L. Transition of care to adult congenital heart centres: what do patients know about their heart condition? Can J 2002;18(2):141–146.
17. Goossens E, Van DK, Zupancic N. Effectiveness of structured patient education on the knowledge level of adolescents and adults with congenital heart disease. Eur J Cardiovasc Nurs. 2014;13(1):63–70.
18. Mora M, Moons P. Assessing the level of evidence on transfer and transition in young people with chronic conditions: protocol of a scoping review. Syst Rev. 2016;5(1):166.
19. Blum RW, Garell D, Hodgman CH, Jorissen TW, Okinow NA, Orr DP, et al. Transition from child-centered to adult health-care systems for adolescents with chronic conditions. A position paper of the Society for Adolescent Medicine. J Adolesc Health. 1993;14(7):570–6.
20. David TJ. Transition from the paediatric clinic to the adult service. J R Soc Med. 2001;94(8):373–4.
21. Goodhand J, Hedin CR, Croft NM, Lindsay JO. Adolescents with IBD: the importance of structured transition care. J Crohns Colitis. 2011;5(6):509–19.
22. Amaria K, Stinson J, Cullen-Dean G, Sappleton K, Kaufman M. Tools for addressing systems issues in transition. Healthc Q. 2011;14 Spec No 3:72–6.
23. Leung Y, Heyman MB, Mahadevan U. Transitioning the adolescent inflammatory bowel disease patient: guidelines for the adult and pediatric gastroenterologist. Inflamm Bowel Dis. 2011;17(10):2169–73.
24. Schwartz LA, Tuchman LK, Hobbie WL, Ginsberg JP. A social-ecological model of readiness for transition to adult-oriented care for adolescents and young adults with chronic health conditions. Child Care Health Dev. 2011;37(6):883–95.
25. Mackner LM, Crandall WV, Szigethy EM. Psychosocial functioning in pediatric inflammatory bowel disease. Inflamm Bowel Dis. 2006;12(3):239–44.
26. Shaw RJ, DeMaso DR. Respiratory illness. Textbook of pediatric psychosomatic medicine. Washington, DC: APA Publishing; 2010.
27. Mahan JD, Betz CL, Okumura MJ, Ferris ME. Self-management and transition to adult health care in adolescents and young adults: a team process. Pediatr Rev. 2017;38(7):305–19.
28. Sable C, Foster E, Uzark K, Bjornsen K, Canobbio M. Best practices in managing transition to adulthood for adolescents with congenital heart disease: the transition process and medical and psychosocial issues. Circulation. 2011;123(13):1454–85.
29. Baumgartner H, Budts W, Chessa M. Recommendations for organization of care for adults with congenital heart disease and for training in the subspecialty of "Grown-up Congenital Heart Disease" in Europe: a position paper of the Working Group on Grown-up Congenital Heart Disease of the European Society of Cardiology. Eur Heart J. 2014;35(11): 686–90.
30. Shaw K, Southwood T, McDonagh J. User perspectives of transitional care for adolescents with juvenile idiopathic arthritis. Rheumatology. 2004;43(6):770–8.
31. Hudsmith LE, Thorne SA. Transition of care from paediatric to adult services in cardiology. Arch Dis Child. 2007;92:927–30.

32. Foster E, Graham TP, Driscoll DJ, Reid GJ, Reiss JG, Russell IA, et al. Task Force 2: special health care needs of adults with congenital heart disease. J Am Coll Cardiol. 2001;37:1176–83.
33. Reiss JG, Gibson RW, Walker LR. Health care transition: youth, family, and provider perspectives. Pediatrics. 2005;115(1):112–20.
34. American Academy of Pediatrics, American Academy of Family Physicians, American College of Physicians-American Society of Internal Medicine. A consensus statement on health care transitions for young adults with special health care needs. Pediatrics. 2002;110(6 Pt 2):1304–6.
35. Wray J, Maynard L. Specialist cardiac services: what do young people want? Cardiol Young. 2008;18(6):569–74.
36. Simko LC, McGinnis KA, Schembri J. Educational needs of adults with congenital heart disease. J Cardiovasc Nurs. 2006;21(2):85–94.
37. Betz CL. Adolescents in transition of adult care: why the concern? Nurs Clin North Am. 2004;39(4):681–713.

Perspectives From Well-Being to Organizational Health in Congenital Heart Disease's Nursing Care

Adelaide Orlando

Abstract

Over the past few decades, many studies have shown that the characteristics of work in the healthcare sector have a deep impact on employee welfare.

Higher health levels for patients with congenital heart disease can be found in presence of a greater concentration of knowledge/expertise and nursing psycho-physical well-being. The human factor is a key element in the production and delivery process of healthcare services, and thus it can influence the outcome. Working well-being is directly related to organizational health. A good work environment creates well-being if it is able to promote, maintain, and improve the quality of individuals' life and the physical, psychological, and social well-being of the community of people working in that context.

17.1 Aid Relationship

In the aid relationship, to abide by impersonality means to fall into the unauthentic [1], and vice versa, being authentically in the aid relationship implies the acceptance of personal involvement, with all the consequences in terms of vulnerability and risk.

The relationship is both heart and substance of the aid relationship, required by the sick person and provided by the attending person, and mainly consists in a communication between two human beings [2].

A. Orlando
Service of Psychology, Associazione Italiana Cardiopatici Congeniti Adulti (AICCA), IRCCS Policlinico San Donato, Milan, Italy

© Springer International Publishing AG, part of Springer Nature 2019
S. F. Flocco et al. (eds.), *Congenital Heart Disease*,
https://doi.org/10.1007/978-3-319-78423-6_17

In the tales of Greek mythology, Chiron the centurion, a master in the medical arts, was struck by a poisoned arrow but, being immortal, he could neither die nor heal himself. The psychologist Henri Nouwen uses this metaphor in his book *The Wounded Healer* [3] and is suited to …healers, that is, anyone who carries out a work involving an aid relationship. In such context, while having to help the sick persons, the attending person also has to carry personal injuries that cannot justify his departure from the profession.

Being employed in the healthcare sector implies a delicate and necessary involvement of emotional life, as the cornerstone of an interpersonal relationship that cannot be reduced to a mere technical performance. Health practitioners, who are on a daily basis in close contact with situations involving the fragility and precariousness of life (congenital heart disease, intensive therapy, oncology, hematology, geriatrics …), know that the scientific expertise is not enough to cope with the suffering. They are well aware of the need to have places, times, and tools to elaborate their emotional experiences. Being prevented from avoiding involvement, which would result in a betrayal of the aid relationship, professional nurses no longer are unemotional and perfectly efficient machines but vulnerable human beings. They claim what they were denied from the beginning: the possibility of taking care of themselves, without which any aid relationship becomes, over time, unsustainable. It is therefore essential to provide health practitioners with tools for the care of their emotional health and the continuous renewal of their professional motivation [4].

17.2   Health Culture Within the Organization

Over the last years, the majority of healthcare organizations have been sensitive to the needs of nurses whose satisfaction is increasingly felt as a priority [5]. The well-being of the organization and the health and quality of life in working environments have become important issues in health management [6].

The human relations movement [7] highlighted the importance of the human factor, and we now started to discuss about the damages that could affect the individual's well-being at work, about the monotonous and repetitive pace of the work, and about the downgrading that hinders the exploitation of individual potentials.

In the 1950s and 1960s, the studies on the occupational stress and its causes—the so-called psychosocial risks—expanded the interest from the knowledge and treatment of the psychophysical health of workers to the investigation of the working mechanisms that affect the health. The worker is now seen in connection with its surrounding environment, although the concept of linear randomness [8] continues to exist.

The following decades, between the 1970s and 1980s, witness the shift from a treatment-oriented approach to one that focuses on prevention. There are interesting studies on the quality of workplace safety (health protection), and new concepts are introduced, such as wellness and occupational health promotion. A new field of action which aims to improve and maintain a state of physical and psychological well-being gradually emerges. The ideas of work, individual, and organization are increasingly and systematically analyzed, taking more aspects into consideration. If environmental conditions were previously conceived as causes of unhealthy effects, now the aim is to change the workers' behaviors which are likely to increase the severity of illnesses or other disabling health conditions [8].

During this period, actions are taken with the aim of improving the individual/environment relationship, thanks to the researches on occupational stress. Today, one of the major social and health problem are stress-related psychological and physiological disorders. Experts believe that 50–80% of workers' illnesses are closely related to stress [9].

Every environmental stimulus requires a reaction of the individual which can be a source of stress (stressor). Individuals react by assessing the situation and the skills they feel to possess in order to deal with the situation: this cognitive assessment determines the stressful power of every environmental stimulus. The cognitive assessment determines the *strain*, that is, the negative impact (which consists in psychological distress and/or illness) that the potentially stressful situation has on the individual [10].

These types of risk may be linked to more typical dysfunctional responses, such as negative feelings, depression, hypertension, cardiovascular disease, or problems that affect the organization, such as job dissatisfaction, high turnover, and marked absenteeism. Working in environments which are deemed to be sources of stress, such as the healthcare sector, facilitates the early exit from the workforce [11].

Managerial nursing culture should aim at managing services with organizational models that consider both users and nurses as care seekers, since they are users of a service that consists in the simultaneous demand for assistance and responsiveness to the need. In this framework, the nursing manager plays a key role. It is a professional figure who places itself above everyone in a healthcare company. Thus it is no longer in line but in staff with it, directly participating in the "government management" at the various levels of the organization [12].

17.3   Care for Others and Care for Themselves

In recent years, the problem of safety and psychophysical well-being of workers received an increasing interest in our country. In particular, greater attention was paid to overall well-being in the work environment, expanding the protection of the worker to psychological, physical, and social well-being.

The nursing profession involves various types of commitment that can be a source of stress and imbalance for both the private and the professional life of them.

On the basis of the concepts outlined by Avallone et al. [12], organizational well-being is "The set of cultural units, processes, and organizational practices that animate the dynamics of coexistence in working environments by promoting, maintaining, and improving the quality of life and the level of physical, psychological, and social well-being of working communities."

The term burnout (burned, burst) is used for the first time in the healthcare sector by Freudenberger [13]. In English sports journalism, the term describes the abrupt decline in performance of an athlete due to the lack of motivation. With this term, Freudenberger indicates a condition of physical and emotional breakdown observed among practitioners engaged in aid professions. This condition is determined by the chronic emotional tension created by the contact and the continuous and intense engagement with suffering people.

The word "burnout" conceives the condition of occupational stress that can be frequently observed among the subjects involved in the aiding activities: it is therefore a professional disease which is particularly relevant in the healthcare sector.

The risk of burnout appears when the healthcare professional, overburdened by environmental and emotional-relational stress, undergoes a crisis and starts to carry out dysfunctional behaviors and attitudes both against patients and colleagues.

The professional has to be trained to recognize and manage all those ambivalent emotional urges that inevitably emerge during the contact with suffering people. This allows him to handle these feelings without being overwhelmed.

In addition to factors common to all professions that may lead to occupational stress conditions (overwork, limited participation in professional decisions, role ambiguity, etc.), in the healthcare sector, due to the specific traits of the profession, there is also the emotional "cost" which derives from the proximity with suffering people.

It is necessary for nurses and other practitioners to first take care of themselves in order to live, to work adequately, and to provide as much aid as possible.

The relationship between the healthcare professional and the patient with congenital heart disease, as in all critical aid activities (oncology, dialysis, burn units, infectious diseases, hospice, intensive care, and intensive therapy), is close, intense, engaging, and long-lasting. In addition, patients and their relatives transfer their feelings of impotence, abandonment, loneliness, pain, anguish, death, etc. into the relationship. They express doubts and pose questions that are sometimes difficult to answer. Over time, this particular state of mind leaves a mark on professionals both on a professional and on a human level.

These sides of the problem add on to the growing number of congenital heart disease patients and to the increasing complexity of protocols for the specific treatment of these patients.

17.4 Wellness or Health?

17.4.1 Organizing Health and Well-Being

Well-being is a word with different meanings. Work well-being is proportionally related to organizational health.

A positive work environment, according to the definition of the International Council of Nurses (2007), fosters high-quality performances and working conditions. In particular, it tends to promote health, safety, and well-being of healthcare professionals, to ensure high-quality medical care, to maintain and increase workers' motivation, and to enhance the performance of individuals and organizations.

A healthy work environment encourages the well-being of its employees and makes organizations more efficient with a comfortable and engaging internal atmosphere.

In presence of poor organizational well-being, we witness a general decline in performances and then absenteeism, low levels of motivation, stress and burnout, reduced work readiness, lack of confidence, lack of commitment, and an increase in claims of the patients [14].

It is increasingly common to hear about organizational health. Scholars such as the psychologist, Roberto Grandis, expert in behavioral issues, and Giuseppe Negro, expert in organization, discuss about developing the culture of organizational health within work environments. Both regard well-being as a positive interface between the individual and the organization and as an investment on the only "tangible" assets that are women and men who put together the organization. In other words, they regard well-being as "people satisfaction" [15].

Therefore, the concept of organizational health refers to the way the individual lives with his work organization [16]. The more the individual feels he belongs to the organization because he shares the values, the practices, and the languages, the more he finds motivation and meaning for his work.

The idea of health in the work environment has different meanings both for the workers and the organization: physical health, emotional and psychological well-being, safety, a low rate of injuries, an open and productive atmosphere, comfortable relationships, engagement and tension toward the goals, etc.

The history of the actions undertaken with the aim of enhancement of health and psychophysical well-being in an organizational environment begins around the 1940s when Elton Mayo started its counseling programs for the employees of Hawthorne's Western Electric in Chicago. These programs were built on the idea that greater attention had to be paid to the emotional elements of the work environment in order to improve its organizational life [12].

Occupational stress is the general term to describe a negative emotional experience (which goes with biochemical, behavioral, and cognitive alterations). The individual perceives it at work as the consequence of the difficulty of coping with burdensome demands, coming from inside and outside the work environment [17].

The factors and variables which make an organization capable of expressing health and maintaining conditions of well-being/malaise are different. Therefore, it is not easy to give a comprehensive definition of organizational well-being.

In addition, the organization should be able to control the causes of stress (we refer to the perceived level of physical and mental fatigue and stress), the features of the task (we refer to the content of the work and to the workload), and discord (we refer to the presence of both manifest and implicit conflicting situations).

17.4.2 Studies and Models

In medical literature, the starting point of the various models related to the "medicine of work" is that work is the result of a balance disorder between the employees' needs and their available resources.

In 1970, Cristina Maslach referred to burnout as "a syndrome of *emotional exhaustion, depersonalization,* and *personal accomplishment* that may arise in those who carry out an aid profession" [18]. This concept led to the identification of the three dimensions of *burnout*, which are examined by the Maslach Burnout Inventory, the world's leading instrument for the assessment of this phenomenon. It uses three scales: *emotional exhaustion*, *depersonalization*, and *personal accomplishment*.

Burnout is the result of chronic stress especially when there exists an excessive pressure and there is a conflict with low levels of emotional recognition.

Healthcare professionals, especially nurses working with congenital heart disease patients, endure a lot of stress since, according to Maslach, they have long working hours, a wide range of activities, and complicated relationships with patients, families, and colleagues. Therefore, healthcare professionals' life quality within the work environment is the new challenge for the organization of healthcare services.

Medical literature provides a lot of examples of researches that sought to identify what the causes and the effects for the employees' are. These researches support the use of models that could explain how and under which conditions individuals experience malaise or well-being in the work environment.

To this regard, we can mention the effort-reward-imbalance model (ERI) by Siegrist [19] and the job demand-control model (JD-C) by Kasarek [19]. They certainly represent the most used models by medical literature in these years. The latter is a model based on situational factors which are considered the main source of occupational stress. However, these models have mainly focused on the negative outcomes such as health problems, stress, and burnout [19].

In the attempt to overcome the abovementioned limits and to use a more comprehensive approach that includes both the negative and positive indicators of work well-being, a new model, the job demands-resources model (JD-R) [19], has been proposed and developed. The basic idea is that a healthy work environment does not only develop through the absence of negative factors but can also be achieved by promoting positive features.

Recently, a growing number of studies has highlighted how individual characteristics and assets can help the worker (in our case the nurse specialized in congenital heart disease) to adapt to work demands, to modify the perception of stress, and to improve the start of the syndrome [20]. It has been also found that the use of coping skills increases the occupational resilience of the individual [21].

In light of the job demand-resources model [21], burnout and stress reflect a stressor-neutral approach [22].

Indeed, the factor influencing the burnout progression is the individual's response to stress.

Therefore, burnout can be understood as the ultimate outcome of nonadaptive coping in response to chronic stress.

The job demand-resources model is gaining an increasing interest both in the academic world and in the intervention programs. The reason beyond this interest lies in the possibility that the model offers an in-depth analysis of the dynamics of work well-being and motivation.

Working on one's own resources and communicative skills becomes an essential step, even to better manage stressful psychosocial events and emotions, such as rabies, significantly associated with burnout levels [23].

References

1. Heidegger M. Essere e tempo. Milano: Longanesi; 1997.
2. Comancini G. Lettera a un medico sulla cura degli uomini. J Sci Commun. 2003;2(3):162.
3. Nouwen HJ, editor. Il guaritore ferito. Brescia: Queriniana; 2010.
4. Bruzzone D, Musi E, editors. Vissuti di cura. Competenze emotive e formazione nelle professioni sanitarie. Milano: Guerini; 2007.
5. Bolognini B. (2007) L'analisi del benessere organizzativo. Roma: Carocci Editore.
6. Camerini D, Conway PM, Lusignani M. Condizioni di lavoro infermieristico e intensione di cambiare: risultati dello studio europeo in Italia. Giornale Italiano di Scienze Infermieristiche. 2005;1:6–11.
7. Mayo E. The social problem of an industrial civilization. Boston: Harvard University Press; 1945.
8. Avallone F, Paplomatas A. Salute organizzativa, psicologia del benessere nei contesti lavorativi. Milano: Raffaello Cortina Editore; 2005.
9. Barbini N, Beretta GG, Minnucci MP, Andrani M. Le principali patologie causa di assenza dal lavoro. Analisi della banca dati INPS. G Ital Med Lav Ergon. 2006;28(1):14–9.
10. Ragazzoni P, Tangolo D, Zotti AM. Stress occupazionale e valorizzazione delle risorse umane in azienda sanitaria: dalla valutazione al processo di cambiamento. G Ital Med Lav Ergon. 2004;26(2):119–26.
11. Houkes I, Janssen PPM, Jonge J, Bakker AB. Specific determinants of intrinsic work motivation, emotional exhaustion and turnover intention: a multisample longitudinal study. J Occup Organ Psychol. 2003;76:427–50.
12. Sili A, vellone E, Fida R, et al. La salute organizzativa degli infermieri. Guida pratica all'utilizzo del Questionario infermieristico sulla salute organizzativa (QISO). Napoli: Edises Editore; 2010.
13. Freudenberger HJ. Staff burnout. J Soc Issues. 1974;30:259–165.
14. Roelen CA, Koopman PC, Notenbomer A, et al. Job satisfaction and sickness absence: a questionnaire survey. J Occup Environ Med. 2008;58:567–71.
15. Avallone F, Paplomatas A. Salute organizzativa. Milano: Raffello Cortina Editore; 2005.
16. Avallone F, Bonaretti M, Rubbettino. Il Benessere Organizzativo, Un approccio per migliorare la qualità del lavoro nelle amministrazioni pubbliche. Soveria Mannelli: Rubbettino; 2003.
17. Kelleher CC, O'Connor M. Lifestyle practices and the health promoting environment of hospital nurses. J Adv Nurs. 1998;28(2):438–47.
18. Baum A. Stress, intrusive imagery, and chronic distress. Health Psychol. 1990;6:653–75.
19. Maslach C. La sindrome del burnout. Il prezzo dell'aiuto agli altri. Assisi: Cittadella; 1982.
20. Bakker AB, Demerouti E. The job demands-resources model: state of the art. J Manag Psychol. 2007;22(3):309–28.
21. Edwars D, Burnard P, Coyle D, Fothergill A, Hanningan B. Stress and burnout in community mental health nursing: a review of the literature. J Psychiatr Ment Health Nurs. 2000;7(1):7–14.
22. Greifer AN. Occupational resilience: protective factors among clinical social workers. Diss Abst Int Sec A Humanit Soc Sci. 2005;65(12-A):4721.
23. Bakker AB, Demerouti E. Job demands-resources theory. In: Chen PY, Cooper CL, editors. Work and wellbeing: wellbeing: a complete reference guide, vol. III. Chichester: Wiley-Blackwell; 2014. p. 37–64.

Self-Care in Congenital Heart Disease Patients

18

Rosario Caruso

Abstract

Self-care is the process of maintaining health through health promoting practices and managing illness. Self-care is very important for patients with CHD, due to its link with medication taking, symptom monitoring, dietary adherence, fluid restriction, alcohol restriction, physical exercise, smoke cessation, all-cause hospitalization, cost of care, and quality of life. However, little research is currently available on CHD patients' self-care. This chapter offers a portrait of what self-care is, and why it is so important.

18.1 What Is Self-Care?

Since the 1970s, self-care has been typically defined as "*the practice of activities that individuals initiate and perform on their own behalf in maintaining life, health, and well-being*" [1]. Considering that definition, self-care was studied in relation to the individual's practice of a range of activities, which are often linked to the diversity of the many clinical, personal, and social nuances of the same individuals. More recently, the attention of researchers is on the self-care process rather than specific self-care activities [2]. For this reason, there is a consensus in literature in defining self-care as a process of maintaining health through health promoting practices and managing illness [2]. This definition allows to study the self-care in both healthy

R. Caruso
Health Professions Research and Development Unit, IRCCS Policlinico San Donato, Milan, Italy
e-mail: rosario.caruso@grupposandonato.it

© Springer International Publishing AG, part of Springer Nature 2019   289
S. F. Flocco et al. (eds.), *Congenital Heart Disease*,
https://doi.org/10.1007/978-3-319-78423-6_18

and ill states. However, terms like self-management, self-regulation, self-monitoring or adherence are often used interchangeably as a synonym of self-care, without a clear definition [3].

Currently, the literature shows how self-care has a close relation with the individual's awareness of their physical and mental health status, including awareness of their current health (e.g., blood sugar, body mass index, blood pressure), which requires receiving regular checks to be assessed or self-assessed. Riegel et al. have identified the elements of self-care in a middle-range theory for chronic diseases [2], which could also be useful to assess self-care for CHD patients.

An underlying process that makes self-care so complex is the need for decision-making, where the naturalistic decision-making is a better description of the process used by patients in self-care [4]. It reflects the automatic, impulsive, and even contextual decisions that people make in complex real-world situations. The middle-range theory for chronic diseases of Barbara Riegel has three main assumptions:

- There are differences between general self-care and illness-specific self-care.
- Decision-making requires the ability to focus attention and to think sufficient capacity for working memory and the ability to understand and weigh information.
- Self-care for patients with multiple comorbid conditions may be conflicting when self-care is considered for each illness separately.

Riegel also distinguishes "self-care intended outcome" and "self-care unintended outcome." Important intended outcomes are illness stability, health, well-being, and quality of life, while unintended outcomes could include a higher burden associated with the need to perform self-care and guilt when one fails to follow treatment advice.

18.2   Why Self-Care Is Important for Patients with CHD?

Self-care is a real approach to living which incorporates behaviors that refresh the person, replenish the personal motivation, and help an individual to grow as a person even when the individual has a CHD. It implies to creating time for ourselves each day to improve energy, concentration, and overall wellness. Meeting one's own needs tends to make a person more able to help and support others, boosting sound peer relationships. Generally, self-care is associated to the achievement of more happiness and fulfillment from life. More specifically self-care was widely studied in people with heart failure [5–8], where a number of positive implication were highlighted for persons with high level of self-care. The main implications are related to *medication taking, symptom monitoring, dietary adherence, fluid restriction, alcohol restriction, physical exercise, smoke cessation, all-cause hospitalization, cost of care,* and *quality of life* [8].

Medication adherence is generally expressed as the percentage of prescribed doses that are actually taken or taken on time, and it is a crucial aspect of the CHD overall management. There are many common reasons for nonadherence to medications which include cost, attitudes about taking medicines, and the effect of certain medicines on sexual function. It is common in the literature to classify patients as adherent when >80% of doses are taken and nonadherent when <80% are taken [9]. Medication adherence is an important component of self-care, being defined as specific self-care behavior. For this reason, people with higher self-care level are likely more adherent with their prescribed medications.

Inability to recognize early symptoms, especially for patients with CHD, could predict negative outcome. Even when symptoms are recognized, their interpretation can be a challenge for afflicted patients, considering that the symptomatology could be diverse or less specific in some situations. Efforts to improve patients' abilities to recognize, interpret, and act on their early symptoms means efforts their self-care, due to symptom monitoring is a specific self-care behavior.

Some CHD patients could have some disorder related to their dietary adherence. For example, some authors described the excess weight is higher of 25% in pediatric and adolescent patients with CHD [10]. Body Mass Index (BMI) should be performed annually, while waist circumference could be considered in overweight or obese adults [11]. Moreover, disordered dietary habits and nonadherents with dietary prescriptions could lead to dyslipidemia, hypertension, or diabetes, which are important modifiable risk factors for developing cardiovascular disease [11]. Patients with higher self-care levels are more adherent with their dietary indications.

Many people with cardiovascular disease believe that drinking water is helpful [12], but fluid intake should be restricted in patients with severe symptoms of heart failure. In those cases adherence to dietary fluid and sodium restrictions can help balance sodium and water and minimize the risk of acute congestive episodes.

Other potential problems for patients with CHD are associated with alcohol intake. Despite alcohol is toxic to the liver, and it has detrimental effects on other organs, decreasing motivation to limit sodium and food intake, being an addictive substance, some authors shows that rates of alcohol intake in patients with CHD were comparable with the general population consumption [13]. At the same way, CHD smoke habits seem to be comparable with the general population habits. However, smoke is often more frequent in patients with CHD expressing depressive symptoms [14]. The behavior of patients with CHD is generally more influenced by their peer relationships rather than their clinical condition [15].

Physical routine exercise is a potent way to improve oxygen delivery and to decrease inflammation. Even patients with severe, symptomatic left ventricular dysfunction could benefit from an individually tailored exercise program based on the results of formal exercise testing [16]. No universal prescription and consensus for a particular exercise regimen for patients with CHD exists, but it is surely a good way to improve the overall well-being, when there are no contraindications. Adults with congenital heart disease have a range of physical activity levels between normal and severely limited. Moreover, most patients showed a willingness to participate in exercise but were uncertain of the safety or benefit [17]. Health fears and misconceptions are common barriers to regular physical activity in patients with CHD, but it is reasonable to link lower functional capacity to poor outcomes; for this reason—with few exceptions—patients with CHD should be counselled to exercise regularly [18].

The readmission rate per 1000 patients with CHD seems to be 12.6% for patients aged ≥65 years, 8.5% for adults, and 8.3% for infants [19]. Increasing comorbidities are an important risk factor for readmission; for this reason the primary and secondary preventions are strategic in patients with CHD. Hence, self-care could be useful to prevent or best manage some comorbidities related to life styles.

Regarding patients' quality of life, the research results seem to be contradictory, while some studies show that congenital heart disease can impact the quality of life, others describe a better perception of quality of life among children and adolescents with CHD when compared with healthy control people [20, 21]. Quality of life is surely related to multiple factors and not solely determined by patients' heart defect and various medical or demographic characteristics [22].

18.3 Patients with CHD and Self-Care

Despite the importance of self-care for people with CHD, literature has paid little attention on this topic. There are many areas, which should be more investigated. Those areas can be summarized as below:

• The development of a specific CHD disease self-care assessment tool.
• Description of self-care levels according to the middle-range theory for chronic diseases.
• The description of which approach could enhance self-care levels.
• The description between self-care and health literary.
• The description between self-care and clinical outcomes among patients with CHD.

18.4 Nursing and Self-Care

To help people improve their self-care behaviors, nurses must have knowledge about the attributes associated with those behaviors in health and in deviations from health status. Nurses need to identify what aspects in the persons' health situations may affect their self-care behaviors, such as the caregiver contribution or some life-style behaviors. For these reasons, the assessment is strategic to plan a realistic and effective care objective. Nurses are historically well suited to play a leadership role in promoting primary healthcare [23, 24]. In this field, knowledge of epidemiology, social, and behavioral science are required in assisting the individual and community to engage in self-care. Moreover, nurses are frequently identified as influential and significant practitioners in health promotion, due to their broad knowledge about all aspects of healthcare which is a priceless resource for patients.

Self-care is a milestone in nursing practice since Dorothea Orem theory, reaching up to the recent middle-range theory for chronic diseases of Riegel. Orem theory has already considered the patient as a person self-reliant and responsible for self-care. This approach is confirmed in the naturalistic definition of Riegel. Nurses have to be aware that self-care involves taking control of political, economic, social, cultural, environmental, behavioral, and biological factors. Their role is paramount in understanding patients' self-care and to advocate for patients' empowerment to achieve best self-care levels.

References

1. Orem D. Nursing concepts of practice. 6th ed. St Louis: Mosby; 1991.
2. Riegel B, Jaarsma T, Strömberg A, Steinbright EC. A middle-range theory of self-care of chronic illness. Adv Nurs Sci. 2012;3:194–204. https://doi.org/10.1097/ANS.0b013e318261b1ba.
3. Ausili D, Masotto M, Dall'Ora C, et al. A literature review on self-care of chronic illness: definition, assessment and related outcomes. Prof Inferm. 2014;67:180–9. https://doi.org/10.7429/pi.2014.673180.
4. Klein G. Naturalistic decision making. Hum Factors. 2008;50:456–60. https://doi.org/10.1518/001872008X288385.
5. Clark AP, McDougall G, Riegel B, et al. Health status and self-care outcomes after an education-support intervention for people with chronic heart failure. J Cardiovasc Nurs. 2015;30:S3–S13. https://doi.org/10.1097/JCN.0000000000000169.
6. Graven LJ, Grant JS. Social support and self-care behaviors in individuals with heart failure: an integrative review. Int J Nurs Stud. 2014;51:320–33. https://doi.org/10.1016/j.ijnurstu.2013.06.013.
7. Moser DK, Watkins JF. Conceptualizing self-care in heart failure. J Cardiovasc Nurs. 2008;23:205–18. https://doi.org/10.1097/01.JCN.0000305097.09710.a5.
8. Riegel B, Moser DK, Anker SD, et al. State of the science: promoting self-care in persons with heart failure: a scientific statement from the American Heart Association. Circulation. 2009;120:1141–63. https://doi.org/10.1161/CIRCULATIONAHA.109.192628.
9. De Geest S, Abraham I, Moons P, et al. Late acute rejection and subclinical noncompliance with cyclosporine therapy in heart transplant recipients. J Heart Lung Transplant. 1998;17:854–63.
10. Barbiero SM, D'Azevedo Sica C, Schuh DS, et al. Overweight and obesity in children with congenital heart disease: combination of risks for the future? BMC Pediatr. 2014;14:271. https://doi.org/10.1186/1471-2431-14-271.
11. Jensen M, Ryan D, Apovian C, Ard J. 2013 AHA/ACC/TOS guideline for the management of overweight and obesity in adults. Circulation. 2014;129:S102–38.
12. van der Wal MHL, Jaarsma T, Moser DK, et al. Compliance in heart failure patients: the importance of knowledge and beliefs. Eur Heart J. 2005;27:434–40. https://doi.org/10.1093/eurheartj/ehi603.
13. Reid GJ, Webb GD, McCrindle BW, et al. Health behaviors among adolescents and young adults with congenital heart disease. Congenit Heart Dis. 2008;3:16–25. https://doi.org/10.1111/j.1747-0803.2007.00161.x.
14. Khan M, Monaghan M, Klein N, et al. Associations among depression symptoms with alcohol and smoking tobacco use in adult patients with congenital heart disease. Congenit Heart Dis. 2015;10:E243–9. https://doi.org/10.1111/chd.12282.
15. Flocco SF, Caruso R, Dellafiore F, et al. Towards the standardization of transition care models for adolescents with congenital heart disease (CHD): a perspective. J Clin Exp Cardiol. 2017;8:1–3. https://doi.org/10.4172/2155-9880.1000495.
16. Fletcher GF, Balady GJ, Amsterdam EA, et al. Exercise standards for testing and training: a statement for healthcare professionals from the American Heart Association. Circulation. 2001;104:1694–740.

17. Dua JS, Cooper AR, Fox KR, Stuart AG. Physical activity levels in adults with congenital heart disease. Eur J Cardiovasc Prev Rehabil. 2007;14:287–93. https://doi.org/10.1097/HJR.0b013e32808621b9.
18. Chaix M-A, Marcotte F, Dore A, et al. Risks and benefits of exercise training in adults with congenital heart disease. Can J Cardiol. 2016;32:459–66. https://doi.org/10.1016/j.cjca.2015.12.007.
19. Islam S, Yasui Y, Kaul P, Mackie AS. Hospital readmission of patients with congenital heart disease in Canada. Can J Cardiol. 2016;32:987.e7–987.e14. https://doi.org/10.1016/j.cjca.2015.12.018.
20. Bertoletti J, Marx GC, Hattge Júnior SP, Pellanda LC. Quality of life and congenital heart disease in childhood and adolescence. Arq Bras Cardiol. 2014;102:192–8.
21. Fteropoulli T, Stygall J, Cullen S, et al. Quality of life of adult congenital heart disease patients: a systematic review of the literature. Cardiol Young. 2013;23:473–85. https://doi.org/10.1017/S1047951112002351.
22. Apers S, Luyckx K, Moons P. Quality of life in adult congenital heart disease: what do we already know and what do we still need to know? Curr Cardiol Rep. 2013;15:407. https://doi.org/10.1007/s11886-013-0407-x.
23. Caruso R, Fida R, Sili A, Arrigoni C. Towards an integrated model of nursing competence: an overview of the literature reviews and concept analysis. Prof Inferm. 2016;69:35–43. https://doi.org/10.7429/pi.2016.691035.
24. Caruso R, Pittella F, Zaghini F, et al. Development and validation of the nursing profession self-efficacy scale. Int Nurs Rev. 2016;63:455–64. https://doi.org/10.1111/inr.12291.

Nursing Research and Quality Improvement Initiatives for Patients with Congenital Heart Disease

19

Federica Dellafiore and Eva Goossens

Abstract

The population of adults with congenital heart disease (CHD) is rapidly growing as extensive improvements in congenital cardiology and heart surgery have created new groups of children surviving into adolescence and adulthood. With improvement of clinical outcomes, involvement of nurses in research and quality initiatives has expanded over the past decades. Such initiatives aim to improve the provision of evidence-based nursing care for patients with CHD along their life span.

The role of a clinical nurse specialist is described to be foundational for the delivery of high-quality, effective, compassionate health care, where provision of interdisciplinary clinical practice is closely linked to the newest research insights. The role of advanced practice nurses (APN) is recognized to be a cornerstone in the provision of holistic patient care. The task set of such advanced nursing roles include performance of comprehensive assessment of patients' needs, counseling activities regarding education, employment, family planning, and supporting the development of self-management and coping strategies.

In order to provide patient-tailored care, a comprehensive understanding of patients' needs is crucial to manage the diversity and complexity of CHD care and to support the unique clinical needs and challenges encountered by this patient population. The main topics investigated by nursing research over the

F. Dellafiore (✉)
Health Professions Research and Development Unit, IRCCS Policlinico San Donato, San Donato Milanese (MI), Italy
e-mail: federica.dellafiore@grupposandonato.it

E. Goossens
Department of Public Health and Primary Care, Academic Center for Nursing and Midwifery, KU Leuven, Leuven, Belgium

Research Foundation Flanders (FWO), Brussels, Belgium
e-mail: eva.goossens@kuleuven.be

© Springer International Publishing AG, part of Springer Nature 2019
S. F. Flocco et al. (eds.), *Congenital Heart Disease*,
https://doi.org/10.1007/978-3-319-78423-6_19

recent years were CHD lived experiences, quality of life, parenting of patients, and transitional care. Although the field of nursing research expanded tremendously over the past decades, important gaps in our knowledge and evidence base remain, however, pertinent. Further empirical investigations are mandatory to gain a full understanding of important aspects of effective nursing care for patients with CHD and enlarge the evidence-base supporting quality improvement initiatives.

19.1 Introduction

Nowadays, a vivid debate is ongoing regarding the organization of healthcare provision for patients with congenital heart disease (CHD) [1]. Discussions are evolving with respect to the organizational characteristics and competencies required for a qualification as a CHD specialist center, as the entire care process for patients with CHD is multidimensional, complex, and challenging [2]. Furthermore, the presence of an interdisciplinary team is defined as the basis for the provision of high-quality care to children, adolescents, and adults with CHD. Such a collaborative practice model, in which a physician-led team of medical doctors, nurse practitioners, and other clinicians collaborate when providing comprehensive, quality patient care, was found to be beneficial for patients and their families but also for the organization of the overall care process [3]. The recent body of literature comprises numerous task forces, consensus statements, and guidelines enabling us to better define and declare the appropriate system(s) of care delivery, evidence-based practice, and the composition of the team providing high-level care to this growing population of adults with CHD [4].

19.2 The Key Role of Nursing Care

In such a collaborative care model, nurses play a key role in the management of expert lifelong care for patients with CHD. As CHD is considered to be a complex chronic condition, continuous specialized care is essential to meet the specific needs of both children, adolescents and adults and to reduce the negative impact this condition might have on patients' lives [5]. The provision of lifelong care requires properly trained healthcare professionals, specifically trained in the management of patients with CHD at every stage of life [6].

Over the past decade, the role for advanced practice nurses (e.g., clinical nurse specialist, nurse practitioner, or nurse consultant) has expanded and gained a prominent role [4]. Advanced practice nurses (APNs) have an expert-level skill set for chronic disease management and are the central coordinating point of care throughout patients' lives. The provision of accessible uninterrupted care is particularly of importance as patients with CHD encounter complex chronic health issues, affecting their everyday life. The role of APNs is multidimensional, as they have a responsibility in providing information and education to patients, troubleshooting in case of patient concerns, and assuring appropriate evidence-based care and ongoing support for patients and families. Additionally, nurses play a vital role in skill training of patients and families, helping them adjust to living with a complex chronic condition after hospital care.

The APN forms a cornerstone for the assessment of patients' needs, counseling activities regarding education, employment, family planning, and fostering of self-management and coping skills in patients. Furthermore, an APN is often considered to act as a care coordinator, facilitating the transfer and transition of adolescents with CHD to adulthood. In many programs, APNs are highly accessible for patients and are reachable from the community, hospital clinics, or during an inpatient stay through telephone or email services [6].

Additionally, an APN is supposed to be actively involved in research studies, quality improvement initiatives, and implementation projects related to CHD care. It is vital for the quality of care that insights gained from scientific research form a basis for quality improvement initiatives and vice versa. This reciprocal relationship between research, innovation, and quality improvement is of great importance to CHD care, as this is considered to be a young specialization within the discipline of cardiology. Nurses, involved in the care for patients with CHD, should be encouraged and supported to become involved in research initiatives in order to create a solid evidence base on which to build strong, high-quality care practices.

In fact, over the past decades, a new generation of nurse researchers made important contributions to the improvement of patient care, supporting nurses in daily work, in acting and working in line with evidence-based practice [7]. In addition, with their knowledge and hands-on experience, nurses can theorize, hypothesize, structure, and collect data and perform research leading to better care. The goal of nursing research is to achieve better care standards, patient-reported outcomes and applications for patients and families [7]. Ultimately, this will benefit not only patients and their families but also the interprofessional and interdisciplinary teams caring for these patients within hospitals.

Some nursing studies performed in the past, focused either on the clinical management of CHD during childhood [8] or on the multiple challenges encountered by patients in the transition to adulthood [9, 10]. The clinical management of CHD from infancy to adulthood is a more complex aspect of treatment and care. The increasing survival of children with CHD challenges healthcare systems in managing the numerous healthcare needs of young patients during their transition to adulthood. A comprehensive understanding of the perspectives of patients, parents, and healthcare providers is required [11].

Nowadays, healthcare providers have access to eminence-based guidelines and recommendations [12], which should help physicians and nurses to make decisions in daily clinical practice [8]. Guidelines summarize and evaluate all currently available evidence on a particular issue with the aim of assisting professionals in selecting the best management strategies for an individual patient, afflicted by a given condition, taking into account the impact on outcome, as well as the risk–benefit ratio of particular diagnostic or therapeutic means [12].

19.3   The Research on CHD Lived Experiences

Another aspect which has been investigated by nurse researchers is the lived experiences of children, adolescents, and adults afflicted with CHD and how they evaluate their quality of life. As medical care and treatment have improved substantially, children affected by CHD have a 90% chance of surviving into adulthood. Hence, they are assumed to live longer and healthier lives [13]. Although life expectancy of these patients is increasing, they may, however, face specific medical, psychosocial, and behavioral problems throughout their life span. Due to medical problems, patients with CHD perceive specific psychosocial concerns that influence their experiences and quality of life [14]. Special attention needs to be given to patients' illness experiences, knowledge and health behavior, employability, and insurability. Hence, comprehensive care by specialized healthcare professionals, addressing the multidimensional problems experienced by patients, is required. Interdisciplinary teams in which nurses guarantee the management beyond typical medical issues are promising [6].

19.4   Research on Quality of Life in Patients with CHD

The investigation of the quality of life in children and adolescents with CHD provides complementary information to clinical data assisting decision-making on the part of health professionals. Overall studies were found to report contradictory findings on the quality of life of patients with CHD. While some studies reported CHD negatively impacting quality of life, other studies described a better perception of quality of life among children and adolescents who suffer from the disease as compared with healthy control subjects [15]. The results of recent literature showed that in most cases adolescents and adults with CHD perceive their health to be good and at a comparable level as their "healthy" peers [12]. Pain or discomfort and anxiety or depression were found to be prevalent health problems, but adults with CHD reported less pain or discomfort than the general population [14]. It was further shown that symptoms might occur even if the adult with a CHD reports to be asymptomatic. Despite limitations in everyday life, adolescents and young adults with a surgically palliated univentricular heart experience satisfaction with their lives and see themselves as exceptional, strong, and healthy [16]. Moreover, the findings from some studies highlighted that CHD is a complex heart disease involving all individual aspects of life of patients with CHD. Such as of chronic diseases, the physical, relational, emotional, and spiritual dimensions, patients with CHD appear to stimulate positive coping mechanisms. A feeling of diversity was a central theme of the patients' lived experience, as they are continually faced with physical limitations and visible signs due to their heart defects. The experienced discordance between their world and healthy individuals' reality implies that patients struggle constantly with themselves and with their environment to be accepted as normal. The feeling of "being different" was influenced by attitudes of the environment, healthcare, and patient's personality. Moreover, it determined the perceived impact of the disease on the patient's daily life [17].

19.5   Research on Parenting of Patients with CHD

The parental role and experience of relatives is a topic of growing interest with nursing research, inasmuch as the congenital heart defect could have an adverse impact on the family members, as well as on the patient [18, 19]. Because of potential complications and the chronic nature of the heart defect, patients are in desperate need of physical, emotional, and social care at different stages of their life. These needs might cause a burden of other family members, especially on parents [20]. On the other hand, fear for an unknown future for the child, treatment program, and prognosis of the disease can lead to emergence of psychological problems, especially in parents. According to the findings of a recent content analysis, with the aim to understand care experiences of mothers of children with CHD, mothers expressed an important burden of the child's care and reported to suffer multiple tensions and problems. Furthermore, three secondary themes appeared: (1) the tension resulting from the disease, (2) involvement with internal thoughts, and (3) difficulties of care process [21]. Moreover, the relationship between parents and adolescents with CHD seems to have some peculiarities, which are recently highlighted in the findings of a meta-synthesis of qualitative studies: from this research emerged how the role of the CHD adolescents' parents is difficult and how they live with continuous contradictions. The search yielded 405 potentially relevant studies for screening, and only seven articles met all the inclusion criteria. These papers were analyzed and discussed, and a qualitative meta-synthesis was performed, according to the Noblit & Hare methodology [22]. The meta-synthesis resulted in the identification of four main themes, exploring four main contradictions characterizing the CHD adolescents' parents experiences: "fear and uncertainty of the future versus positive coping strategies," "parents hyper-responsibility and overprotection versus adolescents' independence desire," "desire to give support, but not to be supported," and "normality desire versus awareness to live with particular conditions" [23].

19.6   Research on Transitional Care for Young People with CHD

Recently, research interest related to the process of transfer and transition of young patients with CHD from pediatric to adult cardiac care increased substantially. In fact, the number of studies exploring various aspects of the transition period from childhood to adulthood in patients with CHD grew rapidly in numbers [24, 25]. The American Academy of Pediatrics defined the main goal of the transfer process as the optimization of lifelong function through high-quality and uninterrupted healthcare services [26]. Transitional care models on the other hand have to orient and encourage a sound health behavior in young patients considering how these patients could be exposed to many psychological issues related to their development of self-identity, self-esteem, and self-image [27].

The main psychological issues faced by adolescents with CHD are (a) modification of their body image (e.g., scars, puberty); (b) social functioning (e.g., family or peer relationships); (c) increased risk of anxiety, diminished self-esteem, and depression, often associated with their personal problems internalizing; and (d) problems concerning smoking, alcohol or illicit drug consumption, and sexual behaviors [14]. Some authors reported that smoking, alcohol, or illicit drug consumption among adolescents with CHD are comparable with consumption among healthy peers, but the impact for their health is, however, not comparable to healthy populations [14, 23, 28, 29].

Additionally, during the past decade, literature is characterized by an increasing number of papers aimed to present different transition care models, including generic, disease-based models, and CHD-specific models. The CHD-specific models consider (a) timing of transition (i.e., the process starting based on individualization, according to each patient's medical and developmental conditions); (b) assessing the disease pattern, where both the unoperated CHD patients (i.e., unrecognized or undiagnosed during childhood) and the CHD patients undergoing corrective or palliative surgery during childhood should be assessed; and (c) care planning, involving local hospitals closely linked to the specialist centers with a transition clinic [14].

19.7 State of the Art of CHD Nursing Research

The role of nurse specialists has expanded over the past years, yet there remains an increased need for providing scientific evidence supporting the components of effective and efficient care provided by nurse specialists. To enable the expansion of this evidence base, the establishment of an international nursing research agenda was performed based on a recent mixed-method study investigating research priorities perceived by nurse specialists and researchers within the field of CHD [4]. This study revealed that based on the opinion of experts, priority must be given to studies investigating knowledge and education of patients, outcomes of advanced practice nursing, quality of life, transfer and transition, illness experiences, and psychosocial issues in adults with CHD. A lower priority score was given to studies assessing postoperative pain, sexual functioning, transplantation in adults with CHD, and healthcare costs and utilization. Focusing on the areas of highest priority, researchers ought to expand and strengthen the body of knowledge in ACHD nursing [4].

The numerous research studies described above are closely linked to quality improvement initiatives of nursing care in patients with CHD. The nursing role is rapidly evolving, expanding, and developing, indicating a pertinent need for clinical implementation and evaluation projects in patients with CHD. Furthermore, European and North-American guidelines for the management of patients with CHD have strongly supported and developed individual healthcare providers and specific clinical and nursing programs for specifically care for these patients [30]. Hence, an increasing number of structured and unstructured programs for adults with CHD have been established worldwide [31].

The European Society of Cardiology (ESC) Working Group on Grown-up Congenital Heart Disease published the results of a survey on the content, structure, and resources invested in CHD care programs. The aim of this survey was to describe the staffing levels, clinical activities being performed, available equipment, training levels of staff, and supportive services for patients with CHD in several hospitals across Europe [30]. International recommendations state that at least one specialist center for the patients with CHD is needed for every 5–10 million inhabitants [32], reflecting that 70–140 centers would be needed for the European population (730 million) [30]. The results of this survey showed that there are 50 specialist centers originated from 18 countries in Europe; the UK, Germany, and Sweden were highly represented. The first clinical care programs dedicated to the patients with CHD were founded in the mid-1970s, and exponential growth in programs was observed in the 1990s. Forty-seven programs (94%) were located in a university hospital [30].

An interesting experience related to the implementation of CHD care programs is developed in a Cardiology Hospital in Northern Italy [14]. The transition care model implementation strategy adopted in this center is closely linked to clinical practice and research activities at national and international level. Hence, there is currently a significant lack of data showing the effectiveness of transitional care models and their impact on health outcomes (e.g., follow-up adherence, medical outcomes, psychosocial outcomes, nursing outcomes). For this reason, the North-Italian care program was established as a research project, investigating adolescents' needs and their main social and health issues. This study aims to assess the model's effectiveness regarding some selected outcomes (e.g., adherence, quality of life, overall health outcomes, satisfaction), linking the transition care model implementation to a research project [14]. This strategy could be an efficient start-up to boost the understanding of the adolescents' care needs, potentially providing evidence to the effectiveness of the transition care models.

Conclusion

As extensively described in the current body of literature, the population of adults with CHD is rapidly growing as extensive improvements in congenital cardiology and heart surgery have created new opportunities for patients with CHD. These patients belong to a new and in several respects unexplored population with understudied healthcare needs. Within the care for patients with CHD, the specialist nurse role plays a key role in the provision of person-centered lifelong care for patients with CHD along their life span. Advanced roles for nurses offer the opportunity to provide expert-level care and to expand the quality of care provided through research and quality improvement projects.

References

1. Iacona G, Giamberti A, Abella R, Pomè G, Agredo J, Mendieta S, et al. Paediatric cardiac surgery in a peripheral European region: is a joint programme a safe alternative to regionalisation? Cardiol Young. 2017;27(2):273–83.
2. Tchervenkov CI, Jacobs JP, Bernier P-L, Stellin G, Kurosawa H, Mavroudis C, et al. The improvement of care for paediatric and congenital cardiac disease across the World: a challenge for the World Society for Pediatric and Congenital Heart Surgery. Cardiol Young. 2008;18(S2):63.

 3. O'Brien P. The role of the nurse practitioner in congenital heart surgery. Pediatr Cardiol. 2007;28(2):88–95.
 4. Goossens E, Fleck D, Canobbio MM, Harrison JL, Moons P. Development of an international research agenda for adult congenital heart disease nursing. Eur J Cardiovasc Nurs. 2012;12(1):7–16.
 5. Moons P, Scholte op Reimer W, De Geest S, Fridlund B, Heikkila J, Jaarsma T, et al. Nurse specialists in adult congenital heart disease: the current status in Europe. Eur J Cardiovasc Nurs. 2006;5(1):60–7.
 6. Moons P, De Geest S, Budts W. Comprehensive care for adults with congenital heart disease: expanding roles for nurses. Eur J Cardiovasc Nurs. 2002;1(1):23–8.
 7. Tingen MS, Burnett AH, Murchison RB, Zhu H. The importance of nursing research. J Nurs Educ. 2009;48(3):167–70.
 8. Kantor PF, Lougheed J, Dancea A, McGillion M, Barbosa N, Chan C, et al. Presentation, diagnosis, and medical management of heart failure in children: Canadian Cardiovascular Society guidelines. Can J Cardiol. 2013;29(12):1535–52.
 9. Ntiloudi D, Giannakoulas G, Parcharidou D, Panagiotidis T, Gatzoulis MA, Karvounis H. Adult congenital heart disease: a paradigm of epidemiological change. Int J Cardiol. 2016;218:269–74.
10. Torok RD, Campbell MJ, Fleming GA, Hill KD. Coarctation of the aorta: management from infancy to adulthood. World J Cardiol. 2015;7(11):765.
11. Chen C-W, Su W-J, Chiang Y-T, Shu Y-M, Moons P. Healthcare needs of adolescents with congenital heart disease transitioning into adulthood: a Delphi survey of patients, parents, and healthcare providers. Eur J Cardiovasc Nurs. 2017;16(2):125–35.
12. Baumgartner H, Bonhoeffer P, De Groot NMS, de Haan F, Deanfield JE, Galie N, et al. ESC guidelines for the management of grown-up congenital heart disease (new version 2010): the task force on the management of grown-up congenital heart disease of the European Society of Cardiology (ESC). Eur Heart J. 2010;31(23):2915–57.
13. van der Bom T, Zomer AC, Zwinderman AH, Meijboom FJ, Bouma BJ, Mulder BJM. The changing epidemiology of congenital heart disease. Nat Rev Cardiol. 2011;8(1):50–60.
14. Flocco SF, Caruso R, Dellafiore F, Orlando A, Magon A, Giamberti A, et al. Towards the standardization of transition care models for adolescents with congenital heart disease (CHD): a perspective. J Clin Exp Cardiol. 2017;8(1):1–3.
15. Bertoletti J, Marx GC, Hattge Júnior SP, Pellanda LC. Quality of life and congenital heart disease in childhood and adolescence. Arq Bras Cardiol. 2014;102(2):192–8.
16. Berghammer M. Living with a congenital heart disease-adolescents' and young adults' experiences. Gothenburg: Komendiet; 2012.
17. Claessens P, Moons P, de Casterlé BD, Cannaerts N, Budts W, Gewillig M. What does it mean to live with a congenital heart disease? A qualitative study on the lived experiences of adult patients. Eur J Cardiovasc Nurs. 2005;4(1):3–10.
18. Connor JA, Kline NE, Mott S, Harris SK, Jenkins KJ. The meaning of cost for families of children with congenital heart disease. J Pediatr Health Care. 2010;24(5):318–25.
19. Harvey KA, Kovalesky A, Woods RK, Loan LA. Experiences of mothers of infants with congenital heart disease before, during, and after complex cardiac surgery. Heart Lung. 2013;42(6):399–406.
20. Rychik J, Donaghue DD, Levy S, Fajardo C, Combs J, Zhang X, et al. Maternal psychological stress after prenatal diagnosis of congenital heart disease. J Pediatr. 2013;162(2):302–7.
21. Sabzevari S, Nematollahi M, Mirzaei T, Ravari A. The burden of care: mothers' experiences of children with congenital heart disease. Int J Community Based Nurs Midwifery. 2016;4(4):374–85.
22. Noblit G, Hare R. Meta-ethnography: synthesizing qualitative studies. Beverly Hills: Sage; 1988.
23. Dellafiore F, Pittella F, Flocco FS, Caruso MP, Bersani V, Cimini A, et al. What about life experiences of congenital heart disease adolescents' parents? A literature review and meta-synthesis. Cardiol Young. 2016;26(Suppl 1):S180.

24. Hays L. Transition to adult congenital heart disease care: a review. J Pediatr Nurs. 2015;30(5):e63–9.
25. Moceri P, Goossens E, Hascoet S, Checler C, Bonello B, Ferrari E, et al. From adolescents to adults with congenital heart disease: the role of transition. Eur J Pediatr. 2015;174(7):847–54.
26. American Academy of Pediatrics, American Academy of Family Physicians, American College of Physicians-American Society of Internal Medicine. A consensus statement on health care transitions for young adults with special health care needs. Pediatrics. 2002;110(6 Pt 2):1304–6.
27. Betz CL. Health care transition for adolescents with special healthcare needs: where is nursing? Nurs Outlook. 2013;61(5):258–65.
28. Reid GJ, Webb GD, McCrindle BW, Irvine MJ, Siu SC. Health behaviors among adolescents and young adults with congenital heart disease. Congenit Heart Dis. 2008;3(1):16–25.
29. Karsdorp PA, Everaerd W, Kindt M, Mulder BJM. Psychological and cognitive functioning in children and adolescents with congenital heart disease: a meta-analysis. J Pediatr Psychol. 2007;32(5):527–41.
30. Moons P, Meijboom FJ, Baumgartner H, Trindade PT, Huyghe E, Kaemmerer H, et al. Structure and activities of adult congenital heart disease programmes in Europe. Eur Heart J. 2010;31(11):1305–10.
31. Hess J, Bauer U, De Haan F, Flesch J. Empfehlungen für Erwachsenen-und Kinderkardiologen zum Erwerb der Zusatz-Qualifikation "Erwachsene mit angeborenen Herzfehlern" (EMAH). Clin Res Cardiol. 2007;2(1):19–26.
32. Landzberg MJ, Murphy DJ, Davidson WR, Jarcho JA, Krumholz HM, Mayer JE, et al. Task force 4: organization of delivery systems for adults with congenital heart disease. J Am Coll Cardiol. 2001;37(5):1187–93.

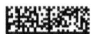